Key Concepts in Pain Management

Key Concepts in
Pain Management

Edited by **Pam Kellner**

FOSTER
A C A D E M I C S

New Jersey

Published by Foster Academics,
61 Van Reypen Street,
Jersey City, NJ 07306, USA
www.fosteracademics.com

Key Concepts in Pain Management
Edited by Pam Kellner

International Standard Book Number: 978-1-63242-251-4 (Hardback)

Printed in the United States of America.

Contents

Preface

This book aims to highlight the current researches and provides a platform to further the scope of innovations in this area. This book is a product of the combined efforts of many researchers and scientists, after going through thorough studies and analysis from different parts of the world. The objective of this book is to provide the readers with the latest information of the field.

International experts and veterans have contributed significant information in this book which encompass several topics regarding the present pain management problems, and provide the readers with a glimpse into the future of pain treatment. This book comprises both original research works as well as clinical information with particular treatment options grouped under five sections namely, chronic pain, cancer pain, non-pharmacological treatments, nursing and pain, and complex regional pain syndrome. The aim of this book is to serve as a valuable source of reference for a broad spectrum of readers including up-to-date pain clinicians as well as the common masses.

I would like to express my sincere thanks to the authors for their dedicated efforts in the completion of this book. I acknowledge the efforts of the publisher for providing constant support. Lastly, I would like to thank my family for their support in all academic endeavors.

Editor

Part 1

Chronic Pain

Chronic Pain in People with Physically Disabling Conditions: A Review of the Application of Biopsychosocial Models

Kathryn Nicholson Perry
University of Western Sydney,
Australia

1. Introduction

There are a wide range of conditions which can result in physical disabilities, affecting more than a billion people or approximately 15% of the population worldwide (World Health Organisation, 2011). Disability is an umbrella term for the restrictions and impairments arising from the interaction between an individual with a health condition and the environment (World Health Organisation, 2011). The physical conditions from which disability arises are diverse and heterogeneous, but include both diseases, such as multiple sclerosis, as well as traumatic and non-traumatic injuries, including spinal cord injury and brain injuries. Research concerning the occurrence of chronic pain (defined as pain persisting beyond the period of healing, usually operationalized as three or six months) among people with physical disabilities, and the impact upon those individuals affected, is relatively limited compared to that focusing on primary pain conditions, such as low back pain. Within the available literature the focus is largely biomedical, with the majority of available research exploring biological factors and medical interventions. A great deal has been gained in the management of primary pain conditions through investigating psychological and social factors, and developing interventions such as cognitive behavioural pain management programs to target these factors. This chapter will describe the current understanding of the role of psychological and social factors in understanding the experience of chronic pain in the context of a physically disabling condition, and the use of interventions addressing these factors in this population.

2. The nature of chronic pain in people with physically disabling conditions

What is known about the nature of chronic pain among those with physically disabling conditions varies depending on the condition of interest. An examination of those publishing in the area suggests that often there are only a small number of groups involved in this research. Most of these research groups only work with one specific condition, with only a very small number working across a range of physically disabling conditions. As a result of these research silos, there are many inconsistencies in the approaches taken in investigating pain in the different conditions. Interpreting the findings of this body of work, particularly attempting to make comparisons across conditions, should therefore be done with caution keeping in mind some important caveats. First, there are variations across studies concerning the nature of the pain conditions which are the subject of investigation, including the duration of the pain condition being explored. Some studies focus on chronic pain (with various criterion applied, commonly either three or six months duration), where others report on episodic, procedural or acute pain or do not specify which type of pain participants are experiencing. Second, some studies restrict their attention to pain thought to be specific to the physically disabling condition in question (such as headaches in those with traumatic brain injury), putting aside those deemed to be general (such as low back pain) which may be overlooked by teams specialising in a specific disabling condition rather than pain itself (Ivanhoe & Hartman, 2004). Finally, studies draw samples from a number of different populations including community samples, membership organisations for people with the physically disabling condition in question, and clinical services, including tertiary services for either pain or a specific physically disabling condition. There are also the usual methodological issues associated with the use of cross-sectional designs and the inevitable reliance upon self-report measures which is a hallmark of this area of research. Despite these issues, there is increasing evidence of a significant prevalence of chronic pain among those with physically disabling conditions.

2.1 Injury related conditions

Injury related conditions for which there is data regarding the nature of chronic pain includes those with a traumatic onset, such as traumatic brain injury and spinal cord injury, and those with a non-traumatic onset, such as cerebral palsy which is thought to be due to an injury to the developing brain. The kinds of traumatic events from which these injuries arise, such as motor vehicle accidents and sporting injuries, may mean that the individual has acquired multiple injuries which may complicate the assessment of the relationship between specific pain conditions and the physically disabling condition of interest.

2.1.1 Traumatic brain injury

Specific pain conditions of interest among those with traumatic brain injury include headaches of various types, but others noted include complex regional pain syndrome (CRPS), heterotopic ossification, and pain due to spasticity (Ivanhoe & Hartman, 2004; Nampiaparampil, 2008). A recent systematic review of chronic pain among those with traumatic brain injury identified 23 studies meeting their criteria, from which they estimated the overall prevalence of chronic pain in people with traumatic brain injury at 51.5% among civilians, with 57.8% reporting chronic headache (Nampiaparampil, 2008). An interesting aspect of findings among this group is that prevalence of chronic headaches differs depending on the severity of the traumatic brain injury (Lahz & Bryant, 1996; Nampiaparampil, 2008), with higher prevalence reported among those with mild traumatic brain injury. It has been observed that those with traumatic brain injury may have other traumatic injuries, and studies regarding the pain conditions in this poly-trauma group are very limited (Dobscha, et al., 2009). The assessment of pain in those with traumatic brain injury, particularly those with severe enough injuries to result in significant impairments to cognition, language or behaviour, may be challenging and so result in less accurate estimates than in some other groups with physically disabling conditions.

2.1.2 Spinal cord injury

Relative to other conditions, there have been a larger number of studies examining chronic pain among those with spinal cord injury. Classifying the pain conditions associated with spinal cord injury has been undertaken by a number of groups, with more concordance among the groups in relation to some pain types than others, such as neuropathic pains (Cardenas, Felix, Cardenas, & Felix, 2009; Finnerup, Baastrup, & Jensen, 2009; Siddall, Yezierski, & Loeser, 2000). A recent systematic review of the prevalence of chronic pain of all causes among those with traumatic spinal cord injury have identified more than forty high quality studies from across the world, but the authors note that despite this there are many contradictions and unanswered questions about the nature of chronic pain in this group (Dijkers, Bryce, & Zanca, 2009). Prevalence rates of the studies included ranged from 26 to 98 percent, but the authors cautioned that the heterogeneity of the studies involved precluded calculation of an overall prevalence rate. It should be noted that co-morbid traumatic brain injury are not uncommon among this group, often within the mild range (Bradbury, et al., 2008). While spinal cord injury has been included in the section on traumatic injuries, some spinal cord injuries develop as a result of disease activity, such as cancer, which may mean the individual experiences other chronic pain conditions. As with many other physically disabling conditions, pain is only one of many troublesome complications. However, a recent study found that relative to others it is the most common and is closely associated with functioning (Jensen, Kuehn, Amtmann, & Cardenas, 2007).

2.1.3 Amputation
Studies of pain post-amputation are largely related to either upper or lower limb amputations. Most studies report on traumatically acquired amputations, although those related to vascular or other conditions are also relatively common. The most common type of pain problems reported in these studies is phantom limb pain and residual (or stump) pain, although it is also possible for people to develop musculoskeletal pain following amputation, for example in the back (Hammarlund, Carlström, Melchior, & Persson, 2011; Kooijman, Dijkstra, Geertzen, Elzinga, & van der Schans, 2000). Prevalence estimates suggest that phantom limb pain occurs in approximately 45 to 80% of people post-amputation, depending partly upon whether those with upper or lower limb amputations are considered, with rates of residual pain similarly high but varying (Behr, et al., 2009; Desmond & Maclachlan, 2010; Dijkstra, et al., 2002; Ehde, et al., 2000; Kooijman, et al., 2000; Schley, et al., 2008).

2.1.4 Cerebral palsy
In contrast to many of the other physically disabling conditions upon which this chapter focuses, research on cerebral palsy related pain is not confined to studies of adults. The common use of registries in a number of countries also means that the populations from which samples are drawn are more complete than in many other conditions. A French study of adults with cerebral palsy found that 75% reported pain of any sort (Gallien, et al., 2007). Musculoskeletal pain has been the subject of most investigation among this population. Prevalence estimates range from approximately one third to two thirds, with the pattern of distribution across the body different depending on the type of cerebral palsy (Engel, Jensen, Hoffman, & Kartin, 2003; Jahnsen, Villien, Aamodt, Stanghelle, & Holm, 2004; Schwartz, Engel, & Jensen, 1999; Vogtle, 2009). Although studies of children are more common in this group, they are limited by a number of factors regarding the measurement of pain and often rely on parental report. However, the available studies suggest 50 to 75 % of children are affected by pain, with approximately one third experiencing moderate to severe pain (Parkinson, Gibson, Dickinson, & Colver, 2010; Russo, Miller, Haan, Cameron, & Crotty, 2008).

2.2 Disease related conditions

Chronic pain has been investigated in the context of a range of diseases which are associated with physical disability. Some of the central pains, such as central post-stroke pain, associated with these conditions have only been recognized relatively recently, and have been subject to intense investigation.

2.2.1 Multiple sclerosis

A range of pain conditions, both general and specific, have been reported in people with multiple sclerosis. These include those related to spasm, neuropathic pains of various types (including trigeminal neuralgia and L'hermitte's sign), back pain and headaches. A recent systematic review of pain among people with multiple sclerosis found twenty-one studies reporting pain prevalence, with an overall range of 29 to 86%, and with few consistent findings related to the relationship between the report of pain and multiple sclerosis characteristics (O'Connor, Schwid, Herrmann, Markman, & Dworkin, 2008). Further, this study reported that between 11 and 23% of people reported pain as a symptom at the onset of their multiple sclerosis. Central pain, including trigeminal neuralgia, has been reported in approximately one third of people with MS (Osterberg, Boivie, & Thuomas, 2005).

2.2.2 Stroke

A number of chronic pain conditions are observed in people who have had a stroke, including shoulder pain, spasticity related pain and headaches, and central post-stroke pain is a uncommon condition particular to stroke. Estimates of the prevalence of chronic pain between studies are variable. Approximately 11 to 21% of people following a first stroke have been reported to have a stroke related pain condition up to 16 months following the stroke (Appelros, 2006; Jonsson, Lindgren, Hallstrom, Norrving, & Lindgren, 2006; Lundstrom, Smits, Terent, & Borg, 2009), whereas 42% of people following stroke attending an out-patient rehabilitation clinic had chronic musculoskeletal pain (Kong, Woon, & Yang, 2004). Neuropathic and central pain conditions occur at a significant level among those who have had a stroke, including estimates of complex regional pain syndrome in 15% of those undergoing inpatient post-stroke rehabilitation and 7% with central poststroke pain (Kitisomprayoonkul, Sungkapo, Taveemanoon, & Chaiwanichsiri, 2010; Klit, Finnerup, Andersen, & Jensen, 2011).

2.2.3 Parkinson's Disease

Relatively little is known about the prevalence and nature of pain in people with Parkinson's Disease, although clinically it is reported to be observed frequently (Beiske & Loge, 2009). Ford (2010) has classified pain problems associated with Parkinson's Disease in five categories: musculoskeletal pain; radicular or neuropathic pain; dystonia-related pain; akathitic discomfort; and central or primary pain. Overall estimates of the prevalence of pain in this group range between and 40 and 83% (Beiske & Loge, 2009; Ford, 2010). Pain has been reported to be the first reported symptom of Parkinson's Disease among a significant minority of those who initially present with non-motor symptoms (O'Sullivan, et al., 2008).

2.2.4 Muscular dystrophy

Duchenne muscular dystrophy, myotonic muscular dystrophy, type I and facioscapulohumeral muscular dystrophy have all been found to be associated with chronic pain (Engel, Kartin, Carter, Jensen, & Jaffe, 2009; Jensen, Abresch, Carter, & McDonald, 2005; Jensen, et al., 2008; Miro, et al., 2009) although there are limited studies with these groups. More than half of the respondents in these studies reported the presence of chronic pain, with pain in the back and legs most commonly reported but with a large number of sites reported to be involved.

2.3 Summary

Although not a comprehensive review of all of those physically disabling conditions which may result in the experience of chronic pain, the above summary suggests that chronic pain is a relatively common but perhaps neglected consequence of physically disabling conditions (Osterberg, et al., 2005). The specific causes and the nature of chronic pain experienced may differ between physically disabling conditions, but its high prevalence indicates that it is a legitimate concern for health practitioners and researchers. Awareness of the likelihood of pain is a necessary, although not sufficient, condition for the effective management of such pain. There is evidence that there are misconceptions among health professionals about the likely occurrence of pain in those with physically disabling conditions (Piwko, et al., 2007). Indeed, studies of people with pain associated with various conditions, including spinal cord injury, cerebral palsy, and multiple sclerosis, indicate that those affected perceive the available treatments and access to them to be inadequate (Cardenas, et al., 2009; Henwood & Ellis, 2004; Kennedy, Lude, & Taylor, 2006; Pollmann, Feneberg, & Erasmus, 2004; Wartan, Hamann, Wedley, & McColl, 1997). In addition, the economic costs of pain among those with physically disabling conditions appears to be large, with a Canadian study estimating that the cost of pain among people multiple sclerosis over a 6 month period was Can$80 million (Piwko, et al., 2007).

3. Psychological and social factors in chronic pain among those with physically disabling conditions

Biopsychosocial models of pain, which are characterized by a focus on the interaction between biological, psychological and social variables in the pain experience, dominate the contemporary understanding of primary pain conditions, such as headache and low back pain (Gatchel, Peng, Peters, Fuchs, & Turk, 2007). The use of biopsychosocial models has also been promoted as the most appropriate framework for the understanding and management of disability of all types (World Health Organisation, 2011).The importance of these models is that they broaden the focus of health professionals to consider psychological and social factors which affect the course of a chronic pain condition. Crucially, where many chronic pain conditions were resistant to the available medical interventions, resulting in a significant proportion of the population living with chronic pain, biopsychosocial models offered a new treatment target focused on reducing the psychological distress and functional disability experienced by those with persisting pain (Blyth, et al., 2001).

Within the broad category of biopsychosocial models, those informed by cognitive behavioural theories are most common. These models particularly address the role of cognitions and behaviours in the development and maintenance of pain, as well as associated pain-related distress and disability. A wide range of cognitive and behavioural constructs have been investigated to determine their relationship with the experience of pain and associated disability and distress (Vlaeyen & Linton, 2000). There is some support for many of these constructs in individual studies. However, among these constructs, pain catastrophizing, pain self-efficacy, and avoidance have all been found to be consistently related to the experience of pain and associated disability or distress across different populations and methodologies. In addition, the presence of altered mood, such as symptoms of depression and anxiety, or the co-existence of psychiatric disorders such as post-traumatic stress disorder, all seem to be important in influencing the course of a chronic pain condition.

The application of biopsychosocial models to chronic pain among those with physically disabling conditions has lagged significantly behind its use among primary pain conditions, where it has long been acknowledged that presence of pain or the intensity of pain does not fully explain pain-related disability or distress (Heneweer, et al., 2007). Among the physically disabling conditions outlined above with documented, significant rates of associated chronic pain there were no peer-reviewed publications available addressing psychosocial variables in the case of Parkinson's Disease. In addition, the investigation of variables has been patchy across the different conditions, and there are few specific models proposed for those with chronic pain in the context of physically disabling conditions. Some of the reasons for this are unclear, although it may be suggested that the obvious presence of pathology among those with physically disabling conditions results in a tendency to discount the possible role of other factors in causing pain-related disability or distress. This is despite repeated findings across a number of diagnoses that condition-related variables, such as severity of injury or illness, are frequently not at all or only weakly related to pain intensity and related disability or distress (Hoffman, et al., 2007).

It is notable that while biopsychosocial models do not dictate that only negative or adverse outcomes are possible following development of pain, much of the available research focuses on factors associated with poor outcomes. In contrast, a study of people with spinal cord injuries or multiple traumas examined factors which differentiated different adjustment trajectories and identified three: the resilience trajectory, characterized by low levels of mental health symptoms at both early and late stage of admission following injury, the recovery trajectory where the individual shows an improving pattern of mental health symptoms, and the distress trajectory, where higher levels of mental health symptoms at the early stage are sustained in the longer term (Quale & Schanke, 2010). The study reports that the latter accounted for only one fifth of the participants in their study, and that maximum pain at admission differentiated those in the resilience vs the distress trajectory.

Studies investigating the relationship between psychosocial factors and chronic pain in people with physically disabling conditions fall into two main categories. First, psychosocial factors are examined as predictors of chronic pain or pain-related disability, for example does a particular way of thinking about pain have an impact on how much pain is experienced. Second, chronic pain is examined as a contributor to adjustment following onset of a physically disabling condition, for example do those with chronic pain as a result of a physically disabling condition have higher levels of depressive symptomatology. The rapid development of theory and research related to biopsychosocial models of chronic pain has led to some overlap of concepts. A good example of this being that pain catastrophizing first appeared as one of many unhelpful coping strategies, but has now been reframed as a belief alongside others such as self-efficacy or helplessness. It is therefore somewhat difficult to categorize the current literature into particular themes. The purpose of this section is to describe the current evidence regarding the relationship between psychological and social factors and chronic pain in people with physically disabling conditions, and to identify gaps in the current literature which require further investigation.

3.1 Psychological factors

Under the category psychological factors, the main variables to consider are mood and mental health, cognitive responses to pain, and behavioural responses to pain. The extent of the literature in these three areas varies markedly across the various physically disabling conditions under consideration.

3.1.1 Mood and mental health

The association between chronic pain and changes in mood and mental health, including symptoms of depression and anxiety, is perhaps the most frequently explored aspect of biopsychosocial models among those with physically disabling conditions. In some physically disabling conditions, a clear relationship between chronic pain and psychological distress has been consistently demonstrated, whereas in others the findings are more mixed. Pain has been found to be associated with psychological distress in most of the studies identified in cerebral palsy, traumatic brain injury, multiple sclerosis, amputation, spinal cord injury, and muscular dystrophy (Engel, et al., 2003; Engel, Schwartz, Jensen, & Johnson, 2000; Hoffman, et al., 2007; Kalia & O'Connor, 2005; Kratz, et al., 2010; Middleton, Tran, & Craig, 2007; Miro, et al., 2009; Motl, McAuley, Snook, & Gliottoni, 2009; Nicholson Perry, Nicholas, & Middleton, 2009; Nicholson Perry, Nicholas, Middleton, & Siddall, 2009; Norrbrink Budh, Hultling, & Lundeberg, 2005; Stormer, et al., 1997; Turner, Jensen, Warms, & Cardenas, 2002), although the strength of the relationship has varied across studies and conditions. In addition, studies in people with spinal cord injury pain found that continuous pain, as opposed to intermittent pain, was associated with higher levels of depression and anxiety, and conversely more stress among women with spinal cord injuries was associated with consistent reports of pain over a ten year period (Norrbrink Budh & Osteraker, 2007; Rintala, Hart, & Priebe, 2004). Negative mood has also been reported to be a trigger to exacerbations in chronic pain among people with spinal cord injury (Widerstrom-Noga & Turk, 2004). Some studies have presented exceptions to this general rule in the case of cerebral palsy, multiple sclerosis and stroke (Hirsh, Gallegos, Gertz, Engel, & Jensen, 2010; Kong, et al., 2004; Newland, Naismith, & Ullione, 2009; Newland, Wipke-Tevis, Williams, Rantz, & Petroski, 2005). Moderators of this relationship include gender, with the relationship not being found in males with multiple sclerosis in one study, and aetiology (traumatic versus non-traumatic) for amputation in one study moderating the relationship at early time points (Kalia & O'Connor, 2005; Kratz, et al., 2010). Physically disabling conditions in which findings are mixed in this regard include those with phantom limb pain and stump pain following amputation (Fisher & Hanspal, 1998). While most of these studies have been conducted with adults with physically disabling conditions, a study with a large sample of older children with cerebral palsy suggests that children with moderate or severe pain are significantly more likely to have higher levels emotional and behavioural problems (Parkes, et al., 2008). One study in people with multiple sclerosis found that affective memory biases, a measure of vulnerability to depression, may mediate the relationship between chronic pain and depressive symptoms in this group (Bruce, Polen, & Arnett, 2007).

Most studies of the relationship between pain and depression in physically disabling conditions solely report on cross-sectional associations. In some studies, however, they specifically examine pain as a predictor of depression, or in other cases the reverse. Determining the direction of the relationship have proved problematic, although there is some evidence among people with spinal cord injury to support the hypothesis than persisting pain is a driver of depression rather than the converse (Cairns, Adkins, & Scott, 1996; Putzke, Richards, Hicken, & DeVivo, 2002).The presence of depression at one time point has been reported to be a risk factor for pain at a later time point among those with multiple sclerosis and spinal cord injury (Buchanan, Wang, Tai-Seale, & Ju, 2003; Putzke, et al., 2002).

Depression is associated with pain-related interference in a number of physically disabling conditions, including amputation, multiple sclerosis and spinal cord injury (Kratz, et al., 2010; Nicholson Perry, Nicholas, & Middleton, 2009; Nicholson Perry, Nicholas, Middleton, et al., 2009; Norrbrink Budh, et al., 2005; Norrbrink Budh & Osteraker, 2007; Osborne, et al., 2006; Turner, et al., 2002). There is evidence of a similar moderating effect of depression upon the relationship between pain and disability among those with spinal cord injury as is seen in other chronic pain populations (Borsbo, Peolsson, & Gerdle, 2009), and a similar but less clear interaction between these variables in those with traumatic brain injury (Hoffman, et al., 2007). The impairment to quality of life attributable to chronic pain has been reported to be related to depressive symptoms among individuals with spinal cord injury (Cruz-Almeida, Alameda, & Widerstrom-Noga, 2009). In addition, negative moods, boredom and stress reported in a large sample of older children with cerebral palsy was found to be significantly predicted by the presence of pain, although only to contribute a relatively small proportion of variation in this aspects of quality of life and interestingly overall quality of life was found to be consistent with other children without cerebral palsy (Dickinson, et al., 2007).

Studies of the relationship between chronic pain and anxiety among people with physically disabling conditions are less common. However, in studies of people with multiple sclerosis, anxiety has been found to be positively associated with pain severity, particularly among women (Kalia & O'Connor, 2005; Motl, et al., 2009). Studies among people with spinal cord injury have also shown a significant relationship between anxiety and pain severity (Nicholson Perry, Nicholas, & Middleton, 2009; Nicholson Perry, Nicholas, Middleton, et al., 2009; Norrbrink Budh, et al., 2005; Norrbrink Budh & Osteraker, 2007). There are a few studies examining the relationship between pain and post-traumatic stress disorder (PTSD). In a study of people with both traumatic and non-traumatic amputation, pain and pain-related interference was positively correlated with PTSD symptoms in both groups (Kratz, et al., 2010). Pain-related anxiety, often measured as a combination of cognitions, behaviours and emotion, has also been found to moderate the relationship between chronic pain and disability among those with spinal cord injury, with those reporting higher levels of pain related anxiety experiencing greater disability (Borsbo, et al., 2009). Anger has been less well investigated, although it has been shown to moderate the perception of pain in people with spinal cord injury (Conant, 1998; Summers, Rapoff, Varghese, Porter, & Palmer, 1991).

3.1.2 Cognitive responses to pain

The relationship between cognitive responses to pain, or beliefs, and pain-related disability and distress has been explored in those with a number of the physically disabling conditions of interest. Pain catastrophizing, characterized by a tendency to negative and unrealistic beliefs in response to pain, and is the cognitive factor with the greatest body of evidence supporting its role. While pain catastrophizing has often been measured in questionnaires designed to measure coping strategies, it is best considered alongside other beliefs, and so will be reported on in this section.

Pain catastrophizing has been found to be associated with pain intensity among people with chronic phantom limb pain post-amputation, multiple sclerosis and spinal cord injury (Hill, Niven, & Knussen, 1995; Nicholson Perry, Nicholas, & Middleton, 2009; Osborne, Jensen,

Ehde, Hanley, & Kraft, 2007; Turner, et al., 2002; Vase, et al., 2011; Wollaars, Post, van Asbeck, & Brand, 2007). In a study of people with phantom limb pain, pain catastrophizing was also shown to significantly contribute to wind-up-like pain when anxiety and depression were controlled for (Vase, et al., 2011)

Pain catastrophizing has been found to be positively associated with pain-related disability among those with spinal cord injury, cerebral palsy, phantom limb pain, muscular dystrophy and multiple sclerosis (Borsbo, et al., 2009; Douglas, Wollin, & Windsor, 2008; Engel, et al., 2000; Hill, et al., 1995; Miro, et al., 2009; Molton, et al., 2009; Nicholson Perry, Nicholas, & Middleton, 2009; Nicholson Perry, Nicholas, Middleton, et al., 2009; Osborne, et al., 2007). Psychological functioning among people with spinal cord injury, multiple sclerosis, phantom limb pain, muscular dystrophy and cerebral palsy has been found to be negatively associated with pain catastrophizing (Douglas, et al., 2008; Engel, Jensen, & Schwartz, 2006; Engel, et al., 2000; Hanley, et al., 2004; Hill, et al., 1995; Miro, et al., 2009; Molton, et al., 2009; Nicholson Perry, Nicholas, & Middleton, 2009; Nicholson Perry, Nicholas, Middleton, et al., 2009; Osborne, et al., 2007; Smedema, Catalano, & Ebener, 2011; Ullrich, Jensen, Loeser, & Cardenas, 2007; Wollaars, et al., 2007). Pain catastrophizing has also been shown to mediate the relationship between pain severity and psychological distress and pain-related disability among people with spinal cord injury (Ullrich, et al., 2007). It has been suggested that pain catastrophizing may, in fact, be a function of disturbed mood. This suggestion is brought into question by findings in both phantom limb pain and spinal cord injury related chronic pain which shows that pain catastrophizing is associated with pain intensity when mood is controlled for (Ullrich, et al., 2007; Vase, et al., 2011). Among the many studies of individuals with spinal cord injury pain, veterans with the condition appear to have higher levels of pain catastrophizing than non-veterans (Ullrich, Jensen, Loeser, Cardenas, & Weaver, 2008).

While most of these studies are cross-sectional in nature, a prospective study of people with spinal cord injury with chronic pain found that over a six month period decreases in pain catastrophizing were associated with decreased pain interference and improved psychological functioning (Hanley, Raichle, Jensen, & Cardenas, 2008). Conversely, a similar study in phantom limb pain found that pain catastrophizing at one month following amputation (that is, before chronic pain had developed) was predictive of decreased depressive symptoms and pain-related interference at both 12 and 24 months (Hanley, et al., 2004). While this may appear counter-intuitive, the authors suggest that the function of pain catastrophizing soon after amputation may be different to that in those with established chronic pain, who are the subject of most other studies on the subject.

Perceived control over pain has also been investigated, and there is less extensive evidence to support its role in relation to psychological functioning and disability in those with chronic pain secondary to physically disabling conditions. A study of people with spinal cord injury related chronic pain found that increases in perceived control over pain in a six month period was related to decreased pain intensity and pain interference, as well as increased psychological functioning, although the former was a non-significant finding (Hanley, et al., 2008). External locus of control in relation to pain as also been positively associated with depression among people with spinal cord injury related pain (Wollaars, et al., 2007). In addition, two studies of people with phantom limb pain, including a prospective study of people with phantom limb pain from one to 24 months, demonstrated some weak evidence for its influence on pain intensity, psychological functioning, and pain-related disability (Hanley, et al., 2004; Hill, et al., 1995).

Other findings related to pain-related beliefs have also been noted but with much less consistency. A belief that pain is constant or enduring has been found to significantly predict both pain intensity and interference to activities due to pain among those with multiple sclerosis (Douglas, et al., 2008). The lower endorsement of the belief that others should be solicitous in response to pain behaviours was associated with better psychological functioning among people with muscular dystrophy (Miro, et al., 2009)

3.1.3 Behavioural responses to pain

Comparison of the use of behavioural responses to pain, also commonly referred to as coping strategies, among people with chronic pain secondary to physically disabling conditions to those with chronic primary pain conditions has revealed both similarities and differences. In people with cerebral palsy, use of behavioural coping strategies such as guarding and rest was reported to be less common and task persistence more common (Engel, et al., 2000). Conversely, cognitive coping strategies, such as diverting attention, reinterpreting sensations, and praying and hoping, were reportedly used more commonly. The authors suggest that some of these differences may be attributable to different background levels of the use of behavioural strategies such as resting and guarding, which may already be employed for non-pain related reasons among those with physically disabling conditions, and increased reliance on cognitive strategies over which they may be hypothesized to have more control.

The association of particular coping strategies with pain intensity or associated psychological distress or disability has been explored in a number of physically disabling conditions, including spinal cord injury, but with few significant relationships detected (Hanley, et al., 2008; Turner, et al., 2002). In some other studies, however, significant relationships have been found. In a study of people with phantom limb pain, behavioural activity was found to be associated with higher levels of pain, in contrast with findings in those with chronic primary pain conditions (Hill, et al., 1995). Passive coping strategies, including guarding, resting, asking for assistance, seeking social support and pacing, were found to be predictive of pain interference but not psychological functioning among people with spinal cord injury and muscular dystrophy (Miro, et al., 2009; Molton, et al., 2009). Reduction of activity, through resting or avoidance, has been associated with positively associated with pain interference in people with cerebral palsy and muscular dystrophy, and with symptoms of depression in people with cerebral palsy (Engel, et al., 2000; Miro, et al., 2009).

Seeking social support has been found to be positively associated with pain-related disability among people with cerebral palsy and muscular dystrophy (Engel, et al., 2006; Miro, et al., 2009), a finding that may initially appear counter-intuitive. The authors of the cerebral palsy study identified the fact that the items on the scale potentially reflect both adaptive and maladaptive aspects of social support seeking (Engel, et al., 2006). However, operant models of chronic pain suggest that pain contingent social support would result in increased disability, which may also provide a parsimonious explanation of the findings.

The extent to which respondents with multiple sclerosis believed they were able to control or decrease their pain through use of their coping strategies has been found to be associated with decreased pain intensity, however no specific coping strategy was predictive (Douglas, et al., 2008). Further, in the same study no coping strategy was found to be predictive of life interference due to pain and only coping by increasing activities was found to be associated with improved psychological functioning.

3.2 Social factors

Although clearly identified as part of the various biopsychosocial models of pain proposed, social factors have been relatively less well represented in the literature. Studies examining social factors most often report on perceived social support and partner responses to pain behaviours.

3.2.1 Social support

Studies examining the associations between social support and pain are available in people with limb loss, spinal cord injury, multiple sclerosis and muscular dystrophy.

Social support was found to be negatively associated with pain in studies among people with traumatic limb loss, whereas no relationship was found in people with spinal cord injury pain (Kratz, et al., 2010; Stroud, Turner, Jensen, & Cardenas, 2006). Studies of people with multiple sclerosis have resulted in mixed findings, with negative associations with pain in one study and no association in the other (Motl, et al., 2009; Osborne, et al., 2007). A study designed to identify factors which were predictive of consistency of pain over ten years among people with spinal cord injury found that among male respondents, receiving less social support during the first phase of the study was predictive of continuing pain over the life of the study (Rintala, et al., 2004)

Associations between lower levels of social support and greater pain-related disability has been found in people with non-traumatic limb loss, multiple sclerosis and muscular dystrophy, but not in people with spinal cord injury (Kratz, et al., 2010; Miro, et al., 2009; Motl, et al., 2009; Osborne, et al., 2007; Stroud, et al., 2006). In one study, greater social support at one month post amputation was predictive of greater reduction in pain interference at 12 and 24 months (Hanley, et al., 2004). In addition, increased social support has been found to be associated with lower levels of anxiety and depression in people with multiple sclerosis and with depression in people with spinal cord injury (Motl, et al., 2009; Stroud, et al., 2006). Among people with muscular dystrophy, social support was associated positively with psychological functioning (Miro, et al., 2009). Hanley et al. (2004) also looked at the relationship between social constraint, which is the need to hide one's feelings about the amputation from others, and pain and pain-related interference. Increased need for social constraint was associated with pain intensity and interference in both those with traumatic and non-traumatic limb loss in the 6 to 12 month period.

3.2.2 Partner responses to pain behaviours

The most common maladaptive form of partner response to pain behaviours reported in the general chronic pain literature is that of solicitous responding, which is a key mechanism in operant models of pain, hypothesized to increase pain-related disability. A study in people with spinal cord injury chronic pain found perceived solicitous responding from partners were unrelated to pain intensity, pain-related disability, or depression (Stroud, et al., 2006). One study in people with limb loss found that less frequent solicitous responding at one month post amputation was predictive of greater reductions in pain interference at 12 and 24 months (Hanley, et al., 2004). Other forms of partner responses to pain behaviour measured in people with spinal cord injury related chronic pain are negative and distracting responses (Stroud, et al., 2006). Negative responses, such as criticism, and distracting responses were both associated with higher depression, but not pain intensity or pain related disability. Most studies which report upon partner responses to pain behaviours in the context of physically disabling conditions provide information about participants perception of their significant others solicitous responses to their pain behaviours. One study in people with spinal cord injury reported on partner's ratings of their own responses to pain behaviour, and it was notable that these were unrelated to pain intensity, depression or pain-related disability in their partner (Stroud, et al., 2006).

3.3 Summary
Reviewing the evidence presented here, a number of issues are apparent. First, that there is a great deal of variation across physically disabling conditions in the extent to which biopsychosocial factors have been investigated. Second, that over all the conditions considered, social factors are relatively less well explored and this remains a significant omission in the literature. Despite this, and the variation in the patterns in each specific physically disabling condition, across the majority of the conditions for which data is available it is clear that there is evidence to suggest that psychological and social factors are broadly related to pain intensity, as well as associated disability and distress. Across all the factors which have been investigated thus far, it appears that the findings related to pain catastrophizing and its association with pain intensity and related disability and distress are the most consistent. This suggests that pain catastrophizing should be explored as part of assessment protocols for people with chronic pain associated with physically disabling conditions. Further research in the area is clearly needed, particularly prospective studies that begin prior to the development of chronic pain, and which are sufficiently large to permit demographic and medical factors to be controlled for in the analyses.

4. Interventions focused on psychological and social factors

There are two major reasons why psychosocial interventions for pain might be considered for people with chronic pain secondary to physically disabling conditions. The first, that psychosocial variables are important contributors to variance in pain itself, as well as pain related distress or disability, and the second, that existing interventions based on biomedical models of pain are insufficient. The evidence presented in the previous section suggests that, while there are gaps in the literature, there is sufficient reason to think that psychosocial variables do make a significant contribution to pain and associated distress and disability. In addition, there is evidence that people with chronic pain secondary to a range of physically disabling conditions, including cerebral palsy, stroke and multiple sclerosis, are unlikely to be receiving treatment for their pain, are dissatisfied with the pain treatment available to them or report limited improvement in pain despite treatment (Engel, et al., 2003; Hirsh, et al., 2010; Kalia & O'Connor, 2005; Kong, et al., 2004).

Psychosocial interventions for people with chronic pain, predominantly behavioural and cognitive behavioural in origin, are well-established and supported by an extensive evidence base (Meldrum, 2007). A series of systematic reviews and meta-analyses attest to the efficacy of these programs among child and adults with primary chronic pain conditions, as well as early interventions designed to reduce the development of pain-related disability (Eccleston, Morley, Williams, Yorke, & Mastroyannopoulou, 2002; Eccleston, Yorke, Morley, Williams, & Mastroyannopoulou, 2003; Linton & Nordin, 2006; Morley, Eccleston, & Williams, 1999).

4.1 The nature of psychosocial interventions
A very small number of studies have been published that specifically report on the use of psychosocial interventions among people with physically disabling conditions. The majority

of these have involved group-based cognitive behavioural pain management programs, but they also include cognitive restructuring and hypnosis. The potential use of such interventions in people with spinal cord injury was identified in the early 1990's (Umlauf, 1992), but a review of the literature concerning the application and evaluation of these programs among any group with a physically disabling condition reveals a disappointingly small number of studies and little translation into standard practice.

4.2 Feasibility and acceptability of psychosocial interventions

A study undertaken in the US specifically examined the issue of the feasibility and acceptability of psychosocial interventions, with a mixed sample of individuals with chronic pain of more than six months duration occurring secondary to multiple sclerosis, amputations, spinal cord injury and cerebral palsy (Ehde & Jensen, 2004). The study found that both the cognitive restructuring intervention, and the control condition which was an educational intervention, were both rated positively by the participants. A study of a cognitive behavioural pain management program for people with spinal cord injury neuropathic pain reported that attendance at the group was high and participants reported that they were very satisfied with the program (Norrbrink Budh, Kowalski, & Lundeberg, 2006). Authors of another study, examining the effectiveness of a cognitive behavioural pain management program for people with spinal cord injury, provide an analysis of the issues encountered in the implementation of the program (Nicholson Perry, Nicholas, & Middleton, 2010; Nicholson Perry, Nicholas, & Middleton, 2011). These findings suggest that these interventions are potentially acceptable, at least to people with spinal cord injury related pain.

4.3 Use and effectiveness of psychosocial interventions

Psychosocial interventions for pain either described for use with or evaluated with people with physically disabling conditions are extremely few. They are mainly cognitive behavioural, group-based pain management programs, but examples of the use of cognitive restructuring alone and hypnosis are also reported.

4.3.1 Cognitive behavioural group-based pain management programs

Four group-based, cognitive behavioural pain management program of various sorts are described in the literature (Cundiff, Blair, & Puckett, 1995; Gironda, 2004; Nicholson Perry, et al., 2010; Norrbrink Budh, et al., 2006). The main components of such interventions are represented in Table 1. The earliest reports in the literature of cognitive behavioural pain management programs in physically disabling conditions were for spinal cord injury pain and were descriptive. Cundiff and colleagues (1995) described the development of a group-based cognitive behavioural pain management program for people with spinal cord injury pain of all types. This involved many of the common components of pain management programs for primary pain diagnoses, including: the explanation of the self-management model, relaxation (including diaphragmatic breathing, guided imagery), the role of self-talk, and pain behaviours and their impact. Gironda (2004) reported on an intervention which was characterized as an interdisciplinary pain management program for spinal cord injury shoulder pain. It was described as a functional preservation approach aimed at enabling individuals to maintain and improve functional capacities where injuries had already been sustained. The program was provided during a two week in-patient stay and comprised of:

medication adjustment; an exercise regimen designed to increase range of motion, endurance and stretch in upper limbs; biomechanical education; a psychoeducational component designed to enhance understanding of the self-management approach, promote problem-solving and implementation of strategies at home, raise awareness of compensatory responses that may be impacting upon psychological or physical well-being; and recreation therapy to encourage return to social and leisure interests. Preliminary data from eight participants in the program suggested improvements across a range of domains, including mood, sleep and pain intensity during shoulder range of motion testing.

Component	Description
Education regarding pain	Information is presented about the underlying pain mechanisms relevant to chronic pain, including central sensitization, as well as the limitations of medical treatment for chronic pain.
Goal-setting	Collaborative goal-setting related to a variety of goals across a wide spread of domains, including physical activities or mood, emphasizing the identification of short-term goals building towards long-term goals that are challenging but achievable in order to increase a sense of mastery.
Activity pacing	Adoption of quota or time based activities, systematically upgraded over time and linked to goals.
Relaxation	Applied relaxation to reduce muscle tension and improve sleep.
Functional exercise	Whole body reconditioning exercise programme related functional physical goals.
Stretch	Whole body daily stretch programme.
Cognitive therapy	Identification and modification of unhelpful thoughts regarding pain, such as catastrophizing.
Medication reduction	Gradual reduction of inappropriate or excessive pain medications using an agreed schedule.
Flare-up management & relapse prevention	Development of a plan to manage temporary increases in pain (flare ups) or other situations likely to trigger relapse.

Table 1. Common components of cognitive behavioural pain management programs

Two controlled studies have been published which have examined the effectiveness of cognitive behavioural group pain management programs for people with physically disabling conditions, both in those with spinal cord injury (Nicholson Perry, et al., 2010; Norrbrink Budh, et al., 2006). The first controlled study in the literature described a cognitive behavioural pain management program for people with neuropathic pain arising from a spinal cord injury (Norrbrink Budh et al., 2006). The program developed was very like the pain management programs described for people with primary pain diagnoses in content, although of shorter duration (totalling 50 hours over ten weeks). Compared with those in the no-treatment control group, those participating in the program showed significant improvements in depression and sense of coherence (a concept comprising comprehensibility, manageability and meaningfulness of the injury) over 12 months. While there were no other significant differences between the groups, the treatment group showed improvements in anxiety symptoms, emotional reaction and sleep from baseline to the 12-month evaluation, but no significant changes over time were observed in the other outcome measures (including pain intensity and unpleasantness, health-related quality of life and life satisfaction). An Australian study compared a cognitive behavioural pain management program with standard care in a tertiary pain management service in Australia. The program was a modification of an existing program, the design and implementation of which is reported in depth elsewhere, which was approximately half of the usual number of contact hours (Nicholson Perry, et al., 2011). The group attending the pain management program showed an overall improved in mood and pain-related disability at the end of the program compared with the controlled group. This was associated with significant decreases in pain catastrophizing and anxiety in the pain management program group. Three-quarters of people completing the pain management program reported a clinically significant improvement, in contrast to less than a third in the usual care comparison group, however long-term follow up data in this group suggested that benefits were not maintained at six months. Both programs were approximately half of the optimal dose (100 hours) recommended for the management of patients with heterogeneous, disabling chronic pain in a pain management program (Guzman, et al., 2001). While it may appear at first sight that there is a degree of inconsistency in providing an intervention incorporating pacing, where other evidence suggests pacing is an unhelpful strategy among those with chronic pain due to physically disabling conditions, this may be a matter of definition; pacing as taught in cognitive behavioural pain management programs takes a systematic approach to continuing to build up quotas of activity which it may be hypothesized is absent in what respondents would endorse as pacing in surveys of pain-related coping strategies. However, the findings from the evaluation of the programs suggested that there was merit in pursuing the use of cognitive behavioural pain management programs in the context of refractive spinal cord injury pain.

4.3.2 Cognitive restructuring

A pilot program exploring the use of a cognitive restructuring intervention targeting catastrophizing for a heterogeneous group of people with disability related chronic pain has recently been reported (Ehde & Jensen, 2004). The authors compared eight 90-minute sessions of cognitive restructuring with an education control intervention among 18 people with disability-related chronic pain (including those with amputations, spinal cord injury, cerebral palsy and multiple sclerosis). The cognitive restructuring intervention included: the role of negative cognitions; how to identify maladaptive thinking; thought-stopping and cognitive restructuring techniques; and use of reassuring self-statements. The education control intervention included pain education (underlying mechanisms and theories of pain), sleep problems in pain and common pain treatments. The authors report that nine of those who attended the first session did not return, but of the eighteen who did continue with their treatment all reported benefiting from the intervention regardless of the group attended. The preliminary results reported by the authors, describing mean pain intensity on a range of 0 to 10 before and after attendance, suggested that whereas pain intensity was unchanged in those attending the education group there was a reduction of approximately 0.2 of a standard deviation among those participating in the cognitive intervention. The authors conclude that a properly powered controlled trial would be required to establish the effectiveness of this approach, but that it was certainly feasible to provide and regarded as acceptable by at least half the patients. Although the literature on the use of psychosocial interventions in people with physically disabling conditions is limited, there is some evidence of similar therapeutic mechanisms operating in these populations as in chronic primary pain conditions (Burns,

Kubilus, Bruehl, Harden, & Lofland, 2003). In particular, the observation of the association between decreased pain catastrophising and improvements in mood and disability in those who participate in the interventions is consistent with findings in other chronic pain populations (Jensen, et al., 2011; Nicholson Perry, et al., 2010). This cognitive restructuring intervention therefore has particular promise as it targets pain catastrophizing, but requires implementation of a smaller range of treatment strategies than traditional cognitive behavioural pain management programs as described above.

4.3.3 Hypnosis
Hypnosis has also been applied to spinal cord injury related pain in a series of studies (Ehde & Jensen, 2007) using individual hypnosis treatments with 10 sessions over four weeks and daily practice. The suggestions used were reported to include imagery, changing sensations and ignoring pain, with associated post-hypnotic suggestions that a relaxed state and the ability to ignore pain will become increasingly easy. The case studies found that a sub-group of individuals with disability-related pain were able to obtain decreases in pain severity, with associated improvements in mood, sleep and general well-being in individual cases. However, in the absence of randomized controlled trials, no firm conclusions can be drawn about the effectiveness of hypnosis in this context.

In a variation of the more common cognitive behavioural interventions reported in the literature, a cognitive restructuring approach combined with self-hypnosis training was reported in people with multiple sclerosis (Jensen, et al., 2011). This intervention was intended to target pain catastrophising as well as pain intensity. When compared with either cognitive restructuring or hypnosis alone, or the control condition, the combined approach resulted in a decrease in the frequency of pain catastrophising and increase in the frequency of reassuring cognitions, as well as improved average and worst pain intensity.

4.4 Barriers to the use of psychosocial interventions
While access to specialist pain management services of any type is problematic, there are some additional reasons to think that access to psychosocial pain interventions will be particularly difficult for those with physically disabling conditions. Broadly, these include the demands of providing such services and accessibility of such services. Health professionals specialising in the provision of psychosocial interventions for chronic pain, such as clinical psychologists, tend to be limited in supply and concentrated in specialist services in major cities. The skills and expertise required to provide psychosocial pain management interventions to those with physically disabling conditions requires expertise in both pain and some of the specific aspects of the physically disabling condition which may impact upon the delivery of the intervention. This includes having an understanding of the physically disabling conditions and its associated symptoms, such as motor function or fatigue, and how these may impact upon the relevance or implementation of the strategies taught. The additional challenges to mobility from having a physically disabling conditions, as well as chronic pain, in combination with environmental barriers which must be overcome to attend a specialist pain management service reduces the chances that an individual with a chronic pain problem due to a physically disabling condition will be able to attend. The costs of living with a physically disabling condition may result in limited financial resources available to fund travel or accommodation in locations where specialist pain management services are available.

Service delivery models which are able to overcome some of these barriers are yet to be designed, and many of the interventions with a research pedigree to support them have not generalized to routine care due to the lack of support to assist with translation into routine clinical practice. The increased availability of high speed internet may permit the use of online interventions to provide at least some access to some of the components of effective psychosocial interventions for chronic pain, either for use alone or with the support of a health professional, and this may be of particular benefit to those with pain secondary to physically disabling conditions.

4.5 Summary

Despite the limited evidence available about the effective of psychosocial interventions in people with physically disabling conditions, the findings suggest that there is merit in further research to evaluate their usefulness in a broader range of conditions. Intervention studies in this area are notoriously difficult, due to the many barriers to participation and retention in trials. National and international collaborations are likely to be necessary to ensure a sufficient sample size for such studies to be adequately powered. Provision of these services is impeded by a number of practical barriers, some of which might at least partially addressed by making more effective use of information technology (World Health Organisation, 2011). While there is currently insufficient evidence to support a wholesale recommendation to use these interventions in all physically disabling conditions, in light of the dissatisfaction with pain treatment among many with chronic pain secondary to physically disabling conditions they may be considered for use on an individual basis.

5. Conclusion

It can be concluded based upon the data presented that the application of biopsychosocial models to the understanding, assessment and management of chronic pain associated with physically disabling conditions is at an early stage of development. There is a well-established body of research in some conditions, such as spinal cord injury, whereas almost nothing is known about the application of these models to other conditions, notably Parkinson's Disease. Many of the patterns observed in primary pain conditions are replicated in these conditions, but the exceptions noted underscore the importance of caution in generalising findings from one condition to another. Relatively, research concerning the use of psychosocial interventions is less well-developed that research examining the relationships between psychosocial and pain variables in physically disabling conditions. Despite this, the findings generally are suggestive of an important role of including psychosocial variables in our conceptualization of individual differences in the experience of chronic pain and its consequences in people with physically disabling conditions, and the possibility of improved outcomes through the use of psychosocial interventions.

6. Acknowledgement

Much of what I have learned about this area has resulted from the conversations I have been privileged to have with people with physically disabling conditions, and I thank them for their willingness to educate me. I am continually grateful for the opportunity to work with many wise colleagues who have taught me a great deal about pain and some of the physically disabling conditions which have formed the subject of this chapter. In particular, I would like to thank Associate Professor Michael Nicholas, Associate Professor James

Middleton, Professor Ashley Craig and Associate Professor Philip Siddall. I would also like to express my gratitude to the School of Psychology, University of Western Sydney for the support provided in the writing of this chapter, particularly the continuing support of Professor Jane Ussher, as well as the able assistance of Rio Yamaguchi.

7. References

Appelros, P. (2006). Prevalence and predictors of pain and fatigue after stroke: a population-based study. *International Journal of Rehabilitation Research, 29*(4), 329-333.

Behr, J., Friedly, J., Molton, I., Morgenroth, D., Jensen, M. P., & Smith, D. G. (2009). Pain and pain-related interference in adults with lower-limb amputation: Comparison of knee-disarticulation, transtibial, and transfemoral surgical sites. *Journal of Rehabilitation Research and Development, 46*(7), 963-972.

Beiske, A., & Loge, J. (2009). Pain in Parkinson's disease: prevalence and characteristics. *Pain, 141*(1-2), 173-177.

Blyth, F. M., March, L. M., Brnabic, A. J., Jorm, L. R., Williamson, M., & Cousins, M. J. (2001). Chronic pain in Australia: a prevalence study. *Pain, 89*(2-3), 127-134.

Borsbo, B., Peolsson, M., & Gerdle, B. (2009). The complex interplay between pain intensity, depression, anxiety and catastrophising with respect to quality of life and disability. *Disability and Rehabilitation, 31*(19), 1605-1613.

Bradbury, C. L., Wodchis, W. P., Mikulis, D. J., Pano, E. G., Hitzig, S. L., McGillivray, C. F., et al. (2008). Traumatic brain injury in patients with traumatic spinal cord injury: Clinical and economic consequences. *Archives of Physical Medicine and Rehabilitation, 89*(12, Supplement 12), S77-84.

Bruce, J. M., Polen, D., & Arnett, P. A. (2007). Pain and affective memory biases interact to predict depressive symptoms in multiple sclerosis. *Multiple Sclerosis, 13*(1), 58-66.

Buchanan, R. J., Wang, S., Tai-Seale, M., & Ju, H. (2003). Analyses of nursing home residents with multiple sclerosis and depression using the Minimum Data Set. *Multiple Sclerosis, 9*(2), 171-188.

Burns, K., Kubilus, A., Bruehl, S., Harden, R., & Lofland, K. (2003). Do changes in cognitive factors influence outcome following multidisciplinary treatment for chronic pain? A cross-lagged panel analysis. *Journal of Consulting and Clinical Psychology, 71*, 81-91.

Cairns, D. M., Adkins, R. H., & Scott, M. D. (1996). Pain and depression in acute traumatic spinal cord injury: Origins of chronic problematic pain? *Archives of Physical Medicine & Rehabilitation., 77*(4), 329-335.

Cardenas, D. D., Felix, E. R., Cardenas, D. D., & Felix, E. R. (2009). Pain after spinal cord injury: a review of classification, treatment approaches, and treatment assessment. *PM and R, 1*(12), 1077-1090.

Conant, L. L. (1998). Psychological variables associated with pain perceptions among individuals with chronic spinal cord injury pain. *Journal of Clinical Psychology in Medical Settings, 5*(1), 71-90.

Cruz-Almeida, Y., Alameda, G., & Widerstrom-Noga, E. G. (2009). Differentiation between pain-related interference and interference caused by the functional impairments of spinal cord injury. *Spinal Cord, 47*(5), 390-395.

Cundiff, G. W., Blair, K. L., & Puckett, M. J. (1995). Group pain management therapy for persons with spinal cord injury. *SCI Psychosocial Process, 8*(2), 61-66.

Desmond, D. M., & Maclachlan, M. (2010). Prevalence and characteristics of phantom limb pain and residual limb pain in the long term after upper limb amputation. *International Journal of Rehabilitation Research, 33*(3), 279-282.

Dickinson, H. O., Parkinson, K. N., Ravens-Sieberer, U., Schirripa, G., Thyen, U., Arnaud, C., et al. (2007). Self-reported quality of life of 8-12-year-old children with cerebral palsy: a cross-sectional European study. *Lancet, 369*(9580), 2171-2178.

Dijkers, M., Bryce, T., & Zanca, J. (2009). Prevalence of chronic pain after traumatic spinal cord injury: a systematic review. *Journal of Rehabilitation Research and Development, 46*(1), 13-29.

Dijkstra, P. U., Geertzen, J. H., Stewart, R., van der Schans, C. P., Dijkstra, P. U., Geertzen, J. H. B., et al. (2002). Phantom pain and risk factors: a multivariate analysis. *Journal of Pain and Symptom Management, 24*(6), 578-585.

Dobscha, S. K., Clark, M. E., Morasco, B. J., Freeman, M., Campbell, R., & Helfand, M. (2009). Systematic review of the literature on pain in patients with polytrauma including traumatic brain injury. *Pain Medicine, 10*(7), 1200-1217.

Douglas, C., Wollin, J. A., & Windsor, C. (2008). Biopsychosocial correlates of adjustment to pain among people with multiple sclerosis. *Clinical Journal of Pain, 24*(7), 559-567.

Eccleston, C., Morley, S., Williams, A., Yorke, L., & Mastroyannopoulou, K. (2002). Systematic review of randomised controlled trials of psychological therapy for chronic pain in children and adolescents, with a subset meta-analysis of pain relief. *Pain, 99*(1-2), 157-165.

Eccleston, C., Yorke, L., Morley, S., Williams, A. C., & Mastroyannopoulou, K. (2003). Psychological therapies for the management of chronic and recurrent pain in children and adolescents. *Cochrane Database of Systematic Reviews, 1*.

Ehde, D. M., & Jensen, M. P. (2004). Feasibility of a cognitive restructuring intervention for treatment of chronic pain in persons with disabilities. *Rehabilitation Psychology, 49*(3), 254-258.

Ehde, D. M., Czerniecki, J. M., Smith, D. G., Campbell, K. M., Edwards, W. T., Jensen, M. P., et al. (2000). Chronic phantom sensations, phantom pain, residual limb pain, and other regional pain after lower limb amputation. *Archives of Physical Medicine & Rehabilitation, 81*(8), 1039-1044.

Ehde, D. M., & Jensen, M. P. (2004). Feasibility of a cognitive restructuring intervention for treatment of chronic pain in persons with disabilities. *Rehabilitation Psychology, 49*(3), 254-258.

Ehde, D. M., & Jensen, M. P. (2007). Psychological treatment for pain management in persons with spinal cord injury: cognitive therapy and self-hypnosis training. *Topics in Spinal Cord Injury Rehabilitation, 13*(2), 72-80.

Engel, J. M., Jensen, M. P., Hoffman, A. J., & Kartin, D. (2003). Pain in persons with cerebral palsy: extension and cross validation. *Archives of Physical Medicine and Rehabilitation, 84*(8), 1125-1128.

Engel, J. M., Jensen, M. P., & Schwartz, L. (2006). Coping with chronic pain associated with cerebral palsy. *Occupational Therapy International, 13*(4), 224-233.

Engel, J. M., Kartin, D., Carter, G. T., Jensen, M. P., & Jaffe, K. M. (2009). Pain in youths with neuromuscular disease. *American Journal of Hospice & Palliative Medicine, 26*(5), 405-412.

Engel, J. M., Schwartz, L., Jensen, M. P., & Johnson, D. R. (2000). Pain in cerebral palsy: the relation of coping strategies to adjustment. *Pain, 88*(3), 225-230.

Finnerup, N. B., Baastrup, C., & Jensen, T. S. (2009). Neuropathic pain following spinal cord injury pain: mechanisms and treatment. *Scandinavian Journal of Pain, 1*(S1), 3-11.

Fisher, K., & Hanspal, R. S. (1998). Phantom pain, anxiety, depression, and their relation in consecutive patients with amputated limbs: case reports. *BMJ (Clinical Research Ed.), 316*(7135), 903.

Ford, B. (2010). Pain in Parkinson's disease. *Movement Disorders, 25*(S1), S98-S103.

Gallien, P., Nicolas, B., Dauvergne, F., Petrilli, S., Houedakor, J., Roy, D., et al. (2007). Pain in adults with cerebral palsy. *Annales de Readaptation et de Medecine Physique, 50*(7), 558-563.

Gatchel, R. J., Peng, Y. B., Peters, M. L., Fuchs, P. N., & Turk, D. C. (2007). The biopsychosocial approach to chronic pain: scientific advances and future directions. *Psychological Bulletin, 133*(4), 581-624.

Gironda, R. J. (2004). An interdisciplinary, cognitive-behavioral shoulder pain treatment program. *SCI Psychosocial Process, 17*(4), 247-252.

Guzman, J., Esmail, R., Karjalainen, K., Malmivaara, A., Irvin, E., & Bombardier, C. (2001). Multidisciplinary rehabilitation for chronic low back pain: systematic review. *British Medical Journal, 322*(7301), 1511-1516.

Hammarlund, C. S., Carlström, M., Melchior, R., & Persson, B. M. (2011). Prevalence of back pain, its effect on functional ability and health-related quality of life in lower limb amputees secondary to trauma or tumour: a comparison across three levels of amputation. *Prosthetics and Orthotics International, 35*(1), 97-105.

Hanley, M. A., Jensen, M. P., Ehde, D. M., Hoffman, A. J., Patterson, D. R., & Robinson, L. R. (2004). Psychosocial predictors of long-term adjustment to lower-limb amputation and phantom limb pain. *Disability & Rehabilitation, 26*(14-15), 882-893.

Hanley, M. A., Raichle, K., Jensen, M., & Cardenas, D. D. (2008). Pain catastrophizing and beliefs predict changes in pain interference and psychological functioning in persons with spinal cord injury. *The Journal of Pain, 9*(9), 863-871.

Heneweer, H., Aufdemkampe, G., van Tulder, M. W., Kiers, H., Stappaerts, K. H., & Vanhees, L. (2007). Psychosocial variables in patients with (sub)acute low back pain: an inception cohort in primary care physical therapy in The Netherlands. *Spine, 32*(5), 586-592.

Henwood, P., & Ellis, J. A. (2004). Chronic neuropathic pain in spinal cord injury: the patient's perspective. *Pain Research and Management, 9*(1), 39-45.

Hill, A., Niven, C. A., & Knussen, C. (1995). The role of coping in adjustment to phantom limb pain. *Pain, 62*(1), 79-86.

Hirsh, A. T., Gallegos, J. C., Gertz, K. J., Engel, J. M., & Jensen, M. P. (2010). Symptom burden in individuals with cerebral palsy. *Journal of Rehabilitation Research and Development, 47*(9), 863-876.

Hoffman, J. M., Pagulayan, K. F., Zawaideh, N., Dikmen, S., Temkin, N., & Bell, K. R. (2007). Understanding pain after traumatic brain injury: impact on community participation. *American Journal of Physical Medicine and Rehabilitation, 86*(12), 962-969.

Ivanhoe, C. B., & Hartman, E. T. (2004). Clinical caveats on medical assessment and treatment of pain after TBI. *Journal of Head Trauma Rehabilitation, 19*(1), 29-39.

Jahnsen, R., Villien, L., Aamodt, G., Stanghelle, J. K., & Holm, I. (2004). Musculoskeletal pain in adults with cerebral palsy compared with the general population. *Journal of Rehabilitation Medicine, 36*(2), 78-84.

Jensen, M. P., Abresch, R. T., Carter, G. T., & McDonald, C. M. (2005). Chronic pain in persons with neuromuscular disease. *Archives of Physical Medicine & Rehabilitation, 86*(6), 1155-1163.

Jensen, M. P., Ehde, D. M., Gertz, K. J., Stoelb, B. L., Dillworth, T. M., Hirsh, A. T., et al. (2011). Effects of self-hypnosis training and cognitive restructuring on daily pain intensity and catastrophizing in individuals with multiple sclerosis and chronic pain. *International Journal of Clinical and Experimental Hypnosis, 59*(1), 45-63.

Jensen, M. P., Hoffman, A. J., Stoelb, B. L., Abresch, R. T., Carter, G. T., & McDonald, C. M. (2008). Chronic pain in persons with myotonic dystrophy and facioscapulohumeral dystrophy. *Archives of Physical Medicine and Rehabilitation, 89*(2), 320-328.

Jensen, M. P., Kuehn, C. M., Amtmann, D., & Cardenas, D. D. (2007). Symptom burden in persons with spinal cord injury. *Archives of Physical Medicine and Rehabilitation, 88*(5), 638-645.

Jonsson, A. C., Lindgren, I., Hallstrom, B., Norrving, B., & Lindgren, A. (2006). Prevalence and intensity of pain after stroke: a population based study focusing on patients' perspectives. *Journal of Neurology, Neurosurgery and Psychiatry, 77*(5), 590-595.

Kalia, L. V., & O'Connor, P. W. (2005). Severity of chronic pain and its relationship to quality of life in multiple sclerosis. *Multiple Sclerosis, 11*(3), 322-327.

Kennedy, P., Lude, P., & Taylor, N. (2006). Quality of life, social participation, appraisals and coping post spinal cord injury: a review of four community samples. *Spinal Cord, 44*(2), 95-105.

Kitisomprayoonkul, W., Sungkapo, P., Taveemanoon, S., & Chaiwanichsiri, D. (2010). Medical complications during inpatient stroke rehabilitation in Thailand: a prospective study. *Journal of the Medical Association of Thailand, 93*(5), 594-600.

Klit, H., Finnerup, N. B., Andersen, G., & Jensen, T. S. (2011). Central poststroke pain: A population-based study. *Pain, 152*(4), 818-824. doi: 10.1016/j.pain.2010.12.030

Kong, K.-H., Woon, V.-C., & Yang, S.-Y. (2004). Prevalence of chronic pain and its impact on health-related quality of life in stroke survivors. *Archives of Physical Medicine and Rehabilitation, 85*(1), 35-40.

Kooijman, C. M., Dijkstra, P. U., Geertzen, J. H. B., Elzinga, A., & van der Schans, C. P. (2000). Phantom pain and phantom sensations in upper limb amputees: an epidemiological study. *Pain, 87*(1), 33-41.

Kratz, A. L., Williams, R. M., Turner, A. P., Raichle, K. A., Smith, D. G., & Ehde, D. M. (2010). To lump or to split? Comparing individuals with traumatic and nontraumatic limb loss in the first year after amputation. *Rehabilitation Psychology, 55*(2), 126-138.

Lahz, S., & Bryant, R. A. (1996). Incidence of chronic pain following traumatic brain injury. *Archives of Physical Medicine and Rehabilitation, 77*(9), 889-891.

Linton, S. J. P., & Nordin, E. M. A. (2006). A 5-year follow-up evaluation of the health and economic consequences of an early cognitive behavioral intervention for back pain: A randomized, controlled trial. *Spine, 31*(8), 853-858.

Lundstrom, E., Smits, A., Terent, A., & Borg, J. (2009). Risk factors for stroke-related pain 1 year after first-ever stroke. *European Journal of Neurology, 16*(2), 188-193.

Meldrum, M. L. (2007). Brief history of multidisciplinary management of chronic pain, 1990-2000. In M. Schatman & A. Campbell (Eds.), *Chronic pain management: guidelines for multidisciplinary program development*: Informa Healthcare.

Middleton, J. W., Tran, Y., & Craig, A. (2007). Relationship between quality of life and self-efficacy in persons with spinal cord injuries. *Archives of Physical Medicine and Rehabilitation, 88*(12), 1643-1648.

Miro, J., Raichle, K. A., Carter, G. T., O'Brien, S. A., Abresch, R. T., McDonald, C. M., et al. (2009). Impact of biopsychosocial factors on chronic pain in persons with myotonic and facioscapulohumeral muscular dystrophy. *American Journal of Hospice & Palliative Medicine, 26*(4), 308-319.

Molton, I. R., Stoelb, B. L., Jensen, M. P., Ehde, D. M., Raichle, K. A., & Cardenas, D. D. (2009). Psychosocial factors and adjustment to chronic pain in spinal cord injury:

replication and cross-validation. *Journal of Rehabilitation Research and Development,* 46(1), 31-42.

Morley, S., Eccleston, C., & Williams, A. (1999). Systematic review and meta-analysis of randomized controlled trials of cognitive behaviour therapy and behaviour therapy for chronic pain in adults, excluding headache. *Pain, 80*(1-2), 1-13.

Motl, R. W., McAuley, E., Snook, E. M., & Gliottoni, R. C. (2009). Physical activity and quality of life in multiple sclerosis: Intermediary roles of disability, fatigue, mood, pain, self-efficacy and social support. *Psychology, Health and Medicine, 14*(1), 111-124.

Nampiaparampil, D. E. (2008). Prevalence of chronic pain after traumatic brain injury: A systematic review. *JAMA: Journal of the American Medical Association, 300*(6), 711-719.

Newland, P. K., Naismith, R. T., & Ullione, M. (2009). The impact of pain and other symptoms on quality of life in women with relapsing-remitting multiple sclerosis. *Journal of Neuroscience Nursing, 41*(6), 322-328.

Newland, P. K., Wipke-Tevis, D. D., Williams, D. A., Rantz, M. J., & Petroski, G. F. (2005). Impact of pain on outcomes in long-term care residents with and without multiple sclerosis. *Journal of the American Geriatrics Society, 53*(9), 1490-1496.

Nicholson Perry, K., Nicholas, M. K., & Middleton, J. W. (2009). Spinal cord injury-related pain in rehabilitation: a cross-sectional study of relationships with cognitions, mood and physical function. *European Journal of Pain: Ejp, 13*(5), 511-517.

Nicholson Perry, K., Nicholas, M. K., & Middleton, J. W. (2010). Comparison of a pain management program with usual care in a pain management center for people with spinal cord injury-related chronic pain. *The Clinical Journal of Pain, 26*(3), 206-216.

Nicholson Perry, K., Nicholas, M. K., & Middleton, J. W. (2011). Multidisciplinary cognitive behavioural pain management programmes for people with a spinal cord injury: design and implementation. *Disability and Rehabilitation, 33*(13-14), 1272-1280. doi: doi:10.3109/09638288.2010.524276

Nicholson Perry, K., Nicholas, M. K., Middleton, J. W., & Siddall, P. (2009). Psychological characteristics of people with spinal cord injury-related persisting pain referred to a tertiary pain management center. *Journal of Rehabilitation Research and Development, 46*(1), 57-67.

Norrbrink Budh, C., Hultling, C., & Lundeberg, T. (2005). Quality of sleep in individuals with spinal cord injury: a comparison between patients with and without pain. *Spinal Cord, 43*(2), 85-95.

Norrbrink Budh, C., Kowalski, J., & Lundeberg, T. (2006). A comprehensive pain management programme comprising educational, cognitive and behavioural interventions for neuropathic pain following spinal cord injury. *Journal of Rehabilitation Medicine, 38*(3), 172-180.

Norrbrink Budh, C., & Osteraker, A. L. (2007). Life satisfaction in individuals with a spinal cord injury and pain. *Clinical Rehabilitation, 21*(1), 89-96.

O'Connor, A. B., Schwid, S. R., Herrmann, D. N., Markman, J. D., & Dworkin, R. H. (2008). Pain associated with multiple sclerosis: systematic review and proposed classification. *Pain, 137*(1), 96-111.

O'Sullivan, S. S., Williams, D. R., Gallagher, D. A., Massey, L. A., Silveira-Moriyama, L., & Lees, A. J. (2008). Nonmotor symptoms as presenting complaints in Parkinson's disease: a clinicopathological study. *Movement Disorders, 23*(1), 101-106.

Osborne, T. L., Jensen, M. P., Ehde, D. M., Hanley, M. A., & Kraft, G. (2007). Psychosocial factors associated with pain intensity, pain-related interference, and psychological functioning in persons with multiple sclerosis and pain. *Pain, 127*(1-2), 52-62.

Osborne, T. L., Turner, A. P., Williams, R. M., Bowen, J. D., Hatzakis, M., Rodriguez, A., et al. (2006). Correlates of pain interference in multiple sclerosis. *Rehabilitation Psychology, 51*(2), 166-174.

Osterberg, A., Boivie, J., & Thuomas, K. A. (2005). Central pain in multiple sclerosis-- prevalence and clinical characteristics. *European Journal of Pain, 9*(5), 531-542.

Parkes, J., White-Koning, M., Dickinson, H. O., Thyen, U., Arnaud, C., Beckung, E., et al. (2008). Psychological problems in children with cerebral palsy: a cross-sectional European study. *Journal of Child Psychology and Psychiatry and Allied Disciplines, 49*(4), 405-413.

Parkinson, K. N., Gibson, L., Dickinson, H. O., & Colver, A. F. (2010). Pain in children with cerebral palsy: a cross-sectional multicentre European study. *Acta Paediatrica, 99*(3), 446-451.

Piwko, C., Desjardins, O. B., Bereza, B. G., Machado, M., Jaszewski, B., Freedman, M. S., et al. (2007). Pain due to multiple sclerosis: analysis of the prevalence and economic burden in Canada. *Pain Research and Management, 12*(4), 259-265.

Pollmann, W., Feneberg, W., & Erasmus, L. P. (2004). Pain in multiple sclerosis--a still underestimated problem. The 1 year prevalence of pain syndromes, significance and quality of care of multiple sclerosis inpatients. *Nervenarzt, 75*(2), 135-140.

Putzke, J. D., Richards, J. S., Hicken, B. L., & DeVivo, M. J. (2002). Interference due to pain following spinal cord injury: important predictors and impact on quality of life. *Pain, 100*(3), 231-242.

Quale, A. J., & Schanke, A. (2010). Resilience in the face of coping with a severe physical injury: A study of trajectories of adjustment in a rehabilitation setting. *Rehabilitation Psychology, 55*(1), 12-22.

Rintala, D. H., Hart, K. A., & Priebe, M. M. (2004). Predicting consistency of pain over a 10-year period in persons with spinal cord injury. *Journal of Rehabilitation Research and Development, 41*(1), 75-88.

Russo, R. N., Miller, M. D., Haan, E., Cameron, I. D., & Crotty, M. (2008). Pain characteristics and their association with quality of life and self-concept in children with hemiplegic cerebral palsy identified from a population register. *Clinical Journal of Pain, 24*(4), 335-342.

Schley, M. T., Wilms, P., Toepfner, S., Schaller, H.-P., Schmelz, M., Konrad, C. J., et al. (2008). Painful and nonpainful phantom and stump sensations in acute traumatic amputees. *Journal of Trauma-Injury Infection & Critical Care, 65*(4), 858-864.

Schwartz, L., Engel, J. M., & Jensen, M. P. (1999). Pain in persons with cerebral palsy. *Archives of Physical Medicine & Rehabilitation, 80*(10), 1243-1246.

Siddall, P. J., Yezierski, R. P., & Loeser, J. D. (2000). Pain following spinal cord injury: clinical features, prevalence and taxonomy. *IASP Newsletter, 3.*

Smedema, S. M., Catalano, D., & Ebener, D. J. (2011). The relationship of coping, self-worth, and subjective well-being: A structural equation model. *Rehabilitation Counseling Bulletin, 53*(3), 131-142.

Stormer, S., Gerner, H. J., Gruninger, W., Metzmacher, K., Follinger, S., Wienke, C., et al. (1997). Chronic pain/dysaesthesiae in spinal cord injury patients: results of a multicentre study. *Spinal Cord, 35*(7), 446-455.

Stroud, M. W., Turner, J. A., Jensen, M. P., & Cardenas, D. D. (2006). Partner responses to pain behaviors are associated with depression and activity interference among persons with chronic pain and spinal cord injury. *The Journal of Pain, 7*(2), 91-99.

Summers, J. D., Rapoff, M. A., Varghese, G., Porter, K., & Palmer, R. E. (1991). Psychosocial factors in chronic spinal cord injury pain. *Pain, 47*(2), 183-189.

Turner, J. A., Jensen, M. P., Warms, C. A., & Cardenas, D. D. (2002). Catastrophizing is associated with pain intensity, psychological distress, and pain-related disability among individuals with chronic pain after spinal cord injury. *Pain, 98*(1-2), 127-134.

Ullrich, P. M., Jensen, M., Loeser, J. D., & Cardenas, D. D. (2007). Catastrophizing mediates associations between pain severity, psychological distress, and functional disability among persons with spinal cord injury. *Rehabilitation Psychology, 52*(4), 390-398.

Ullrich, P. M., Jensen, M. P., Loeser, J. D., Cardenas, D. D., & Weaver, F. M. (2008). Pain among veterans with spinal cord injury. *Journal of Rehabilitation Research and Development, 45*(6), 793-800.

Umlauf, R. L. (1992). Psychological interventions for chronic pain following spinal cord injury. *Clinical Journal of Pain, 8*, 111-118.

Vase, L., Nikolajsen, L., Christensen, B., Egsgaard, L. L., Arendt-Nielsen, L., Svensson, P., et al. (2011). Cognitive-emotional sensitization contributes to wind-up-like pain in phantom limb pain patients. *Pain, 152*(1), 157-162.

Vlaeyen, J. W., & Linton, S. J. (2000). Fear-avoidance and its consequences in chronic musculoskeletal pain: a state of the art. *Pain, 85*(3), 317-332.

Vogtle, L. K. (2009). Pain in adults with cerebral palsy: impact and solutions. *Developmental Medicine and Child Neurology, 51 Suppl 4*, 113-121.

Wartan, S. W., Hamann, W., Wedley, J. R., & McColl, I. (1997). Phantom pain and sensation among British veteran amputees. *British Journal of Anaesthesia, 78*(6), 652-659.

Widerstrom-Noga, E. G., & Turk, D. C. (2004). Exacerbation of chronic pain following spinal cord injury. *Journal of Neurotrauma, 21*(10), 1384-1395.

Wollaars, M. M., Post, M. W. M., van Asbeck, F. W. A., & Brand, N. (2007). Spinal cord injury pain: the influence of psychologic factors and impact on quality of life. *Clinical Journal of Pain, 23*(5), 383-391.

World Health Organisation. (2011). World report on disability 2011. Geneva: World Health Organisation.

Epidural Lysis of
Adhesions and Percutaneous Neuroplasty

Gabor B. Racz[1], Miles R. Day[1], James E. Heavner[1],
Jeffrey P. Smith[1], Jared Scott[2], Carl E. Noe[3], Laslo Nagy[4] and Hana Ilner[1]

[1]Texas Tech University Health Sciences Center, Lubbock, Texas
[2]Advanced Pain Medicine Associates, Wichita, Kansas
[3]University of Texas Southwestern Medical Center, Dallas, Texas
[4]Texas Tech University Health Sciences Center and
Covenant Medical Center, Department of Pediatric Neurosurgery
USA

1. Introduction

Chances are relatively high that each of us will experience low back pain at some point in our lives. The usual course is rapid improvement with 5% to 10% developing persistent symptoms.[1] In the 1990s the estimated cost of low back pain to the health industry was in the billions of dollars, and with a larger proportion of our population now reported to be older, this number can only be expected to increase. [2, 3] Treatment typically begins with conservative measures such as medication and physical therapy and may even include minimally and highly invasive pain management interventions. Surgery is sometimes required in patients who have progressive neurologic deficits or those who do not respond to conservative treatment sometimes chose surgery. A quandary sometimes arises, following a primary surgery, as to whether repeat surgery should be attempted or another alternative technique should be tried. This is the exact problem that the epidural adhesiolysis procedure was designed to address. Failed back surgery or postlaminectomy syndrome led to the development of the epidural adhesiolysis procedure.

It was shown to be effective in many patients with chronic pain after back surgery presumably by freeing up nerves and breaking down scar formation, delivering site-specific corticosteroids and local anesthetics, and reducing edema with the use of hyaluronidase and hypertonic saline. Epidural adhesiolysis has afforded patients a reduction in pain and neurologic symptoms without the expense and occasional long recovery period associated with repeat surgery, and often prevents the need for surgical intervention. Epidural adhesiolysis was given an evidence rating of strong correlating to a 1B or 1C evidence level for post–lumbar surgery syndrome in the most recent American Society of Interventional Pain Physicians evidence-based guidelines. The therapy is supported by observational studies and case series along with randomized-control trials. The recommendation was also made that this therapy could apply to most patients with post laminectomy syndrome or failed back syndrome in many circumstances with informed consent.[4] Additionally, current procedural terminology (CPT) codes have been assigned to the two different kinds of adhesiolysis: CPT 62263 for the three-times injections over 2 to 3 days, usually done in an inpatient hospital setting, and CPT 62264 for the one-time injection series surgery-center model that may need to be repeated 3 to 3.5 times in a 12-month period.

2. Pathophysiology of epidural fibrosis (scar tissue) as a cause of low back pain with radiculopathy

The etiology of chronic low back pain with radiculopathy after appropriate surgery is not well understood. Kuslich et al[5] addressed this issue when they studied 193 patients who had undergone lumbar spine operations given local anesthesic int the epidural space. It was postulated that sciatica could only be produced by stimulation of a swollen, stretched, restricted (i.e., scarred) or compressed nerve root.[5] Back pain could be produced by stimulation of several tissues, but the most common tissue of origin was the outer layer of the annulus fibrosus and the posterior longitudinal ligament. Stimulation for pain generation of the facet joint capsule rarely generated low back pain, and facet synovium and cartilage surfaces of the facet or muscles were never tender.[6]

The contribution of fibrosis to the etiology of low back pain has been debated.[7-9] There are many possible etiologies of epidural fibrosis, including surgical trauma, an annular tear, infection, hematoma, or intrathecal contrast material.[10] These etiologies have been well documented in the literature. LaRocca and Macnab[11] demonstrated the invasion of fibrous connective tissue into postoperative hematoma as a cause of epidural fibrosis, and Cooper et al[12] reported periradicular fibrosis and vascular abnormalities occurring with herniated intervertebral disks. McCarron et al[13] investigated the irritative effect of nucleus pulposus on the dural sac, adjacent nerve roots, and nerve root sleeves independent of the influence of direct compression on these structures. Evidence of an inflammatory reaction was identified by gross inspection and microscopic analysis of spinal cord sections after homogenized autogenous nucleus pulposus was injected into the lumbar epidural space of four dogs. In the control group consisting of four dogs injected with normal saline, the spinal cord sections were grossly normal. Parke and Watanabe[14] showed significant evidence of adhesions in cadavers with lumbar disk herniation.

It is widely accepted that postoperative scar renders the nerve susceptible to injury by a compressive phenomena.[9] It is natural for connective tissue or any kind of scar tissue to form fibrous layers (scar tissue) as a part of the process that transpires after disruption of the intact milieu.[15] Scar tissue is generally found in three components of the epidural space. Dorsal epidural scar tissue is formed by reabsorption of surgical hematoma and may be involved in pain generation.[16] In the ventral epidural space, dense scar tissue is formed by ventral defects in the disk, which may persist despite surgical treatment and continue to produce low back pain and radiculopathy past the surgical healing phase.[17] The lateral epidural space includes the epiradicular structures outside the root canals, known as the lateral recesses or "sleeves," which are susceptible to lateral disk defects, facet hypertrophy, and neuroforaminal stenosis.[18]

Although scar tissue itself is not tender, an entrapped nerve root is. Kuslich et al[5] surmised that the presence of scar tissue compounded the pain associated with the nerve root by fixing it in one position and thus increasing the susceptibility of the nerve root to tension or compression. They also concluded that no other tissues in the spine are capable of producing leg pain. In a study of the relationship between peridural scar evaluated by magnetic resonance imaging (MRI) and radicular pain after lumbar diskectomy, Ross et al[19] demonstrated that subjects with extensive peridural scarring were 3.2 times more likely to experience recurrent radicular pain.

This evidence also parallels a new study by Gilbert et al[20] in which lumbosacral nerve roots were identified as undergoing less strain than previously published during straight leg raise and in which hip motion greater than 60 degrees was determined to cause displacement of the nerve root in the lateral recess.

3. Fluid foraminotomy: Foraminal adhesiolysis or disentrapment

Relative or functional foraminal root entrapment syndrome secondary to epidural fibrosis with corresponding nerve root entrapment is frequently evident after an epidurogram and signified by lack of epidural contrast flow into epidural finger projections at those levels. The lysis procedure effectively serves as a fluid foraminotomy reducing foraminal stenosis caused by epidural fibrosis. In addition to increasing foraminal cross-sectional area, adhesiolysis serves to decompress distended epidural venous structures that may exert compression at nearby spinal levels (Fig. 1) and inevitably cause needle stick related epidural hematomas. Adhesiolysis has led to the development of flexible epiduroscopy that is being pioneered by, primarily initiated, pursued and to this day supported by Dr. James Heavner.[21,22]

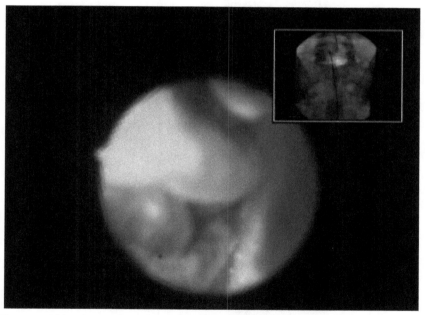

Fig. 1. Engorged blood vessels in the epidural cavity as observed during epiduroscopy. Insert in upper right corner is fluoroscopy showing location for epiduroscopy tip (left anterior border of L5)

4. Diagnosis and radiologic diagnosis of epidural fibrosis

As with any patient, a thorough musculoskeletal and neurologic examination should be performed. In addition to standard dural tension provocative tests, we recommend a provocative test called 'dural tug'. To perform the test, the patient should be instructed to sit up with a straight leg, bend forward flexing the lumbar spine until their back pain starts to become evident, and the head and neck flexed rapidly forward. During this maneuver, the dura is stretched cephalad and if adhered to structures such as the posterior longitudinal ligament, the most heavily innervated spinal canal structure, the movement of the dura will elicit back pain that is localized to the pain generator. A positive dural tug maneuver has been observed to resolve after percutaneous neuroplasty. (Fig 2 A-E)

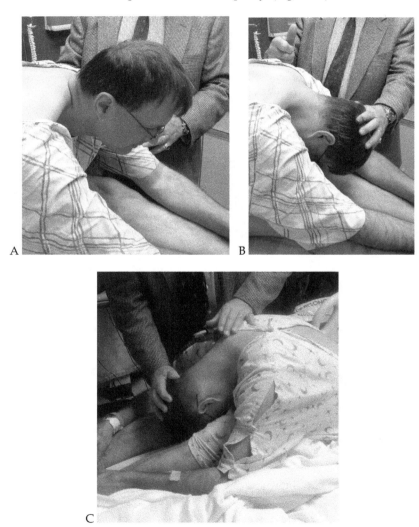

Fig. 2. A-C. A) The 'dural tug' maneuver being performed prior to percutaneous neuroplasty. B) Note pain reproduction prior to full neck flexion secondary to dural adhesions. C) Patient after percutaneous neuroplasty with pain free neck and back flexion due to treatment of dural adhesions.

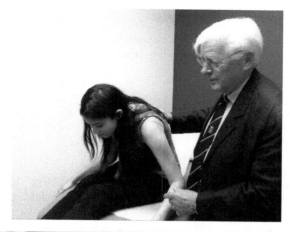

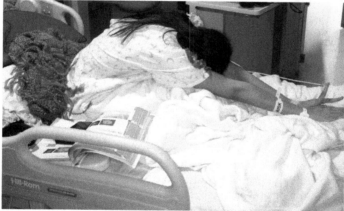

Fig. 2. D-E. D) There is decreased spine flexion prior to treatment secondary to dural adhesions. E) After treatment, the same patient demonstrates increased painless flexion of the spine.

MRI and computed tomography (CT) are diagnostic tools; sensitivity and specificity are 50% and 70%, respectively.[15] CT myelography may also be helpful, although none of the aforementioned modalities can identify epidural fibrosis with 100% reliability. In contrast, epidurography is a technique used with considerable success and it is believed that epidural fibrosis is best diagnosed by performing an epidurogram.[23-26] It can detect filling defects in good correlation with a patient's symptoms in real time.[26] A combination of several of these techniques would undoubtedly increase the ability to identify epidural fibrosis.

5. Current Procedural Terminology or CPT codes

The American Medical Association has developed Current Procedural Terminology codes for epidural adhesiolysis, which include 62264 for a single infusion and 62263 for a staged three-series infusion.

6. Indications for epidural adhesiolysis

Although originally designed to treat radiculopathy secondary to epidural fibrosis following surgery, the use of epidural adhesiolysis has been expanded to treat a multitude of pain etiologies. These include the following[27]:
1. Failed back surgery syndrome
2. Postlaminectomy syndrome of the neck and back after surgery
3. Disk disruption
4. Metastatic carcinoma of the spine leading to compression fracture
5. Multilevel degenerative arthritis
6. Facet pain
7. Spinal stenosis
8. Pain unresponsive to spinal cord stimulation and spinal opioids
9. Thoracic disk related chest wall and abdominal pain (after mapping)

7. Contraindications

The following are absolute contraindications for performing epidural adhesiolysis:
1. Sepsis
2. Chronic infection
3. Coagulopathy
4. Local infection at the procedure site
5. Patient refusal
6. Syrinx formation

A relative contraindication is the presence of arachnoiditis. With arachnoiditis, the tissue planes may be adherent to one another, increasing the chance of loculation of contrast or medication. It may also increase the chance of spread of the medications to the subdural or subarachnoid space, which can increase the chance of complications. Practitioners with limited experience with epidural adhesiolysis should consider referring these patients to a clinician with more training and experience.

8. Patient preparation

When epidural adhesiolysis has been deemed an appropriate treatment modality, the risks and benefits of the procedure should be discussed with the patient and informed consent obtained. The benefits are pain relief, improved physical function, and possible reversal of neurologic symptoms. Risks include, but are not limited to, bruising, bleeding, infection, reaction to medications used (i.e., hyaluronidase, local anesthetic, corticosteroids, hypertonic saline), damage to nerves or blood vessels, no or little pain relief, bowel/bladder incontinence, worsening of pain, and paralysis. Patients with a history of urinary incontinence should have a urodynamic evaluation by a urologist before the procedure to document the preexisting urodynamic etiology and pathology.

9. Anticoagulant medication

Medications that prolong bleeding and clotting parameters should be withheld before performing epidural adhesiolysis. The length of time varies depending on the medication taken. A consultation with the patient's primary physician should be obtained before stopping any of these medications, particularly in patients who require chronic anticoagulation such as those with drug-eluting heart stents or prosthetic heart valves. Nonsteroidal anti-inflammatory drugs and aspirin, respectively, should be withheld 4 days and 7 to 10 days before the procedure. Although there is much debate regarding these medications and neuraxial procedures, we tend to be on the conservative side. Clopidogrel (Plavix) should be stopped 7 days before, whereas ticlopidine (Ticlid) is withheld 10 to 14 days before the adhesiolysis.[28] Warfarin (Coumadin) stoppage is variable but 5 days is usually adequate.[27] Patients on subcutaneous heparin should have it withheld a minimum of 12 hours before the procedure, whereas those on low-molecular-weight heparin require a minimum of 24 hours.[28] Over-the-counter homeopathic medications that prolong bleeding parameters should also be withheld. These include fish oil, vitamin E, gingko biloba, garlic, ginseng, and St. John's Wort. Adequate coagulation status can be confirmed by the history, INR, prothrombin time, partial thromboplastin time, and a platelet function assay or bleeding time. The tests should be performed as close to the day of the procedure as possible. Tests performed only a few days after stopping the anticoagulant medication may come back elevated because not enough time has elapsed to allow the anticoagulant effects of the medication to resolve. The benefits of the procedure must be weighed against the potential sequelae of stopping the anticoagulant medication and this should be discussed thoroughly with the patient.

10. Preoperative laboratory

Before the procedure, a complete blood count and a clean-catch urinalysis are obtained to check for any undiagnosed infections. An elevated white count and/or a positive urinalysis should prompt the physician to postpone the procedure and refer the patient to the primary care physician for further workup and treatment. In addition, history of bleeding, abnormalities a prothrombin time, partial thromboplastin time, and platelet function assay or bleeding time, are obtained to check for coagulation abnormalities. Any elevated value warrants further investigation and postponement of the procedure until those studies are complete.

11. Technique

This procedure can be performed in the cervical, thoracic, lumbar, and caudal regions of the spine. The caudal and transforaminal placement of catheters will be described in detail, whereas highlights and slight changes in protocol will be provided for cervical and thoracic catheters. Our policy is to perform this procedure under strict sterile conditions in the operating room. Prophylactic antibiotics with broad neuraxial coverage are given before the procedure. Patients will receive either ceftriaxone 1 g intravenously or Levaquin 500 mg orally in those allergic to penicillin. The same dose is also given on day 2. An anesthesiologist or nurse anesthetist provides monitored anesthesia care.

12. Caudal approach

The patient is placed in the prone position with a pillow placed under the abdomen to correct the lumbar lordosis and a pillow under the ankles for patient comfort. The patient is asked to put his or her toes together and heels apart. This relaxes the gluteal muscles and facilitates identification of the sacral hiatus. After sterile preparation and draping, the sacral hiatus is identified via palpation just caudal to the sacral cornu or with fluoroscopic guidance. A skin wheal is raised with local anesthetic 1-inch lateral and 2 inches caudal to the sacral hiatus on the side opposite the documented radiculopathy. A distal subcutaneous approach theoretically provides some protection from meningitis, as a local skin infection would be much preferred over infection closer to the caudal epidural space. The skin is nicked with an 18-gauge cutting needle, and a 15- or 16-gauge RX Coudé (Epimed International) epidural needle is inserted through the nick at a 45-degree angle and guided fluoroscopically or by palpation to the sacral hiatus (Figs. 3 and 4).

When the needle is through the hiatus, the angle of the needle is dropped to approximately 30 degrees and advanced. The advantages of the RX Coudé needle over other needles are the angled tip, which enables easier direction of the catheter, and the tip of the needle is less sharp. The back edge of the distal opening of the needle is designed to be a noncutting surface that allows manipulation of the catheter in and out of the needle. A Touhy needle has the back edge of the distal opening, which is a cutting surface and can more easily shear a catheter. A properly placed needle will be inside the caudal canal below the level of the S3 foramen on anteroposterior (AP) and later fluoroscopic images. A needle placed above the level of the S3 foramen could potentially puncture a low-lying dura. The needle tip should cross the midline of the sacrum toward the side of the radiculopathy.

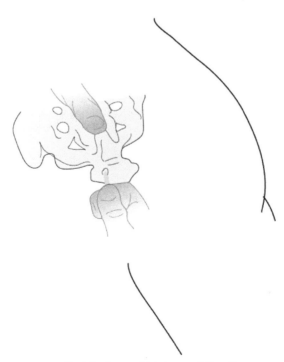

Fig. 3. Caudal lysis sequence—first find sacral hiatus and tip of coccyx.

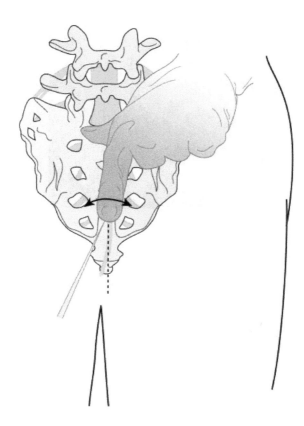

Fig. 4. Roll palpating index finger to identify the sacral cornu and thus the target sacral hiatus.

An epidurogram is performed using 10 mL of a non-ionic, water-soluble contrast agent. Confirm a negative aspiration for blood or cerebrospinal fluid before any injection of the contrast or medication. Omnipaque and Isovue are the two agents most frequently used and are suitable for myelography.[29, 30] Do not use ionic, water-insoluble agents such as Hypopaque or Renografin or ionic, water-soluble agents such as Conray. [31,32] These agents are not indicated for myelography. Accidental subarachnoid injections can lead to serious untoward events such as seizure and possibly death. Slowly inject the contrast agent and observe for filling defects. A normal epidurogram will have a "Christmas tree" pattern with the central canal being the trunk and the outline of the nerve roots making up the branches. An abnormal epidurogram will have areas where the contrast does not fill (Fig. 5). These are the areas of presumed scarring and typically correspond to the patient's radicular complaints. If vascular uptake is observed, the needle needs to be redirected.

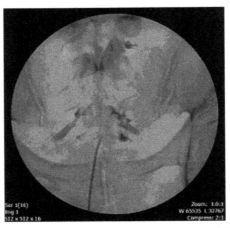

Fig. 5. Initial dye injection Omnipaque 240 (10 mL) showing sacral S3 runoff and filling defects at S2, S1, and right L5

After turning the distal opening of the needle ventral lateral, insert a TunL Kath or TunL-XL (stiffer) catheter (Epimed International) with a bend on the distal tip through the needle (Figs. 6 and 7). The bend should be 2.5 cm from the tip of the catheter and at a 30-degree angle. The bend will enable the catheter to be steered to the target level (Fig 8). Under continuous AP fluoroscopic guidance, advance the tip of the catheter toward the ventral-lateral epidural space of the desired level. The catheter can be steered by gently twisting catheter in a clockwise or counterclockwise direction. Avoid "propellering" the tip (i.e., twisting the tip in circles) because this makes it more difficult to direct the catheter. Do not advance the catheter up the middle of the sacrum because this makes guiding the catheter to the ventral-lateral epidural space more difficult. Ideal location of the tip of the catheter in the AP projection is in the foramen just below the midportion of the pedicle shadow (Figs 9 and 10). Check a lateral projection to confirm that the catheter tip is in the ventral epidural space.

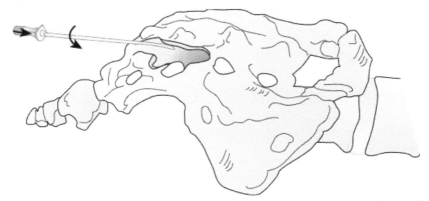

Fig. 6. The needle is placed through the sacral hiatus into the sacral canal and rotated in the direction of the target. Do not advance beyond the S3 foramen.

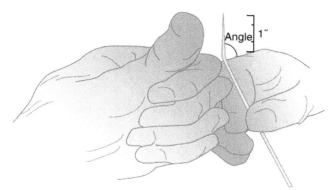

Fig. 7. The Epimed Racz catheter is marked for the location of the bend, or use the thumb as reference for the 15-degree angle bend

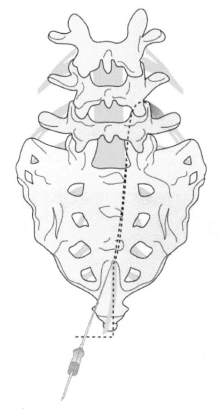

Fig. 8. The direction of the catheter is just near the midline; direct the curve under continuous fluoroscopic guidance to the ventral lateral target site. The needle rotation, as well as the catheter navigation, may need to be used to reach the target

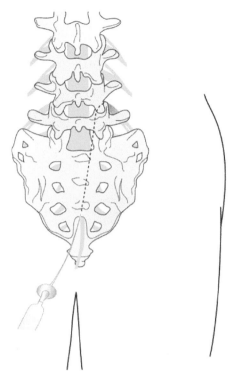

Fig. 9. The needle is removed, and the catheter is placed in the ventral lateral epidural space ventral to the nerve root

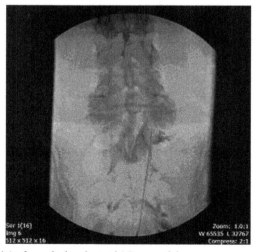

Fig. 10. Catheter (24xL) is threaded to lateral L5 neural foramen

Under real-time fluoroscopy, inject 2 to 3 mL of additional contrast through the catheter in an attempt to outline the "scarred in" nerve root (Fig 11). If vascular uptake is noted, reposition the catheter and reinject contrast. Preferably there should not be vascular runoff, but infrequently secondary to venous congestion, an epidural pattern is seen with a small amount of vascular spread. This is acceptable as long as the vascular uptake is venous in nature and not arterial. Extra caution should be taken when injecting the local anesthetic to prevent local anesthetic toxicity. Toxicity is volume and dose related and so far there has not been any reported complications from small volume venous spread. Any arterial spread of contrast always warrants repositioning of the catheter. We have never observed intra-arterial placement in 25 years of placing soft, spring-tipped catheters.

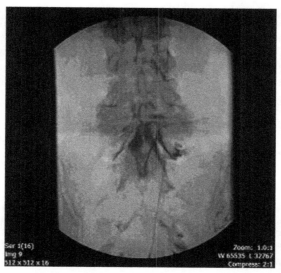

Fig. 11. Contrast injection Omnipaque 240, additional 5 mL opening right L5, S1, S2, and S3 perineural spaces; also left L5, S1, S2, and S3 in addition to right L4 spread in cephalad direction

Inject 1500 U of hyaluronidase dissolved in 10 mL of preservative-free normal saline. A newer development is the use of Hylenex or human-recombinant hyaluronidase, which carries the advantage of a reportedly increased effectiveness at the body's normal pH compared to bovine-recombinant hyaluronidase.[33] This injection may cause some discomfort, so a slow injection is preferable. Observe for "opening up"(i.e. visualization) of the "scarred in" nerve root (Figs 12 and 13 ; see also Fig. 11). A 3 mL test dose of a 10 mL local anesthetic/steroid (LA/S) solution is then given. Our institution used 4 mg of dexamethasone mixed with 9 mL of 0.2% ropivacaine. Ropivacaine is used instead of bupivacaine for two reasons: the former produces a preferential sensory versus a motor block, and it is less cardiotoxic than a racemic bupivacaine. Doses for other corticosteroids commonly used are 40 to 80 mg of methylprednisolone (Depo-Medrol), 25 to 50 mg of triamcinolone diacetate (Aristocort), 40 to 80 mg of triamcinolone acetonide (Kenalog), and 6 to 12 mg of betamethasone (Celestone Solu span). If, after 5 minutes, there is no evidence of intrathecal or intravascular injection of medication, inject the remaining 7 mL of the LA/S solution.

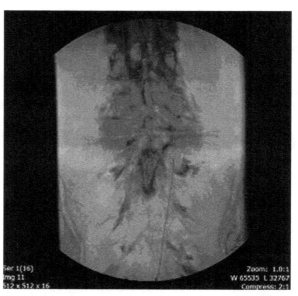

Fig. 12. Additional contrast and hyaluronidase injection opens up bilaterally formerly scarred areas. The Christmas tree appearance is obvious.

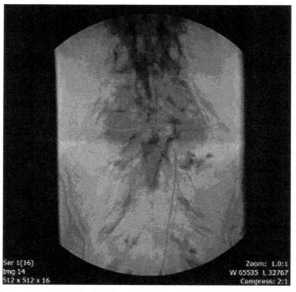

Fig. 13. Catheter advances to the desired symptomatic level of right L5 in the ventral lateral epidural space. Injection of contrast followed by 10 mL hyaluronidase 1,500 units opens up bilaterally L3-5, S1, S2, and S3 neural foramina.

Remove the needle under continuous fluoroscopic guidance to ensure the catheter remains at the target level (Fig 14). Secure the catheter to the skin using nonabsorbable suture and coat the skin puncture site with antimicrobial ointment. Apply a sterile dressing and attach a 0.2 µ m filter to the end of the catheter. Affix the exposed portion of the catheter to the patient with tape and transport the patient to the recovery area.

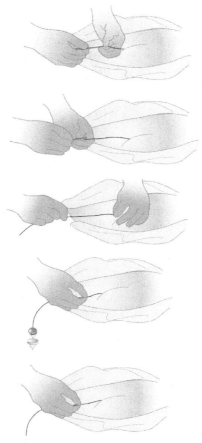

Fig. 14. Five picture sequence of removal of the needle to prevent dislodging the catheter from target site before suturing and application of dressing.

A 20- to 30-minute period should elapse between the last injection of the LA/S solution and the start of the hypertonic saline (10%) infusion. This is necessary to ensure that a subdural injection of the LA/S solution has not occurred. A subdural block mimics a subarachnoid block but it takes longer to establish, usually 16 to 18 minutes. Evidence for subdural or subarachnoid spread is the development of motor block. If the patient develops a subarachnoid or subdural block at any point during the procedure, the catheter should be removed and the remainder of the adhesiolysis canceled. The patient needs to be observed to document the resolution of the motor and sensory block and to document that 10 mL of the hypertonic saline is then infused through the catheter over 15 to 30 minutes. If the patient complains of discomfort, the infusion is stopped and an additional 2 to 3 mL of 0.2% ropivacaine is injected and the infusion is restarted. Alternatively, 50 to 75 μ g of fentanyl can be injected epidurally in lieu of the local anesthetic. After completion of the hypertonic saline infusion, the catheter is slowly flushed with 2 mL of preservative-free normal saline and the catheter is capped.

Our policy is to admit the patient for 24-hour observation status and do a second and a third hypertonic saline infusion the following day. On post–catheter insertion day 2, the catheter is twice injected (separated by 4- to 6-hour increments) with 10 mL of 0.2% ropivacaine without steroid and infused with 10 mL of hypertonic saline (10%) using the same technique and precautions as the day 1 infusion. At the end of the third infusion, the catheter is removed and a sterile dressing applied. The patient is discharged home with 5 days of oral cephalexin at 500 mg twice a day or oral levofloxacin (Levaquin) at 500 mg once a day for penicillin-allergic patients. Clinic follow-up is in 30 days.

13. Transforaminal catheters

Patients with an additional level of radiculopathy or those in whom the target level cannot be reached by the caudal approach may require placement of a second catheter. The second catheter is placed into the ventral epidural space via a transforaminal approach.

After the target level is identified with an AP fluoroscopic image, the superior endplate of the vertebra that comprises the caudal portion of the foramina is "squared," that is, the anterior and posterior shadows of the vertebral endplate are superimposed. The angle is typically 15 to 20 degrees in a caudocephalad direction. The fluoroscope is then oblique approximately 15 degrees to the side of the radiculopathy and adjusted until the spinous process is rotated to the opposite side. This fluoroscope positioning allows the best visualization of the superior articular process (SAP) that forms the inferoposterior portion of the targeted foramen. The image of the SAP should be superimposed on the shadow of the disk space on the oblique view. The tip of the SAP is the target for the needle placement (Fig 15). Raise a skin wheal slightly lateral to the shadow of the tip of the SAP. Pierce the skin with an 18-gauge needle and then insert a 15- or 16-gauge RX Coudé needle and advance using gun-barrel technique toward the tip of the SAP. Continue to advance the needle medially toward the SAP until the tip contacts bone. Rotate the tip of the needle 180 degrees laterally and advance about 5 mm (Fig 16). Rotate the needle back medially 180 degrees (Fig 17).

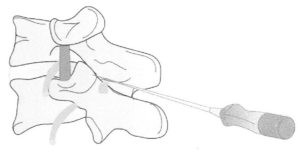

Fig. 15. Transforaminal lateral-oblique view. Target the SAP with the advancing RX Coude needle.

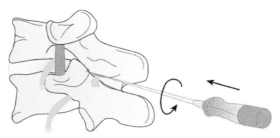

Fig. 16. Following bony contact with SAP. Lateral rotation of 180 degrees to allow passage toward the target.

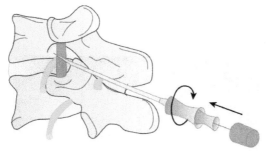

Fig. 17. Note the intertransverse ligament. The needle tip with the RX Coude 2 that has 1 mm protruding blunt stylet will pass through the ligament and will be less likely to damage the nerve.

As the needle is advanced slowly, a clear "pop" is felt as the needle penetrates the inter transverse ligament. Obtain a lateral fluoroscopic image. The tip of the needle should be just past the SAP in the posterior foramen. In the AP plane, the tip of the needle under continuous AP fluoroscopy, insert the catheter slowly into the foramen and advance until the tip should be just short of the middle of the spinal canal (Fig 18 to 20).

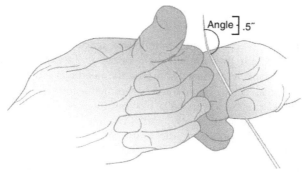

Fig. 18. The distal tip of the catheter may be bent 15-degrees, 3/4 inch length.

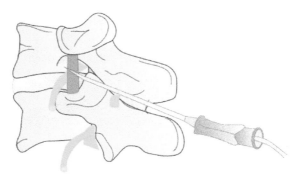

Fig. 19. Once the intertransverse ligament is perforated, the catheter is steered to the ventral lateral epidural space (lateral view).

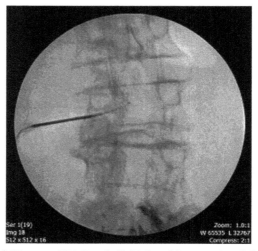

Fig. 20. Transforaminal 15-gauge RX-Coude 2 (Epimed International, Johnstown, NY) catheter at left L3-4 threaded almost to near *midcanal* position (anteroposterior view).

Confirm that the catheter is in the anterior epidural space with a lateral image (Fig 21). Anatomically, the catheter is in the foramen above or below the exiting nerve root (Fig 22). If the catheter cannot be advanced, it usually means the needle is either too posterior or too lateral to the foramen. It can also indicate that the foramen is too stenotic to allow passage of the catheter. The needle can be advanced a few millimeters anteriorly in relation to the foramen, and that will also move it slightly medial into the foramen. If the catheter still will not pass, the initial insertion of the needle will need to be more lateral. Therefore the fluoroscope angle will be about 20 degrees instead of 15 degrees. The curve of the needle usually facilitates easy catheter placement. The final position of the catheter tip is just short of the midline.

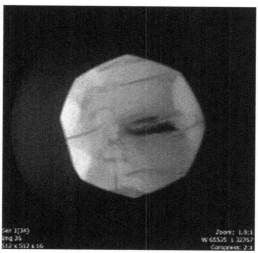

Fig. 21. Lateral view of Fig. 169-13 . Transforaminal-ventral-anterior catheter dye spread to epidural and L3-4 intradiscal area (through annular tear).

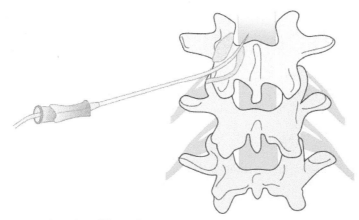

Fig. 22. Anteroposterior view. The catheter is in optimal position near midline via the transforaminal placement.

Inject 1 to 2 mL of contrast to confirm epidural spread. When a caudal and a transforaminal catheter are placed, the 1500 U of hyaluronidase are divided evenly between the two catheters (5 mL of the hyaluronidase/saline solution into each). The LA/S solution is also divided evenly, but a volume of 15 mL (1 mL steroid and 14 mL 0.2% ropivacaine; of the total volume, 5 mL is transforaminal and 10 mL is caudal) is used instead of 10 mL. Remove the needle under fluoroscopic guidance to make sure the catheter does not move from the original position in the epidural space. Secure and cover the catheter as described previously. The hypertonic saline solution is infused at a volume of 4 to 5 mL per transforaminal and 8 to 10 mL per caudal catheter over 30 minutes. The hypertonic saline injection volume should always be less than or equal to the local anesthetic volume injected to avoid pain from injection. It behooves the practitioner to check the position of the transforaminal catheter under fluoroscopy before performing the second and third infusions. The catheter may advance across the epidural space into the contralateral foramen or paraspinous muscles or more commonly back out of the epidural space into the ipsilateral paraspinous muscles.

This results in deposition of the medication in the paravertebral tissue rather than in the epidural space. As with the caudal approach, remove the transforaminal catheter after the third infusion. A recent development is the R-X Coude 2 needle in which a second protruding stylet may allow closer needle placement and less chance of nerve injury.

14. Cervical lysis of adhesions

The success of the caudal approach for lysis of adhesions led to the application of the same technique to the cervical epidural space. The indications and preprocedure workup are the same as those for the caudal lysis technique, but there are a few differences in technique and volumes of medication used.

The epidural space should be entered via the upper thoracic interspaces using a paramedian approach on the contralateral side. The most common levels are T1-2 and T2-3. Entry at these levels allows for a sufficient length of the catheter to remain in the epidural space after the target level has been reached. If the target is the lower cervical nerve roots, a more caudal interspace should be selected. We place the patient in the left lateral decubitus position, but use a prone approach in larger patients.

A technique referred to as the "3-D technique" is used to facilitate entry into the epidural space. The "3-D" stands for *direction, depth,* and *direction.* Using an AP fluoroscopic image, the initial *direction* of the 15- or 16-gauge RX Coudé needle is determined. Using a modified paramedian approach with the skin entry one and a half levels below the target interlaminar space, advance and direct the needle toward the midpoint of the chosen interlaminar space with the opening of the needle pointing medial. Once the needle engages the deeper tissue planes (usually at 2 to 3 cm), check the depth of the needle with a lateral image. Advance the needle toward the epidural space and check repeat images to confirm the *depth.* The posterior border of the dorsal epidural space can be visualized by identifying the junction of the base of the spinous process of the vertebra with its lamina. This junction creates a distinct radiopaque "straight line." Once the needle is close to the epidural space, obtain an AP fluoroscopic image to recheck the *direction* of the needle. If the tip of the needle has crossed the midline as defined by the spinous processes of the vertebral bodies, pull the needle back and redirect. The "3-D" process can be repeated as many times as is necessary to get the needle into the perfect position.

Using loss-of-resistance technique, advance the needle into the epidural space with the tip of the RX-Coudé needle, pointed caudally. Once the tip is in the epidural space, rotate the tip cephalad, and inject 1 to 2 mL of contrast to confirm entry. Rotation or movement of any needle in the epidural space can cut the dura. This technique has been improved with the advent of the RX Coudé 2 needle, which has a second interlocking stylet that protrudes slightly beyond the tip of the needle and functions to push the dura away from the needle tip as it is turned 180 degrees cephalad (Fig. 23 A-E).

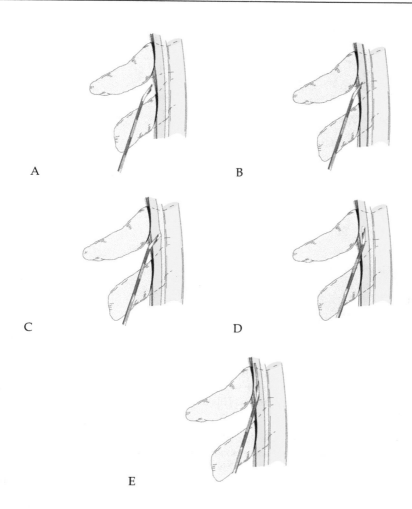

Fig. 23. Sequence of stages to place a catheter using the R-X Coude. **A** and **B.** The needle is inserted into the epidural space with the tip directed as shown. **C.** The protruding stylet is inserted. **D.** Then the needle is rotated so the tip is parallel to the dura. **E.** The catheter is inserted.

Inject an additional small volume as needed to complete the epidurogram. If there is no free flow of injected contrast, pressure may build up in the lateral epidural space. Characteristic fluid spread by the path of least resistance can be recognized as *perivenous counter spread* (PVCS). Presence of PVCS means pressure builds up in the lateral epidural space that is unable to spread laterally to decompress. The dye spread picks the path of least resistance to the opposite side. Pressure may build up and lead to ischemic spinal cord injury. Flexion and rotation of the head and neck can open up lateral runoff and release the pressure through the enlarged neural foramina (Fig 24)[34]

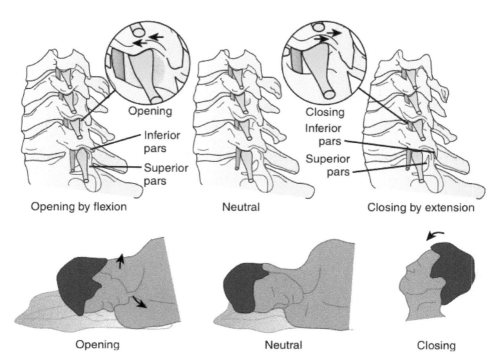

Fig. 24. Flexion rotation, left to right regardless patient position. The neural foramen enlarges on flexion rotation and gets smaller with extension. The inferior pars slides forward over the superior pars to enlarge the foramen. This allows lateral run off and pressure release with PVCS.

As with the caudal epidurogram, look for filling defects. It is extremely important to visualize spread of the contrast in the cephalad and caudal directions. Loculation of contrast in a small area must be avoided as this can significantly increase the pressure in the epidural space and can compromise the already tenuous arterial blood supply to the spinal cord. Place a bend on the catheter as previously described for the caudal approach and insert it through the needle (Fig 23E). The opening of the needle should be directed toward the target side. Slowly advance the catheter to the lateral gutter and direct it cephalad. Redirect the catheter as needed and once the target level has been reached, turn the tip of the catheter toward the foramen (Fig 25A). Inject 0.5 to 1 mL of contrast to visualize the target nerve root. Make sure there is runoff of contrast out of the foramen (Fig 25B). Slowly instill 150 U of Hylenex dissolved in 5 mL of preservative-free normal saline. Follow this with 1 to 2 mL of additional contrast and observe for "opening up" of the "scarred in" nerve root. Give a 2 mL test dose of a 6 mL solution of LA/S. Our combination is 5 mL of 0.2% ropivicaine and 4 mg of dexamethasone. If after 5 minutes there is no evidence of intrathecal or intravascular spread, inject the remaining 4 mL. Remove the needle, and secure and dress the catheter as previously described. Once 20 minutes have passed since the last dose of LA/S solution and there is no evidence of a subarachnoid or subdural block, start an infusion of 5 mL of hypertonic saline over 30 minutes. At the end of the infusion, flush the catheter with 1 to 2 mL of preservative-free normal saline and cap the catheter.

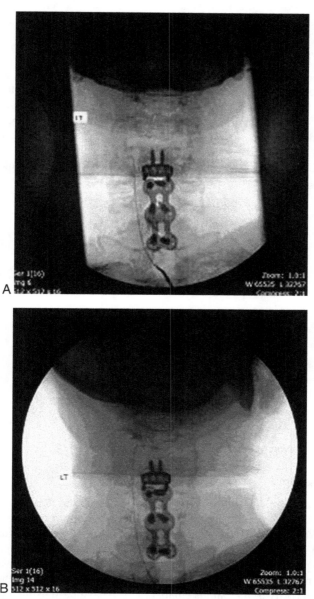

Fig. 25. A & B. **A** Cervical left ventral lateral catheter to the upper level of fusion C5-7. **B** Cervical-left ventral lateral catheter threaded to above level of fusion of C4. The dye injection spreads cephalad and lateral.

The second and third infusions are performed on the next day with 6 mL of 0.2% ropivacaine without spread and 5 mL of hypertonic saline using the same technique and precautions described for the first infusion. The catheter is removed and prophylactic antibiotics are prescribed. Clinic follow-up is 30 days.

15. Thoracic lysis of adhesions

The technique for entry into the thoracic epidural space for adhesiolysis is identical to that for the cervical region. Always remember the 3-D technique. Make sure to get a true lateral when checking the depth of the needle. This can be obtained by superimposing the rib shadows on one another. The target is still the ventrolateral epidural space with the tip of the catheter in the foramen of the desired level. The major difference for thoracic lysis compared to the caudal and cervical techniques is the volumes of the various injectates. Volumes of 8 mL are used for the contrast, Hylenex, LA/S, and hypertonic saline. (Table 1) lists typical infusion volumes for epidural adhesiolysis.

	Contrast	Hyaluronidase and Normal Saline	Local Anesthetic and Steroid	10% Hypertonic Saline Infusion
Caudal	10 mL	10 mL	10 mL	10 mL
Caudal and transforaminal	5 mL in each catheter	5 mL in each catheter	5 mL in each catheter	8 mL in caudal catheter and 4 mL in transforaminal catheter
Thoracic	8 mL	8 mL	8 mL	8 mL
Cervical	5 mL	6 mL	6 mL	5 mL

Table 1. Typical Infusion Volumes for Epidural Adhesiolysis

16. Neural flossing

The protocol for epidural adhesiolysis has been aided by neural flossing exercises that were designed to mobilize nerve roots by "sliding" them in and out of the foramen (Fig 26). This breaks up weakened scar tissue from the procedure and prevents further scar tissue deposition. If these exercises are done effectively three to four times per day for a few months after the procedure, the formation of scar tissue will be severely restricted.

In patients with multilevel radiculopathy and complex pain, it can be difficult to determine from where the majority of the pain is emanating. We have been using a technique that we have termed *mapping* to locate the most painful nerve root with stimulation and then carry out the adhesiolysis at that level. There are several references in the literature regarding the use of stimulation to confirm epidural placement of a catheter and for nerve root localization.[35] The TunL Kath and the TunL-XL catheter can be used as stimulating catheters to identify the nerve root(s).

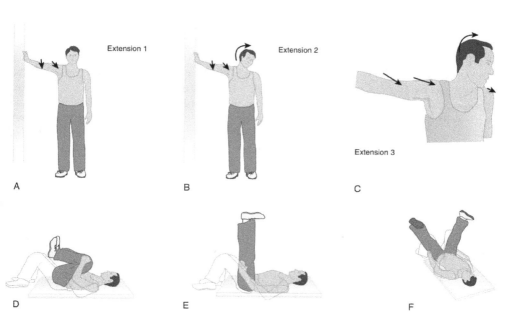

Fig. 26. **A-F Neural flossing exercises. A,** Standing erect, firmly grasp a stable surface (e.g., a door frame) with outstretched arm. Press elbow and shoulder forward. **B,** Next, slowly tilt head in opposite direction from outstretched arm to achieve gentle tension. **C,** Finally, rotate chin toward opposite shoulder as is comfortable. Hold this final position for approximately 20 to 30 seconds. **D,** Lay down supine on an exercise mat without a pillow. Slowly bring both knees close to the chest with bent legs and hold this position for 20 seconds. Release and assume a neutral position. **E,** Again in supine position, raise both legs to 90 degrees, with knees straight while laying flat on a firm surface. Hold for 20 seconds. Assume a neutral position and rest briefly. **F,** Bring both legs to a 90-degree angle while lying supine. Slowly spread legs in a V shape, as much as is comfortable, and hold for 20 seconds.**Epidural Mapping**

After entering the epidural space, advance the catheter into the ventrolateral epidural space past the suspected target level. Make sure the tip of the catheter is pointing laterally toward the foramina, just below the pedicle. Pull the catheter stylet back approximately 1 cm. Using alligator clips, attach the cathode to the stylet and ground the anode on the needle or ground pad or a 22-gauge needle inserted into the skin. Apply electrical stimulation with a stimulator box with a rate of 50 pulses per second and a pulse width of 450 milliseconds, dialing up the amplitude until a paresthesia is perceived in small increments, usually less than 2 or 3 volts. Inquire of the patient as to whether or not the paresthesia is felt in the area of the patient's recognized greatest pain. This process is repeated at each successive level until the most painful nerve root is identified. Once identified, the adhesiolysis is carried out at that level. The mapping procedure is also useful to identify the optimal site of surgery either before the first surgery or when surgery has failed one or more times.

17. Complications

As with any invasive procedure, complications are possible. These include bleeding, infection, headache, damage to nerves or blood vessels, catheter shearing, bowel/bladder dysfunction, paralysis, spinal cord compression from loculation of the injected fluids or hematoma, subdural or subarachnoid injection of local anesthetic or hypertonic saline, and reactions to the medications used. We also include on the consent form that the patient may experience an increase in pain or no pain relief at all. Although the potential list of complications is long, the frequency of complications is very rare. However, there is clearly a learning curve, and recent studies reflect this by the significantly improved long-term outcome and the very rare publications of complications and medicolegal consequences when one considers the ever-increasing clinical experience.

Subdural spread is a complication that should always be watched for when injecting local anesthetic. During the caudal adhesiolysis, particularly if the catheter is advanced along the midline, subdural catheter placement is a risk (Figs 27 and 28). Identification of the subdural motor block should occur within 16 to 18 minutes. Catheters used for adhesiolysis should never be directed midline in the epidural space.

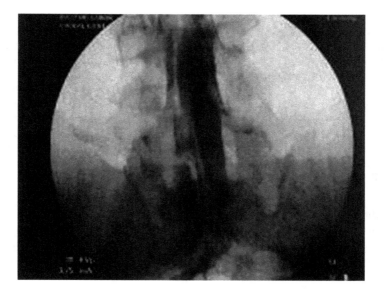

Fig. 27. Midline catheter placement enters subdural space. There is also some epidural dye spread. But the patient starts to complain of bilateral leg pain.

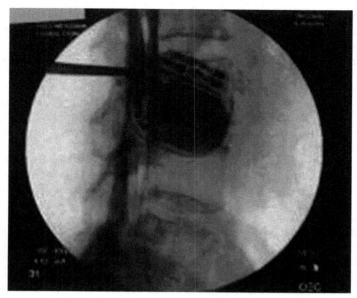

Fig. 28. A 22-gauge spinal needle and extension set with syringe placed in the subdural space and 12 mL fluid aspirated. The patient reported immediate reversal of bilateral leg pain. Note the dye in the extension tubing and syringe at the 7-o'clock position.

18. Outcomes

Initially in the early 1980s the protocol was designed to direct site-specific medication onto the dorsal root ganglion; however, after performing a number of the procedures, it was found that the dorsal root ganglion was exceptionally hard to reach secondary to developing scar tissue or adhesions. In the early days, our understanding was coming from the use of local anesthetics for surgery giving a 2- to 4-hour block for the surgeon to operate. It was gratifying to see chronic pain patients get months and years of pain relief following the placement of the new steerable x-ray visible catheter. The early report in 1985 by Racz et al[36] described the use of phenol at the dorsal root ganglion followed by an observational listing of outcomes that were clearly not as good as the latest studies on failed back surgery and spinal stenosis showing 75% to 80% improvement at 12 months' follow-up by Manchikanti.[34] Initially we were pleased to see some patients getting 3 to 4 months of relief and report seeing recovery of footdrops. This philosophy still proves to be true even in studies in 2008 by Sakai et al [37] in which they found that adhesiolysis with catheter-directed steroid and local anesthetic injection during epiduroscopy alleviated pain and reduced sensory nerve dysfunction in patients with chronic sciatica. The evolution of these findings has changed the process into what it is today.[38] Racz and Holubec first reported on epidural adhesiolysis in 1989.[39] There were slight variations in the protocol compared to today's protocol, namely the dose of local anesthetic and the fact that hyaluronidase was not used. Catheter placement was lesion-specific (i.e., the tip of the catheter was placed in the foramen corresponding to the vertebral level and side of the suspected adhesions). The retrospective analysis conducted 6 to 12 months after the procedure reported initial pain relief in 72.2% of patients (N = 72) at time of discharge. Relief was sustained in 37.5% and 30.5% of patients at 1 and 3 months, respectively. Forty-three percent decreased their frequency and dosage of medication use and 16.7% discontinued their medications altogether. In total, 30.6% of patients returned to work or returned to daily functions. In April 1990, at a presentation of the 7th IASP World Congress on Pain in Adelaide, Austraila, Arthur et al[40] reported on epidural adhesiolysis in 100 patients, 50 of whom received hyaluronidase as part of the procedure. In the hyaluronidase group, 81.6% of the participants had initial pain relief, with 12.3% having persistent relief; 68% of the no hyaluronidase group had relief of pain, with 14% having persistent relief at the end of the 3-year follow-up period from which the study sample was randomly selected.

In 1994 Stolker et al[41] added hyaluronidase to the procedure, but omitted the hypertonic saline. In a study of 28 patients, they reported greater than 50% pain reduction in 64% of patients at 1 year. They stressed the importance of the patient selection and believed that the effectiveness of adhesiolysis was based on the effect of the hyaluronidase on the adhesions and the action of the local anesthetic and steroids on the sinuvertebral nerve.

Devulder et al[42] published a study of 34 patients with failed back surgery syndrome in whom epidural fibrosis was suspected or proved with MRI.[42] An epidural catheter was inserted via the sacral hiatus to a distance of 10 cm into the caudal canal. Injections of contrast dye, local anesthetic, corticosteroid, and hypertonic saline (10%) were carried out daily for 3 days. No hyaluronidase was used. Filling defects were noted in 30 of 34 patients, but significant pain relief was noted in only 7 patients at 1 month, 2 patients at 3 months, and no patients at 12 months. They concluded that epidurography may confirm epidural filling defects for contrast dye in patients with filling defects, but a better contrast dye spread, assuming scar lysis does not guarantee sustained pain relief. This study was criticized for lack of lesion-specific catheter placement resulting in nonspecific drug delivery.[43] The catheter was never directed to the ventral lateral epidural space where the dorsal root ganglion is located and the lateral recess scarring occurs.

Heavner et al[44] performed a prospective randomized trial of lesion-specific epidural adhesiolysis on 59 patients with chronic intractable low back pain. The patients were assigned to one of four epidural adhesiolysis treatment groups: (1) hypertonic (10%) saline plus hyaluronidase, (2) hypertonic saline, (3) isotonic (0.9%) saline, or (4) isotonic saline plus hyaluronidase. All treatment groups received corticosteroid and local anesthetic. Overall, across all four treatment groups, 83% of patients had significant pain relief at 1 month compared to 49% at 3 months, 43% at 6 months, and 49% at 12 months. The hyaluronidase and the hypertonic saline study group had a much lower incidence of additional need for pain procedures than the placebo groups, showing that site-specific catheter placement is important. Active substances and preservative free normal saline were blinded for the placebo effect.

Manchikanti et al[45] performed a retrospective randomized evaluation of a modified Racz adhesiolysis protocol in 232 patients with low back pain. The study involved lesion specific catheter placement, but the usual 3-day procedure was reduced to a 2-day (group 1) or a 1-day (group 2) procedure. Group 1 had 103 patients and group 2 had 129 patients. Other changes included changing the local anesthetic from bupivacaine to lidocaine, substituting methylprednisolone acetate or betamethasone acetate and phosphate for triamcinolone diacetate, and reduction of the volume of injectate. Of the patients in groups 1 and 2, 62% and 58% had greater than 50% pain relief at 1 month, respectively, with these percentages decreasing to 22% and 11% at 3 months, 8% and 7% at 6 months, and 2% and 3% at 1 year. Of significant interest is that the percentage of patients receiving greater than 50% pain relief after four procedures increased to 79% and 90% at 1 month, 50% and 36% at 3 months, 29% and 19% at 6 months, and 7% and 8% at 1 year for groups 1 and 2, respectively. Short-term relief of pain was demonstrated, but long-term relief was not.

Manchikanti, in 1999, evaluated two groups of randomly pulled, 150 patients for a 2-day reinjection procedure, and a second 150 patients for a one-day procedure out of a pool of 536 patients. It was concluded that repeat use of the one-day procedure is also cost effective when evaluated on a 12-month follow-up. The cost effectiveness indicated the lysis procedure to be superior to surgery or the rehabilitation activity program.[45]

In a randomized, prospective study, Manchikanti et al[46] evaluated a 1-day epidural adhesiolysis procedure against a control group of patients who received conservative therapy. Results showed that cumulative relief, defined as relief greater than 50% with one to three injections, in the treatment group was 97% at 3 months, 93% at 6 months, and 47% at 1 year. The study also showed that overall health status improved significantly in the adhesiolysis group. Conservative therapy consisted of physical therapy and medications.

In 2004 Manchikanti et al[47] published their results of a randomized, double-blind, controlled study on the effectiveness of 1-day lumbar adhesiolysis and hypertonic saline neurolysis in treatment of chronic low back pain. Seventy-five patients whose pain was unresponsive to conservative modalities were randomized into one of three treatment groups. Group 1 (control group) underwent catheterization where the catheter was in the sacral canal without adhesiolysis, followed by injection of local anesthetic, normal saline, and steroid. Group 2 consisted of catheterization with site-specific catheter placement being ventral-lateral for adhesiolysis, followed by injection of local anesthetic, normal saline, and steroid. Group 3 consisted of site-specific catheter placement for adhesiolysis, followed by injection of local anesthetic, hypertonic saline, and steroid. Patients were allowed to have additional injections based on the response, either after unblinding or without unblinding after 3 months. Patients without unblinding were offered either the assigned treatment or another treatment based on their response. If the patients in group 1 or 2 received adhesiolysis and injection and injection of hypertonic saline, they were considered withdrawn, and no subsequent data were collected. Outcomes were assessed at 3, 6, and 12 months using visual analog scale pain scores, Oswestry Disability Index, opioid intake, range-of-motion measurement, and P-3. Significant pain relief was defined as average relief of 50% or greater. Seventy-two percent of patients in group 3, 60% of patients in group 2, and 0% of patients in group 1 showed significant pain relief at 12 months. The average number of treatments for 1 year was 2.76 in group 2 and 2.16 in group 3. Duration of significant relief with the first procedure was 2.8 + 1.49 months and 3.8 + 3.37 months in groups 2 and 3, respectively. Significant pain relief (>50%) was also associated with improvement in Oswestry Disability Index, range of motion, and psychologic status.

Manchikanti et al[48,49,] furthered this research using comparisons of percutaneous adhesiolysis versus fluoroscopically guided caudal epidural steroid injections. The first study involved a population of patients with chronic low back pain and known spinal stenosis. The results showed a 76% reduction in pain relief at 1 year with epidural adhesiolysis compared to 4% in the control group. The second study performed in a population of patients with post–lumbar surgery syndrome showed a reduction in pain and improvement in functional status in 73% of the epidural adhesiolysis group compared to 12% in the control group.

In 2006 a study by Veihelmann et al[50] evaluated patients with a history of chronic low back pain and sciatica. Inclusion criteria were radicular pain with a corresponding nerve root compressing substrate found on MRI or CT. All patients were randomized to receive physiotherapy, analgesics, or lysis of adhesions. The lysis group had statistically significantly better outcome than the physical therapy treatment group.

Two other prospective evaluations by Chopra et al and Gerdesmeyer et al[51, 52] evaluated patients with monosegmental radiculopathy of the lumbar spine. All the patients suffered from chronic disk herniations or failed back syndrome. All these randomized trials showed positive short-term and long-term relief. Two prospective evaluations also showed positive short- and long-term relief.[51,52]

19. Conclusion

Epidural adhesiolysis has evolved over the years as an important treatment option for patients with intractable cervical, thoracic, and low back and leg pain. Studies show that patients are able to experience significant pain relief and restoration of function. Manchikanti's studies show that the amount and duration of relief can be achieved by repeat procedures. Recent prospective randomized double-blind studies on failed back surgery and spinal stenosis show 75% and 80% improvement in visual analog scale scores and functional improvements at 12 months' follow-up. There have been no negative studies to date where the lysis target was the ventral-lateral epidural space. The one negative study used a 10 cm sacral mid-canal catheter placement which was non-target specific.[43] This negative study was subsequently used as the placebo group in a study performed by Manchikanti.[47] Manchikanti's study consisted of 3 treatment groups: placebo (sacral mid-canal catheter placement), target specific ventral-lateral epidural without hypertonic saline and target specific ventral-lateral epidural with hypertonic saline . The later two treatment groups had positive outcomes with the hypertonic saline group superior; whereas, the placebo group did not. [47] The evolution in the recognition of the site-specific importance of the catheter and medication delivery together with the fact that physicians need to acquire the skills to be able to carry out the procedure led to the improved outcomes seen in recent prospective randomized studies.

The management of failed back surgery syndrome and post laminectomy syndrome will likely continue to be controversial among the multitude of practitioners who treat these patients. However, in experienced hands, it is established as a reasonable option for many patients.

Percutaneous neuroplasty via a transforaminal approach evolved from the caudal approach. Lysis of adhesions via the caudal approach involves introducing a catheter through the sacral hiatus and advancing it to the affected nerve root in the ventral-lateral epidural space. On the other hand, transforaminal percutaneous neuroplasty achieves a midline catheter placement in the epidural space that is able to target the two most heavily innervated structures in the spine—the posterior annulus fibrosus and the posterior longitudinal ligament.[5] Apart from a surgical approach, the ventral epidural structures have been otherwise inaccessible.

Endoscopy offers direct visualization of the affected nerve roots in addition to mechanical adhesiolysis, and may become more mainstream as the technique is refined.

Facet pain is commonly associated with the postlysis period or after provocative testing a month or so later if two-facet diagnostic blocks show efficacy. In addition to epidural lysis of adhesions, the combined use of radiofrequency facet denervation gives us the best long-term outcome.

Epidural adhesiolysis has been accepted as a treatment for post laminectomy syndrome, failed back syndrome, and cervical and thoracic radicular syndromes. Additional studies are underway to further refine the technique and indications. The combined use of long term patient education for neural flossing exercises and the inclusion of the facet delayed treatment in the algorithm further improves patient outcome. The identification of back pain provocation by saline injection and the successful use of percutaneous neuroplasty in the treatment represents hopeful promise for a cost effective treatment of back pain.

20. Acknowledgements

Racz GB, Day MR, Heavner JE, Scott J. *Lysis of Epidural Adhesions.* In: Waldman S, ed. *Pain Management, 2nd Edition.* Elsevier; 2011: 1258-1272.

Racz GB, Day MR, Heavner JE, Smith JP. The Racz Procedure: Lysis of Epidural Adhesions (Percutaneous Neuroplasty). In: Deer T, ed. The AAPM Text of Pain Medicine. Springer; 2011. The authors would also like to thank Marzieh N. Brown and Paula Brashear for their assistance in the editing of this chapter.

21. References

[1] Lawrence R., Helmick C., Arnett F., et al: Estimates of the prevalence of arthritis and selected musculoskeletal disorders in the United States. *Arthritis Rheum* 1998; 41(5):778-799.

[2] Straus B.: Chronic pain of spinal origin: the costs of intervention. *Spine* 2002; 27(22):2614-2619.

[3] National Center for Health Statistics : *National hospital discharge survey,* Washington, DC, US Department of Health and Human Services, Centers for Disease Control and Prevention, 1990. Report no. PB92-500818

[4] Van Zundert J.: *Personal communication.* 2005.

[5] Kuslich S., Ulstrom C., Michael C.: The tissue origin of low back pain and sciatica. *Orthop Clin North Am* 1991; 22:181-187.

[6] Racz G., Noe C., Heavner J.: Selective spinal injections for lower back pain. *Curr Rev Pain* 1999; 3:333-341.

[7] Anderson S.: A rationale for the treatment algorithm of failed back surgery syndrome. *Curr Rev Pain* 2000; 4:396-406.

[8] Pawl R.: Arachnoiditis and epidural fibrosis: the relationship to chronic pain. *Curr Rev Pain* 1998; 2:93-99.

[9] Cervellini P., Curri D., Volpin L., et al: Computed tomography of epidural fibrosis after discectomy: a comparison between symptomatic and asymptomatic patients. *Neurosurgery* 1988; 23(6):710-713.

[10] Manchikanti L., Staats P., Singh V.: Evidence-based practice guidelines for interventional techniques in the management of chronic spinal pain. *Pain Phys* 2003; 6:3-81.

[11] LaRocca H., Macnab I.: The laminectomy membrane: studies in its evolution, characteristics, effects and prophylaxis in dogs. *J Bone Joint Surg* 1974; 5613:545-550.

[12] Cooper R., Freemont A., Hoyland J., et al: Herniated intervertebral disc–associated periradicular fibrosis and vascular abnormalities occur without inflammatory cell infiltration. *Spine* 1995; 20:591-598.

[13] McCarron R., Wimpee M., Hudkins P., et al: The inflammatory effects of nucleus pulposus; a possible element in the pathogenesis of low back pain. *Spine* 1987; 12:760-764.

[14] Parke W., Watanabe R.: Adhesions of the ventral lumbar dura: an adjunct source of discogenic pain?. *Spine* 1990; 15:300-303.

[15] Viesca C., Racz G., Day M.: Special techniques in pain management: lysis of adhesions. *Anesthesiol Clin North Am* 2003; 21:745-766.

[16] Songer M., Ghosh L., Spencer D.: Effects of sodium hyaluronate on peridural fibrosis after lumber laminectomy and discectomy. *Spine* 1990; 15:550-554.

[17] Key J., Ford L.: Experimental intervertebral disc lesions. *J Bone Joint Surg Am* 1948; 30:621-630.

[18] Olmarker K., Rydevik B.: Pathophysiology of sciatica. *Orthop Clin North Am* 1991; 22:223-233.

[19] Ross J., Robertson J., Frederickson R., et al: Association between peridural scar and recurrent radicular pain after lumbar discectomy; magnetic resonance evaluation. *Neurosurgery* 1996; 38:855-863.

[20] Gilbert K., Brismee J., Collins D., et al: Lumbosacral nerve roots displacements and strain: part 1. A novel measurement technique during straight leg raise in unembalmed calavers. *Spine* 2007; 32(14):1513-1520.Phila Pa 1976

[21] Heavner JE, Chokhavatia S, Kizelshteyn G: Percutaneous evaluation of the epidural and subarachnoid space with a flexible fiberscope, *Reg Anesth* 1991;15:85.

[22] Bosscher HA, Heavner JE: Incidence and severity of epidural fibrosis after back surgery: an endoscopic study, *Pain Pract* 2010; 10: 18-24.

[23] Hatten Jr H.: Lumbar epidurography with metrizamide. *Radiology* 1980; 137:129-136.

[24] Stewart H., Quinnell R., Dann N.: Epidurography in the management of sciatica. *Br J Rheumatol* 1987; 26(6):424-429.

[25] Devulder J., Bogaert L., Castille F., et al: Relevance of epidurography and epidural adhesiolysis in chronic failed back surgery patients. *Clin J Pain* 1995; 11:147-150.

[26] Manchikanti L., Bakhit C., Pampati V.: Role of epidurography in caudal neuroplasty. *Pain Digest* 1998; 8:277-281.

[27] Day M., Racz G.: Technique of caudal neuroplasty. *Pain Digest* 1999; 9(4):255-257.

[28] Horlocker T., Wedel D., Benzon H., et al: Regional anesthesia in the anticoagulated patient: defining the risks (the second ASRA Consensus Conference on Neuraxial Anesthesia and Anticoagulation). *Reg Anesth Pain Med* 2003; 28:172-197.

[29] *Omnipaque product insert*, Princeton, NJ, Nycomed, Inc.

[30] *Isovue product insert*, Princeton, NJ, Bracco Diagnostics, Inc.

[31] *Hypaque product insert*, Princeton, NJ, Amersham Health, Inc.

[32] *Conray product insert*, Phillipsburg, NJ, Mallinckrodt, Inc.

[33] Racz G., Day M., Heavner J., et al: Hyaluronidase: a review of approved formulations, indications and off-label use in chronic pain management. *Expert Opin Biol Ther* 2010; 10(1):127-131.

[34] Racz G.B., Heavner J.E.: Cervical spinal canal loculation and secondary ischemic cord injury — PVCS — perivenous counter spread — danger sign!!. *Pain Pract* 2008; 8:399-403.

[35] Larkin T., Carragee E., Cohen S.: A novel technique for delivery of epidural steroids and diagnosing the level of nerve root pathology. *J Spinal Disord Tech* 2003; 16(2):186-192.

[36] Racz G.B., Sabonghy M., Gintautas J., et al: Intractable pain therapy using a new type of epidural catheter. *JAMA* 1985; 248:579-580.

[37] Sakai T., Aoki H., Hojo M., et al: Adhesiolysis and targeted steroid/local anesthetic injection during epiduroscopy alleviates pain and reduces sensory nerve dysfunction in patients with chronic sciatica. *J Anesth* 2008; 22(3):242-247.

[38] Anderson S., Racz G., Heavner J.: Evolution of epidural lysis of adhesions. *Pain Physician* 2000; 3(3):262-270.

[39] Racz G., Holubec J.: *Lysis of adhesions in the epidural space*. In: Raj P., ed. *Techniques of neurolysis*, Boston: Kluwer Academic; 1989:57-72.

[40] Arthur J., Racz G., Heinrich R., et al: *Epidural space: identification of filling defects and lysis of adhesions in the treatment of chronic painful conditions*. Abstracts of the 7th World Congress on Pain, Paris: IASP Publications; 1993.

[41] Stolker R., Vervest A., Gerbrand J.: The management of chronic spinal pain by blockades: a revew. *Pain* 1994; 58:1-19.

[42] Devulder J., Bogaert L., Castille F., et al: Relevance of epidurography and epidural adhesiolysis in chonic failed back surgery patients. *Clin J Pain* 1995; 11:147-150.

[43] Racz G., Heavner J.: In response to article by Drs. Devulder et al. *Clin J Pain* 1995; 11:151-154.

[44] Heavner J., Racz G., Raj P.: Percutaneous epidural neuroplasty: prospective evaluation of 0.9% saline versus 10% saline with or without hyaluronidase. *Reg Anesth Pain Med* 1999; 24:202-207.

[45] Manchikanti L., Pakanati R., Bakhit C., et al: Role of adhesiolysis and hypertonic saline neurolysis in management of low back pain: evaluation of modification of the Racz protocol. *Pain Digest* 1999; 9:91-96.

[46] Manchikanti L., Pampati V., Fellow B., et al: Role of one day epidural adhesiolysis in management of chronic low back pain: a randomized clinical trial. *Pain Phys* 2001; 4:153-166.

[47] Manchikanti L., Rivera J., Pampati V., et al: One day lumbar adhesiolysis and hypertonic saline neurolysis in treatment of chronic low back pain: a randomized, double-blinded trial. *Pain Phys* 2004; 7:177-186.

[48] Manchikanti L., Cash K., McManus C., et al: The preliminary results of a comparative effectiveness of adhesiolysis and caudal epidural injections in managing chronic low back pain secondary to spinal stenosis. *Pain Phys* 2009; 12(6):E341-E354.

[49] Manchikanti L., Singh V., Cash K., et al: A comparative effectiveness evaluation of percutaneous adhesiolysis and epidural steroid injections in managing lumbar post surgery syndrome. *Pain Phys* 2009; 12(6):E355-E368.

[50] Veihelmann A., Devens C., Trouiller H., et al: Epidural neuroplasty versus physiotherapy to relieve pain in patients with sciatica: a prospective randomized blinded clinical trial. *J Orthop Sci* 2006; 11(4):365-369.

[51] Gerdesmeyer L., Lampe R., Veihelmann A., et al: Chronic radiculopathy: use of minimally invasive percutaneous epidural neurolysis according to Racz. *Der Schmerz* 2005; 19:285-295.

[52] Gerdesmeyer L., Rechl H., Wagenpfeil S., et al: Minimally invasive epidural neurolysis in chronic radiculopathy: a prospective controlled study to prove effectiveness. *Der Orhopade* 2003; 32:869-876.

3

Risk Factors in Opioid Treatment of Chronic Non-Cancer Pain: A Multidisciplinary Assessment

Renata Ferrari, Michela Capraro and Marco Visentin
Hospital Psychology Service, Pain Relief and Palliative Care Unit, Vicenza Hospital,
Italy

1. Introduction

When pain becomes chronic it assumes an almost absolute central role in the disease experience: it characterises and qualifies it, and constantly interferes with the daily life of the patient (Bonica, 1992). It could be said that chronic pain becomes a disease in itself in the patient's perception; daily activities, interpersonal relationships, feelings, are profoundly disturbed by living with pain (Loeser, 2000).

While modern medicine has made notable progress in understanding, diagnosing and treating chronic pain, it continues to be a very widespread problem that significantly compromises the professional, social and family life of the patient, and is often not adequately managed (Manchikanti et al., 2010).

The problem of inadequately managed pain is still a considerable one (Breivik et al., 2006), although the World Health Organization [WHO] (1990) has stated that to be pain free should be considered a right of every patient. The consequences of inadequately treated pain not only have an impact in terms of the physical and psychological suffering of the patient and his family, they also have an enormous economic impact on society as a whole (Brennan et al., 2007; van Leeuwen et al., 2006).

Options for the treatment of chronic pain include both pharmacological treatments (e.g. non steroidal anti-inflammatory drugs, opioids) and non-pharmacological treatments (e.g. physical therapies, acupuncture, cognitive-behavioural therapy, surgical procedures). Choice of treatment should be guided by a complex initial assessment of the patient, which includes the collection of historical information (e.g. pain history and treatments tried, surgical procedures, psychosocial and family history), a physical examination and appropriate diagnostic tests (Passik, 2009).

Opioids are considered one of the most efficacious groups of drugs in treating medium-severe pain (Portenoy, 2000), and their use can result in a significant improvement in the patient's quality of life (Dillie et al., 2008); while there is unanimous agreement on their use in acute and cancer pain, their long-term use for non-cancer chronic pain remains controversial (Dews & Mekhail, 2004; Manchikanti et al., 2010; Rosenblum et al., 2008). The discovery of the properties of these substances, and their use as analgesics, is lost in the mists of time: the Sumerians were starting to cultivate poppies as early as 3400 B.C. (Booth, 1986, as cited in Dews & Mekhail, 2004). In 1803, Friedrich Serturner, a German pharmacist, isolated an alkaloid from opium that he named morphine, and in 1853 Scottish physician Alexander Wood introduced the hypodermic needle and successfully used injections of morphine to treat neuralgia. As Way (1982, as cited in Dews & Mekhail, 2004) highlighted, morphine was the "mainstay" of medical treatment in the United States throughout the nineteenth century, used to treat pain, anxiety and respiratory problems as well as "consumption" and "women's ailments". Opium cultivation was legal in some states, and opium-based products could be bought over the counter (Dews & Mekhail, 2004). Between 1875 and 1877, German physician Eduard Levinstein published a series of articles calling attention to the problem of morphine dependence: his was one of the first studies on the risk of dependence on narcotics, which he estimated to be 75% (White et al., 2001a). In 1914 Kennedy Foster wrote, in New York Medical Journal, "...morphinism is a disease, in the majority of cases, initiated, sustained and left uncured by members of the medical profession" (White et al., 2001b); in the same year the US Congress approved the Harrison Anti-Narcotic Act, the first federal law to limit the sale of any drug. Opioids and cocaine were included in the list of drugs that could only be obtained from a physician or authorised pharmacist. Physicians were authorised to prescribe these substances, but not to patients with dependence problem; given the likelihood of arrest or prosecution, physicians became increasingly cautious in prescribing opioids even for chronic pain (Dews & Mekhail, 2004). In 1969, the WHO abandoned the belief that the medical use of morphine led inevitably to dependence; the WHO clarified that tolerance and physical dependence did not in itself constitute "drug dependence", a diagnosis characterised by typical behaviours, including difficulty in controlling the assumption of drugs, compulsive use of the substance and inappropriate social behaviours (WHO, 1986). In 1970 the Harrison Anti-Narcotic Act and the other federal laws on drugs were replaced by the Comprehensive Drug Abuse and Control Act, which divided substances into six categories, according to their risk of addiction: category I includes heroin and marijuana, category II includes cocaine, opium and morphine, category III includes codeine, category IV includes diazepam and alprazolam, category V includes drugs with small quantities of codeine and category VI includes penicillin and ibuprofen (Dews & Mekhail, 2004). This law established that there were no impediments to prescribing drugs in categories II, III or IV provided there were indications for their use, including chronic non-cancer pain. There was a further development when the WHO Expert Committee on Essential Drugs recognised morphine, codeine and other opioids as "essential drugs," defining them as: "those that satisfy the health care needs of the majority of the population; they should therefore be available at all times in adequate amounts and in the appropriate dosage forms..." (WHO, 1998). The WHO also introduced the "pain analgesia scale" (figure 1) which distinguishes between strong and weak opioids, and establishes their clear roles in pain relief. In Italy, which is one of the countries with the lowest morphine consumption in Europe, several measures have been developed to eliminate the bureaucratic obstacles to the use of opioid analgesics, starting with Law no. 12 of 2001. With Law no. 38 of 2010, opioids may finally be prescribed for pain relief in the same way as other prescription-only drugs.

As illustrated, the use of opioids has historically been subject to cycles of liberalisation and prohibition in clinical practice that account for their still-limited use today (WHO, 1998).

The potential barriers to treatment with opioids may be due to inadequate beliefs of both medical personnel and the patients themselves (Garcia & Altman, 1997).

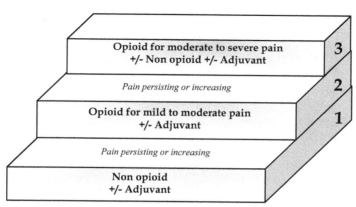

Fig. 1. The WHO pain analgesia scale

Physicians may not prescribe opioids at adequate doses because they do not know how to use them effectively, because they do not assess the pain or effects of treatment systematically, because of fear of sanctions by medical commissions. But some data lead one to believe that the overestimation of the risk of addiction is a significant problem (Dews & Mekhail, 2004); in this respect, the term *opiophobia* has been coined, to refer to the practice of under-prescription of opioid medication due to the fear of inducing addiction in patients (Collett, 1998). By interviewing over 248 US physicians, Bhamb et al. (2006) recently reported that just over half of those interviewed (55.9%), had specific clinical protocols for the prolonged use of opioids in patients with chronic non-cancer pain. 35.1% believed they prescribed opioids less frequently than their colleagues; while the most frequent concerns about starting treatment with opioids were the fear of abuse (84.2%) and addiction (74.9%). Concerns of patients should also be considered: they may not communicate their pain symptoms to their physicians, or may not take the drugs as instructed for fear of becoming dependent on "narcotics" (Dews & Mekhail, 2004). Furthermore, both physicians and patients may develop unjustified anxiety about the side effects of opioid use, believing that these drugs must therefore be reserved for cancer pain (Brennan et al., 2007). Finally, a further barrier to the use of these drugs may be due to overly restrictive national control laws and regulations. Because of this, the WHO has issued guidelines on legislative policies that enable Governments to check if their national laws ensure the availability of opioid analgesics to treat severe pain (WHO, 2002).

Given the importance of these drugs in pain management, as well as the concerns about their use, a series of investigations were carried out in the last twenty years to identify the risk factors that promote or exacerbate opioid misuse. In fact, for physicians, determining the patient's risk of addiction to opioids is of fundamental importance, so that a series of measures can be taken to limit the negative consequences of this (such as constantly monitoring the patient during treatment, planning interdisciplinary treatment or scheduling regular urine toxicology screening).

The intention of this chapter is to examine the principal risk factors for opioid misuse in patients with chronic non-cancer pain. It will also describe the principal tools for selecting patients who are candidates for opioid treatment and for stratifying the risk of misuse. This will be followed by a presentation of the preliminary results of our experience using a diagnostic protocol for patients undergoing long-term treatment with opioids in a multidisciplinary pain relief unit.

2. Risk factors in opioid treatment of patients with chronic pain: Theoretical and research aspects

Over the last twenty years, opioids have been used increasingly to treat chronic non-cancer pain (Ballantyne & Shin, 2008). A broad US investigation fund that, between 1980 and 2000, prescriptions of opioids for musculoskeletal pain doubled from 8% to 16%. Over the same two decades, the use of more powerful opioids for chronic pain (hydrocodone, oxycodone, morphine) increased from 2% to 9% (Caudill-Slosberg et al., 2004). However, if some patients benefit from such treatment in terms of reduction of pain and improvement in quality of life (Dillie et al., 2008), others do not (Ballantyne, 2007; Trescot et al., 2008). Side effects, the absence of any improvement in physical function, the excessive use of opioids, abuse and addiction are common problems that may present during the administration of opioid analgesics (Manchikanti et al., 2010). So in recent years experts and researchers have sought to answer many questions regarding risk factor for opioid misuse, selection of patients, efficacy of treatment particularly over time, whether opioids are able to improve physical function and quality of life. The clear and urgent need to answer these questions is reflected in the considerable increase in studies on this topic in the last decade (Ballantyne & Shin, 2008). Moreover, many guidelines for the use of opioids in patients with chronic non-cancer pain have been produced, which recommend their use for those patients who have not benefited from other pharmacological and non-pharmacological treatments (Chou, 2009; Chou et al, 2009a; Chou et al, 2009b; Chou et al, 2009c; Kalso et al., 2003; Trescot et al., 2006; Trescot at al., 2008).

The following section will provide some notes on pain, on the recommendations contained in the guidelines for the prolonged use of opioids and on the terminology used. The intention is to offer adequate context for the subsequent discussion of the risk factors related to abuse of opioids and the tools that have been developed to select patients to treat with these drugs.

Finally, the preliminary data of our experience using two of these tools, the *Pain Medication Questionnaire* (PMQ; Adams et al., 2004) and the *Diagnosis Intractability Risk and Efficacy Score* (DIRE; Belgrade et al., 2006) in the Italian population are presented.

2.1 The definition and classification of pain

Pain is an extremely complex and subjective phenomenon, defined by the International Association for the Study of Pain [IASP] as *"an unpleasant sensory and emotional experience, associated with real or potential tissue damage or described in terms of such damage"* (Merskey, 1986a). Whether acute or chronic, pain is above all a subjective and multidimensional experience, influenced by biological, psychological and socio-environmental factors.

Pain may be distinguished as acute or chronic based on its duration in time and underlying pathology. Acute pain is produced by lesions to body tissues and the activation of the nociceptive transducers at the site of the tissue damage. It may be consequent on a trauma, a surgical procedure or an inflammatory process, and generally lasts for a relatively short period of time (hours, days or weeks) and stops when the underlying pathology is resolved. Chronic pain lasts for a long period of time (continuously or recurring at intervals of months or years), and is generally accompanies by a low level of underlying pathology which fully explains neither the presence nor the intensity of the pain (Bonica, 1992). Disputes remain about the interval of time that needs to have elapsed since the trauma for pain to be defined as chronic; in clinical practice, a pain is generally described as chronic when it persists for more than 3-6 months (Bonica, 1991; Loeser & Melzack, 1999; Merskey, 1986b; Merskey & Bogduk, 1994).

From a pathogenic perspective, pain may be classified as nociceptive, neuropathic or mixed. Nociceptive pain (somatic or visceral pain) is determined by the activation of nociceptors located in the somatic and visceral structures. It may be further classified as superficial or deep, according to the structure involved, and is due to a tissue lesion that is often evident. Neuropathic pain is typically caused by a change or alteration in the transmission of impulses along the somato-sensorial pathways and is indicative of damage to the conduction systems or to the integration and transmission systems of the central or peripheral nervous system; often it is not accompanied by tissue damage. Finally, when these two types of pain (nociceptive and neuropathic) are both present, this is referred to as mixed pain (Mannion & Woolf, 2000).

Pain is physiological, i.e. it is a vital sign, and a defence system when it constitutes an alarm signal for tissue damage. It becomes pathological when it maintains itself, losing its initial meaning and becoming an illness in itself (pain syndrome) (Mannion & Woolf, 2000).

In biopsychosocial terms, the experience of pain and its impact on the individual are due to the complex interaction of somatic inputs (nociception), psychological processes (e.g. thoughts, coping strategies and emotions) and social contingencies (e.g. social context, significant others, roles and expectations) (Turk & Okifuji, 2002). In persistent pain syndromes, the weight of these three factors can change at different moments of the illness, and none alone can explain the pain situation as a whole. The biological factors can origin, maintain and modulate the physical disorder, the psychological factors influence perception and evaluation of body signals and the social factors give form to the patients' behavioural responses and their perception of their physical condition. Given this complexity, an adequate approach to chronic pain requires multidisciplinary intervention; the treatment aims in these patients are not only pharmacological treatment but also reduction of affective/emotional discomfort, functional recovery, return to work and improvement in family and social relationships.

2.1.1 The prevalence of chronic pain and its socio-economic impact

Chronic pain is a common and persistent problem in society, with a relatively high incidence and a low remission rate (Elliott et al., 2002). Verhaak et al. (1998), after reviewing 15 epidemiological studies on chronic pain in the adult population, concluded that its prevalence varied from 2% to 40%, with a mean value of 15%. Back pain is one of the most frequent forms of chronic pain, with a prevalence rate of approximately 48% (Gureje et al., 1998). Based on interviews of 2305 subjects aged between 35 and 45, Linton et al. (1998) showed that the prevalence of back pain is 66% with slightly higher incidence in women; in particular, 56% of the subjects complained of low back pain, 44% complained of neck pain, and 15% complained of pain in the thoracic spine.

A recent epidemiological study about the prevalence of chronic pain in European countries involving 46,394 subjects found that approximately 19% of adults suffer continuous pain of medium-high intensity that seriously compromises quality of their emotional, social and working life. The prevalence of chronic pain varies from 12% to 20%, and is highest in Norway, Poland and Spain. In Italy, people who suffer from chronic pain syndromes account for approximately 27% of the population. It also emerged that: 59% of those interviewed had been experiencing pain for at least 2-15 years, 21% had been diagnosed with depression consequent on pain, 61% reported great difficulty or incapacity in working outside home, 19% had lost their job and 13% had been forced to change jobs because of the pain. Just 2% of patients reported they were being treated by pain specialists, and about half of these were receiving inadequate treatment (Breivik et al., 2006).

Therefore chronic pain has serious negative effects on the quality of life of the millions of people who experience it, and on the quality of life of their families. In the absence of adequate treatments, patients with chronic pain are often unable to work or even to carry out their normal daily activities.

As well as causing unspeakable suffering to millions of people all over the world, chronic pain has high social cost too. Analysing data from the 1997 Medical Expenditures Panel Survey, which involved 14,147 families, Yelin et al.(2004) found that expenditure by patients with rheumatic disorders was US $ 4,865 per head, for a total of US $ 186.9 million. In 1998, US healthcare expenditure on lower back pain was US $ 90.7 billions (Luo et. al., 2004). A similar investigation found that in 2003 overall spending in the US on care for arthritis and other rheumatic disorders was approximately US $ 128 billion, equivalent to 1.2% of the US gross domestic product in 2003 (Centers for Disease Control and Prevention, 2007).

So far as Europe is concerned, a study of the socio-economic costs of pain syndromes in the United Kingdom estimated that the cost of direct healthcare was £ 1.6 billion in 1998. But this direct cost is insignificant compared to the indirect costs (e.g. days of work lost and loss of productivity) associated with back pain, totalling 10.7 billion (Maniadakis & Gray, 2000). Winkelmann et al. (2011) estimated the annual costs per fibromyalgia patient for 2008 as € 7,900 in France (of which €960 direct costs, €6,990 indirect costs), and € 7,256 in Germany (€ 1,756 direct costs, € 5,491 indirect costs).

2.2 Opioid treatment of chronic non-cancer pain

In recent years, many guidelines for the use of opioids in patients with chronic non-cancer pain have been drawn up. In general the objectives of such documents are: to bring consistency in opioid prescribing to the many diverse groups involved; to provide analysis of evidence to treat a chronic pain patient with opioids, thus, maintaining reasonable patient access while reducing the risk of drug diversion; to provide practical prescribing guidelines for physicians to reduce the risk of legal and regulatory sanctions; and to emphasize the need for systematic evaluation and ongoing care of patients with chronic or persistent pain (Trescot et al., 2006). The perceived benefits of these guidelines include: increased physician awareness about the current issues involving opioids and non-cancer pain; improved patient access; reduced level of opioid abuse; improved ability to manage patient expectations; reduced diversion; improved understanding by law enforcement about proper prescribing patterns; improved cooperation among patients, providers, and regulatory agencies; improved understanding by patients regarding their rights as well as their responsibilities when taking opioid medications (Trescot et al., 2008). These guidelines should be applied flexibly: every physician must establish a treatment plan that takes account of the specific medical conditions of the patient and his personal preferences and needs, and of the physician's own professional experience (Trescot et al., 2006; 2008). Based on a systematic review of the efficacy of treatment with opioids in chronic non-cancer pain by a multidisciplinary group of experts, the American Academy of Pain Medicine formulated a series of recommendations for: patient selection and the stratification of risk of abuse, informed consent to treatment with opioids, initiation and titration of chronic opioid therapy, the use of methadone, patient monitoring, the use of opioids in high risk patients, the assessment of the effectiveness of the drug and the aberrant drug-related behaviours, dose escalation and high dose therapy, opioid rotation, indications for discontinuation of therapy, prevention and management of opioid-related side effects and issues about driving and work safety during treatment with such drugs (Chou, 2009; Chou et al, 2009a; Chou et al, 2009b; Chou et al, 2009c). The recommendations of the American Pain Society and the American Academy of Pain Medicine are shown in table 1.

TOPIC AREA	RECOMMENDATIONS
Patient selection and risk stratification	Prior to initiating chronic opioid therapy, clinicians should conduct a history, physical examination and appropriate testing, including an assessment of risk of substance abuse, misuse, or addiction (strong recommendation, low-quality evidence).
	Clinicians may consider a trial of chronic opioid therapy as an option if chronic non-cancer pain is moderate or severe, pain is having an adverse impact on function or quality of life, and potential therapeutic benefits outweigh or are likely to outweigh potential harms (strong recommendation, low-quality evidence).
	A benefit-to-harm evaluation including a history, physical examination, and appropriate diagnostic testing, should be performed and documented prior to and on an ongoing basis during chronic opioid therapy (strong recommendation, low-quality evidence).
Informed consent and opioid management plans	When starting chronic opioid therapy, informed consent should be obtained. A continuing discussion with the patient regarding chronic opioid therapy should include goals, expectations, potential risks, and alternatives to chronic opioid therapy (strong recommendation, low-quality evidence).
	Clinicians may consider using a written chronic opioid therapy management plan to document patient and clinician responsibilities and expectations and assist in patient education (weak recommendation, low-quality evidence).
Initiation and titration of chronic opioid therapy	Clinicians and patients should regard initial treatment with opioids as a therapeutic trial to determine whether chronic opioid therapy is appropriate (strong recommendation, low-quality evidence).
	Opioid selection, initial dosing, and titration should be individualized according to the patient's health status, previous exposure to opioids, attainment of therapeutic goals, and predicted or observed harms (strong recommendation, low-quality evidence). There is insufficient evidence to recommend short-acting versus long-acting opioids, or as-needed versus around-the-clock dosing of opioids.
Methadone	Methadone is characterized by complicated and variable pharmacokinetics and pharmacodynamics and should be initiated and titrated cautiously, by clinicians familiar with its use and risks (strong recommendation, moderate-quality evidence).
Monitoring	Clinicians should reassess patients on chronic opioid therapy periodically and as warranted by changing circumstances. Monitoring should include documentation of pain intensity and level of functioning, assessments of progress towards achieving therapeutic goals, presence of adverse events, and adherence to prescribed therapies (strong recommendation, low-quality evidence).
	In patients on chronic opioid therapy who are at high risk or who have engaged in aberrant drug-related behaviours, clinicians should periodically obtain urine drug screens or other information to confirm adherence to the chronic opioid therapy plan of care (strong recommendation, low-quality evidence).
	In patients on chronic opioid therapy not at high risk and not known to have engaged in aberrant drug-related behaviors, clinicians should consider periodically obtaining urine drug screens or other information to confirm adherence to the chronic opioid therapy plan of care (weak recommendation, low-quality evidence).

TOPIC AREA	RECOMENDATIONS
High-risk patients	Clinicians may consider chronic opioid therapy for patients with chronic non-cancer pain and history of drug abuse, psychiatric issues, or serious aberrant drug-related behaviours only if they are able to implement more frequent and stringent monitoring parameters. In such situations, clinicians should strongly consider consultation with a mental health or addiction specialist (strong recommendation, low-quality evidence).
Aberrant drug-related behaviours	Clinicians should evaluate patients engaging in aberrant drug-related behaviours for appropriateness of chronic opioid therapy or need for restructuring of therapy, referral for assistance in management, or discontinuation of chronic opioid therapy (strong recommendation, low-quality evidence).
Dose escalations and high-dose therapy	When repeated dose escalations occur in patients on chronic opioid therapy, clinicians should evaluate potential causes and re-assess benefits relative to harms (strong recommendation, low-quality evidence).
	In patients who require relatively high doses of chronic opioid therapy clinicians should evaluate for unique opioid-related adverse effects, changes in health status, and adherence to the chronic opioid therapy treatment plan on an ongoing basis, and consider more frequent follow-up visits (strong recommendation, low-quality evidence).
Opioid rotation	Clinicians should consider opioid rotation when patients on chronic opioid therapy experience intolerable adverse effects or inadequate benefit despite dose increases (weak recommendation, low-quality evidence).
Indications for discontinuation of therapy	Clinicians should taper or wean patients off of chronic opioid therapy who engage in repeated aberrant drug-related behaviours or drug abuse/diversion, experience no progress towards meeting therapeutic goals, or experience intolerable adverse effects (strong recommendation, low-quality evidence).
Opioid-related adverse effects	Clinicians should anticipate, identify, and treat common opioid-associated adverse effects (strong recommendation, moderate-quality evidence).
Use of psychotherapeutic co-interventions	As chronic noncancer pain is often a complex biopsychosocial condition, clinicians who prescribe chronic opioid therapy should routinely integrate psychotherapeutic interventions, functional restoration, interdisciplinary therapy, and other adjunctive non-opioid therapies (strong recommendation, moderate-quality evidence).
Driving and work safety	Clinicians should counsel patients on chronic opioid therapy about transient or lasting cognitive impairment that may affect driving and work safety. Patients should be counselled not to drive or engage in potentially dangerous activities when impaired or if they describe or demonstrate signs of impairment (strong recommendation, low-quality evidence).
Identifying a medical home and when to obtain consultation	Patients on chronic opioid therapy should identify a clinician who accepts primary responsibility for their overall medical care. This clinician may or may not prescribe chronic opioid therapy, but should coordinate consultation and communication among all clinicians involved in the patient's care (strong recommendation, low-quality evidence).
	Clinicians should pursue consultation, including interdisciplinary pain management, when patients with chronic non-cancer pain may benefit from additional skills or resources that they cannot provide (strong recommendation, moderate-quality evidence).
Breakthrough pain	In patients on around-the-clock chronic opioid therapy with breakthrough pain, clinicians may consider as-needed opioids based upon an initial and ongoing analysis of therapeutic benefit versus risk (weak recommendation, low-quality evidence).

Table 1. Guidelines recommended by the American Pain Society and the American Academy of Pain Medicine for the long-term treatment with opioids of patients with chronic non-cancer pain (adapted from Chou, 2009).

Trescot et al. (2006, 2008) confirmed the importance of an overall patient assessment (physical and psychological) before initiating long-term opioid therapy; this assessment must include an appropriate assessment of treatment efficacy at regular intervals (in terms of both pain reduction and recovery of physical function), the identification and treatment of side effects and the monitoring of any abuse or misuse of the drug. The authors proposed a ten step algorithm that physicians could use for this purpose during treatment with opioids.

2.2.1 Terminology of opioid abuse: Dependence, tolerance, addiction

To ensure effective communication between physicians, researchers and legislators, a clear common terminology is needed. Many drugs, including opioids, play an important role in the treatment of pain. However, as shown earlier, the use of opioids is often limited by concerns about abuse, dependence and their possible use for non-medical reasons. Addiction, tolerance and physical dependence are distinct and different phenomena that are often used in a confused way. Since their clinical implications and management are clearly different, it is important to establish uniform definitions based on current scientific and clinical knowledge, to improve the care of patients with chronic pain and encourage appropriate policies for the regulation and control of drugs. For this purpose, the American Academy of Pain Medicine, the American Pain Society and the American Society of Addiction Medicine (American Society of Addiction Medicine, 2001) have recognised the following definitions, and recommend their use:

Addiction is a primary, chronic, neurobiologic disease, with genetic, psychosocial, and environmental factors influencing its development and manifestations. It is characterized by behaviours that include one or more of the following: impaired control over drug use, compulsive use, continued use despite harm, and craving.

Physical dependence is a state of adaptation that is manifested by a drug class specific withdrawal syndrome that can be produced by abrupt cessation, rapid dose reduction, decreasing blood level of the drug, and/or administration of an antagonist.

Tolerance is a state of adaptation in which exposure to a drug induces changes that result in a diminution of one or more of the drug's effects over time.

Pseudoaddiction is a term that has been used to describe behaviour that can occur when the pain is undertreated. Patients with inadequately managed pain may in fact become excessively focused on obtaining drugs. In their intent to obtain relief, patients may also resort to trickery and the use of unlawful substances. Pseudoaddiction may be distinguished from true addiction by the fact that the behaviour disappears when the pain is treated efficaciously.

Misuse is defined as the use of any psychoactive substance in a way other than that for which it has been indicated or prescribed (Wasan et al., 2007). In practical terms, opioid misuse means: inadequate pain management, ineffective treatment, excessive focus on the drug and its effects which does not allow the patient to use other strategies efficaciously to cope with the pain, and finally, worsening of quality of life and altered social, working and psychological functioning.

The term *aberrant drug-related behaviours* has been used to indicate the broad array of problematic nonadherence behaviours (Passik et al., 2006), the nature of which is uncertain until a diagnosis can be developed based on astute clinical assessment (Rosenblum et al., 2008). Portenoy (1996; 2004) has listed a series of behaviours that should engender suspicion of addiction in patients with pain being treated with opioids (table 2). Moreover, Savage

(1993), suggested that the following aspects should also be considered: frequent cancellation of appointments; asking for medicines at the end of every appointment; a history of non-responsiveness to treatment, apart from opioids; a history of negative relationships with many physicians; many "drug allergies" that limit treatment options; finally, a degree of disability that is disproportionate to the basic disorder.

As described above, the use of opioids has raised many concerns; in fact, the use of analgesics without medical prescription, or just to test their effects ("non medical use") represents the second most frequent form of illicit substance use in the United States, after marijuana use (Office of Applied Studies, Substance Abuse and Mental Health Services Administration [SAMHSA], 2008). The National Survey on Drug Use and Health (Office of Applied Studies, SAMHSA, 2009) report on the use of opioids for non-medical purposes in the United States from 2002 to 2007 showed that: in 2007 approximately 5.2 million people of 12 years of age or more had used prescription-only analgesics for non-medical purposes in the previous month; from 2002 to 2007 the use of opioids for non-therapeutic purposes decreased among young people between 12 and 17 years of age (from 3.2% to 2.7%) , while it increased in young adults between 18 and 25 years of age (4.1% to 4.6%) and in adults over 26 (from 1.3% to 1.6%).

Behaviours probably more predictive of addiction
Selling prescriptions drugs
Prescription forgery
Stealing or "borrowing" drugs from others
Injection oral formulations
Obtaining prescription drugs from non-medical sources
Concurrent abuse of alcohol or illicit drugs
Multiple dose escalation or other non-compliance with therapy despite warnings
Multiple episodes of prescription "loss"
Repeatedly seeking prescription from other clinicians or from emergency rooms without informing prescriber or after warning to desist
Evidence of deterioration in the ability to function in work, in the family, or socially that appear to be related to the drug use
Repeated resistance to changes in therapy despite clear evidence of adverse physical or psychological effect from the drug
Behaviours probably less predictive of addiction
Aggressive complaining about the need for more drug
Drug hoarding during periods of reduced symptoms
Requesting specific drugs
Openly acquiring similar drugs from other medical sources
Unsanctioned dose escalation or other non-compliance with therapy on one or two occasions
Reporting psychic effects not intended by the clinician
Resistance to change in therapy associated with "tolerable" adverse effects with expression of anxiety related to the return of severe symptoms

Table 2. Behaviours predictive of addiction (adapted from Portenoy 1996, 2004).

Many studies have been carried out about the prevalence of opioid addiction in patients with chronic pain, but one of the limitations in interpreting their results is the fact that the researchers have used different criteria to establish problematic opioid use; some studies are based on behavioural observations, others on the results of urine toxicology screening, others again on the criteria Diagnostic and Statistical Manual of mental disorders – III or IV [DSM-III-IV] and yet other studies are based on definitions established by the authors themselves.

Based on an extensive literature review, Højsted & Sjøgren (2007) estimated that the prevalence of addiction in the population with chronic non-cancer pain varies from 0% to 50%. In particular, in the studies based on urine toxicology screening the prevalence varies from 17.2% to 39%; in the studies using the DSM-III or DSM-IV criteria it varied from 1.9% to 37%; and, finally, in the studies based on the various behavioural indicators, the prevalence varied from 0% to 50%. In a study of 100 patients with chronic pain in treatment with opioids, Manchikanti et al. (2001) found a prevalence of drug abuse, defined as the occurrence of obtaining a prescription of a controlled substance at least once a month from another physician without approval of the pain physician signing the controlled substance contract, of 24%. Fleming et al. (2007), considering 801 patients with non-cancer pain in chronic treatment with opioids, reported that 9.7% of the sample met the DSM-IV diagnostic criteria for opioid use disorder; the prevalence found by the authors was four times the prevalence in the general population.

Finally, a recent review of the prolonged use of opioids in patients with non-cancer pain estimated the prevalence of addiction indicators as 0.27% of the total number of patients examined (Noble et al., 2010); the authors also observed that minor unwanted effects (e.g. nausea, headache) are frequent during treatment with opioids, but more serious adverse events, such as addiction, are rare.

The hypothesis that short acting drugs such as hydrocodone may make patients more liable to ineffective pain management and misuse or abuse of the drugs than long acting drugs such as methadone was investigated by Manchikanti et al. (2005), who analysed 200 patients with chronic pain, half being treated with hydrocodone and the remainder with methadone. The study found no significant differences in the use of illegal substances and/or opioid abuse in patients treated with short- or long-acting drugs.

So addiction is a well documented problem in pain patients, although it is difficult to estimate its exact prevalence. It is therefore important that clinicians consider the risk of opioid addiction without this prejudicing their use where indicated. In fact, those who use opioids constitute a heterogeneous category that includes extreme cases of patients who abuse medical and non-medical substances, and patients who adhere to treatment (Passik, 2009). For adequate management and treatment of pain, physicians must balance the costs and benefits of opioid treatment; to maximise the benefits they can use different strategies, such as risk assessment and stratification, using specific tools, constant monitoring of treatment and any aberrant drug behaviours, regular urine screening and the possible involvement of another specialist (e.g. psychotherapist, addiction expert).

2.3 Risk factors for opioid abuse

Risk factors for opioid abuse and addiction may be divided into three categories: psychosocial factors, substance-related factors and genetic factors (figure 2). The risk of addiction is highest when the various categories of risk factor are combined. Pain patients without a genetic predisposition, without psychiatric comorbidity who take a stable dose of opioids for the treatment of severe pain in a controlled clinical setting are most unlikely to develop addiction. In contrast, patients with a personal or family history of substance abuse, and with one or more psychosocial issues are at greater risk of developing addiction, especially if the treatment is not carefully structured (Ballantyne, 2007).

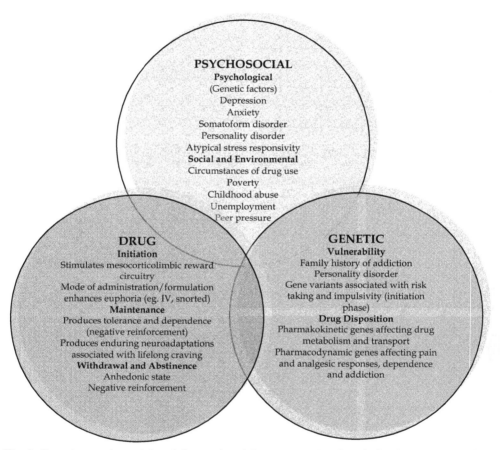

Fig. 2. Genetic, psychosocial and drug-related factors associated with the development of addiction. Adapted from Ballantyne (2007).

The psychosocial factors considered to be most predictive of opioid abuse are the presence of psychiatric disorders (Compton et al., 1998; Sullivan et al., 2006) and a personal and/or family history of substance abuse or drug abuse (Dunbar & Katz, 1996; Schieffer et al., 2005). A significant correlation has been found between chronic pain, mood disorders and aberrant drug use: patients with chronic pain report higher levels of anxiety and depression than patients with other medical conditions, and the incidence of mood disorders has been shown to be higher in patients at high risk of opioid misuse or dependence (Bair et al., 2003; Dersh et al., 2002; Fishbain, 1999).

Using logistic regression, the authors showed that panic attacks, high trait anxiety and the presence of a personality disorder are able to explain the 38% variance in potential abuse of prescribed opioids. To investigate the role of psychological adjustment and psychiatric symptoms in aberrant drug behaviours in pain patients, Wasan et al. (2007) divided the 228 patients enrolled into high-psychiatric and low-psychiatric morbidity, based on the responses to the psychiatric subscale of the Prescription Drug Use Questionnaire (PDUQ; Compton et al., 2008; see § 2.4.). Patients with high psychiatric comorbidity were significantly younger, with a longer mean opioid assumption time (p<0.05); altered urine toxicology screening results were also more frequent among these patients (p<0.01), and they often displayed aberrant drug-related behaviours.

Edlund et al. (2007) conducted a broad prospective study of the risk factors for opioid abuse and addiction using the South Central Veterans Affairs Health Care Network databank. The sample included 15.160 chronic users of opioids in 2002; 45.3% of the sample had a psychiatric diagnosis and 7.6% had a non-opioid substance abuse diagnosis. The results show that prior abuse of non-opioid substances is a strong predictor of abuse/addiction to opioid drugs, while mental disorders are moderately strong predictors. The authors also found that the risk of abuse decreases uniformly with age. Other risk factors for opioid abuse/addiction were male gender, being divorced/separated or single and, finally, being in treatment with opioids for longer. A broad retrospective cohort study that involved 704 patients with chronic pain being treated with opioids was carried out by Banta-Green et al. (2009a) to further comprehend the complex interaction between pain, mental health and addiction. The patients were initially assessed using a structured interview based on DSM-IV criteria for abuse and dependence on opioids, misuse of opioids, anxiety and depression. By regression analysis, the authors identified three distinct categories of patients which they called: a) Typical group (characterised by moderate pain symptoms and limited psychiatric problems); b) Addictive Behaviours group (high psychiatric symptoms, misuse of opioids and moderate pain symptoms); c) Pain Dysfunction group (high intensity and interference of pain, high psychiatric symptoms and consistent misuse of opioids). The patients in the last two groups took an average daily dose of opioids that was three times that of the typical group. The authors suggest that the use of high doses of drugs could constitute a simple indicator to identify those patients that might benefit from further medical or psychiatric assessment, or assessment of drug misuse behaviours.

To determine the incidence of opioid addiction, and the factors predictive for abuse, Ives et al. (2006) carried out a prospective cohort study of 196 patients with chronic pain being treated with opioids. Patients were monitored at regular intervals for an entire year. Opioid abuse was defined based on the presence of: negative urine toxicology screening for prescribed opioids; positive urine toxicology screening for non-prescribed drugs or opioids; supplies of opioids obtained from more than one provider; diversion of opioids, prescription forgery and positive urine toxicology screening for narcotics (cocaine or amphetamines). Opioid abuse was observed in 32% of patients; the most common form of misuse was the detection of cocaine or amphetamine in urine (40.3% of misusers). Abusers were found to be significantly younger (p<0.001); male (p= 0.023); with a history of abuse of alcohol (p= 0.004) and cocaine (p<0.001) than non-abusers. Ethnicity, income, education, levels of depression or disability and pain intensity were not found to be associated with drug misuse. Manchikanti et al. (2006) carried out a prospective longitudinal study of 500 patients with chronic pain to evaluate and correlate multiple variables with the abuse of opioids and illegal substances. Patients who obtained opioid drugs from sources other than the physicians at the clinic where the study was carried out were considered abusers; use of narcotics was ascertained through urine toxicology screening. Opioid abuse was observed in 9% of patients, while the use of illegal substances (e.g. cocaine, marijuana, metamphetamines) was detected in 16% of the sample. Opioid abuse was found to be more frequent in patients with pain due to road traffic accidents, pain in more than one region of the body and subjects with prior substance abuse. The use of illegal substances was more frequent among women and in patients under 45 years of age. The onset of pain after a road traffic accident and the presence of pain in more than one part of the body were also risk factors for narcotic substance abuse. To investigate the effect of gender on aberrant drug-related behaviours, Back et al. (2009) carried out a study on 121 patients (49 make and 72 female), who had to complete a set of tests designed to collect personal and clinical information and data on aberrant drug behaviours (e.g. prescription fraud, using other drug administration routes) and the use of nicotine, alcohol, marijuana, cocaine and hallucinogens. The results show that men were taking the prescribed drug significantly more regularly than women (91.7% v 77.8%, p<0.05), while women tend to keep unused drugs (67.6% v 47.7%; p=0.04) and to use other drugs (e.g. sedatives) to enhance the efficacy of analgesics (38.8% v 20%; p=0.04) more than men. Men tend to use other drug administration routes (e.g. crushing and snorting pills) than women, although this difference was not statistically significant. For men, there was an association between alcohol abuse, use of oxycodone or morphine and aberrant drug behaviours, while in women the aberrant drug behaviours were associated with the use of hydrocodone.

In conclusion, the presence of psychiatric disorders and a personal and/or family history of substance abuse seem to be the most predictive factors of risk of opioid misuse in patients with chronic pain. Other variables such as gender, age and marital status may influence the risk of abuse, although the relationship is less clear, and further investigation is required (Savage, 2002).

2.4 Tools to assess the risk of addiction and dependence

Guidelines suggest that the use of opioids in patients with chronic non-cancer pain must be preceded by an initial stratification of the risk of drug misuse; this evaluation should include even a psychological and psychiatric assessment (Chou, 2009; Chou et al, 2009a; Chou et al, 2009b; Chou et al, 2009c; Kalso et al., 2003; Trescot et al., 2006; Trescot at al., 2008). In recent years, many tools have been developed and examined for this purpose; most investigate the presence of a family and/or personal history of addiction and other factors correlated with opioid misuse, such as age, history of childhood sexual abuse and the presence of mental distress. Some of these tools, were created specifically for use in a population of patients with chronic pain, while others assess the addiction risk factors in general. Table 3 summarises the tools that will then be described in greater detail; however, it is important to bear in mind that none is able to produce an accurate diagnosis about the presence of addiction, abuse or dependence. Besides, many of these are self-assessment tools, and therefore potentially at risk of falsification by the respondent. It is therefore advisable to supplement the information obtained with such tools with data obtained from direct observation of the patient during medical appointments. Anyhow, for patients who are found to be at high risk of misuse of the drug from the initial assessment with one of these scales, it is advisable to provide for constant monitoring of treatment, with regular urine toxicology screening.

Name	Abbreviated name	Authors	Year	Method of administration	Number of items
a	*CAGE- questions Adapted to Include Drugs*	CAGE-AID	Brown & Rounds	1995	Self-administered	4
b1	*Prescription Drug Use Questionnaire*	PDUQ	Compton et al.	1998	Interview	42
b2	*Prescription Drug Use Questionnaire – patient version*	PDUQp		2008	Self-administered	31
c	*Screening Tool for Addiction Risk*	STAR	Friedman et al.	2003	Self-administered	14
d	*Pain Medication Questionnaire*	PMQ	Adams et al.	2004	Self-administered	26
e1	*Screener and Opioid Assessment for Patients with Pain*	SOAPP	Butler et al.	2004	Self-administered	14
e2	*Screener and Opioid Assessment for Patients with Pain – Revised*	SOAPP-R		2008		24
f	*Opioid Risk Tool*	ORT	Webster et al.	2005	Self-administered	5
g	*Addiction Behaviour Checklist*	ABC	Wu et al.	2006	Interview	20
h	*Diagnosis Intractability Risk and Efficacy Score*	DIRE	Belgrade et al.	2006	Team assessment	7
i	*Drug Abuse Screening Test*	DAST	Yudko et al	2007	Self-administered	28

Table 3. Principal tools for the stratification of the risk of opioid addiction and abuse.

a. The *CAGE questions Adapted to Include Drugs* (CAGE-AID; Brown & Rounds, 1995) is an adaptation of the CAGE questionnaire, used for a short screening for alcohol abuse, which also includes substance use. The name CAGE is derived from 4 key words: "cut", "annoyed", "guilty" and "eye-opener". The questionnaire consists of the following 4 questions, to which the subject must reply "yes" or "no": 1) Have you felt you ought to cut down your drinking or drug use?; 2) Have people annoyed you by criticizing your drinking or drug use?; 3) Have you felt bad or guilty about your drinking or drug use?; 4) Have you ever had a drink or used drugs first thing in the morning to steady your nerves or to get rid of a hangover (eye-opener)?. The addiction screening is positive with at least 2 affirmative responses. The CAGE-AID has been validated on a sample of 124 pain patients, demonstrating high values of sensitivity (0.70) and specificity (0.85).

b1. *Prescription Drug Use Questionnaire* (PDUQ, Compton et al., 1998) is a tool, consisting of 42 items to be administered in the form of an interview, that assesses the degree of abuse / misuse of the drug in patients with chronic pain. Care staff trained in the use of the tool take about twenty minutes to complete the interview. The patient must answer yes/no to questions that investigate: pain condition (e.g. "Has the patient explored and/or tried non-opioid or non-pharmacological pain management techniques?"), the ways in which they use drugs (e.g. "Does the patient have more than one prescription provider?"), social/family factors (e.g. "Have family members expressed concerns that the patient is addicted?"), family history of chronic pain and/or addiction (e.g. "Is there a positive history of chronic pain in the patient's mother, father, sibling or blood relative?"), personal history of substance abuse (e.g. "Has the patient ever been diagnosed with addiction to any drug or alcohol") and psychiatric history (e.g. "Has the patient ever been diagnosed with a psychiatric disorder?"). The tool has good internal consistency (Cronbach's α = 0.79). To identify a cut-off, the 52 patients with chronic pain who participated in the pilot study to validate the PDUQ were initially classified as addicted or non-addicted based on criteria developed by the American Society of Addiction Medicine (see § 2.2.2.). Patients with scores of less than 11 did not meet the criteria for a substance abuse disorder, while patients with scores of 15 or more reflected the criteria for a substance abuse disorder. So those who achieved scores of less than 11 use the drug in a suitable way. Moreover, positive answers to 3 specific items of the tool (notably "patient believes he/she is addicted"; "increases analgesic dose/frequency"; "specific drug or route of administration preference") have been identified as more predictive of addiction, with a 92.9% of correct classification. Banta-Green et al. (2009b) carried out a study of 704 patients who had been prescribed long-term treatment with opioids, aimed to examine the factorial structure of the PDUQ. The results show that the items may be grouped into three distinct types of factor "addictive behaviours", "addiction concerns" and "pain treatment problems". The limits of the PDUQ concern the fact that it relies solely on the sincerity of the patient and is difficult to use in an overloaded clinical context.

b2. The *Prescription Drug Use Questionnaire – patient version* (PDUQp) was created by Compton et al. (2008) to obviate the difficulty mentioned above. The PDUQp is a self-administered instrument which consists of 31 items and the total score can vary from 0 to 30. Analysis of the psychometric properties of the new self-administered version was carried out on 135 patients with chronic pain being treated with opioids, monitored for 12 months. The PDUQp proved to have good concurrent validity, calculated by comparing the scores obtained with the scores obtained with the PDUQ (r = 0.64). The tool also proved to have good test-retest reliability, assessed at 4, 8 and 12 months after its first administration (r = 0.67, r = 0.61 and r = 0.40 respectively). A cut-off of 10 is suggested as indicative of drug misuse.

c. The *Screening Tool for Addiction Risk* (STAR, Friedman et al., 2003) consists of 14 questions with true/false responses that investigate potential risk factors for drug. The items were developed based on a literature review carried out by a team of specialists in pain and addiction. Validation of the questionnaire was carried out on 48 patients with chronic pain, 14 of whom had a diagnosis of addiction based on the DSM-IV criteria. The authors found a close correlation between addiction and prior treatment in a rehabilitation unit for alcohol or drug dependence, smoking, and intensity of nicotine craving. In particular, the item on prior experience of alcohol and/or substance detoxification was able to identify correctly 93% of the patients who met the addiction criteria.

d. The Pain Medication Questionnaire (PMQ, Adams et al., 2004) is a self-administered questionnaire that describes a series of dysfunctional behaviours and characteristics that underlie the use of drugs for the treatment of pain. The tool consists of 26 items, for each of which the subject must indicate his degree of agreement or disagreement on a 5 point Likert scale, and a score is attributed to the selected response (disagree = 0, somewhat disagree = 1, neutral = 3, somewhat agree = 4, agree = 5). The sum of the scores of the single items gives a total score, which can vary from a minimum of 0 to a maximum of 104. High scores are correlated with a high risk of opioid misuse. In particular, scores of 25 or more are indicative of opioid misuse, while scores of 30 or more suggest that the patient should be constantly monitored during treatment (Dowling et al., 2007). The validity of the tool was investigated by Adams et al. (2004) on 184 patients with chronic pain, comparing the results obtained with the PMQ with a series of assessment of substance abuse, degree of psychosocial distress, and some indicators of psychological and physical functioning; the test-retest reliability coefficient is 0.85 and the internal consistency is acceptable (Cronbach's α = 0.73). A further study to examine the psychometric characteristics of the PMQ in greater depth was carried out by Buelow et al. (2009). One of the aims was to examine the accuracy of the short form of the PMQ (from which items 5, 10 and 23 had been eliminated, since they had the lowest correlation coefficients) in predicting opioid misuse. Examining 4.182 subjects, of whom 1.813 were involved in an interdisciplinary treatment programme (that included physical, pharmacological and psychological therapy) the authors confirmed the adequate internal consistency of the abbreviated form (Cronbach's α = 0.70) e and of test-retest reliability (r= 0.77). Significant differences also emerged in the mean PMQ score of patients with a history of substance abuse (mean = 24.39) and of patients without a history of abuse (mean = 21.95). Moreover, those patients who interrupted the treatment had mean scores that were significantly higher than those of patients who displayed good compliance. By logistic regression, the authors showed that early request of opioids is the only factor able to predict high or low questionnaire scores of those assessed (age, history of alcohol and/or substance abuse).

e1. The Screener and Opioid Assessment for Patients with Pain (SOAPP, Butler et al., 2004) is a self-administered tool with 14 items that investigate potential risk factors for opioid misuse (e.g. "How often do you take more medications than you are supposed to?"; "How often have others expressed concerns over your use of medication?"). These items were proposed and voted on by a team of experts; the patient must indicate the frequency of each behaviour on a 5 point Likert scale (0 = "never"; 4 = "very often"). The tool was administered to 175 patients with chronic pain and readministered 6 months later to 95 of these patients, to test its reliability over time. The SOAPP proved to have adequate internal consistency (Cronbach's α= 0.74) and good test-retest reliability six months after its first administration (r = 0.71). Scores of 8 or more are indicative of high risk of abuse (sensitivity: 0.91; specificity: 0.69). In a study investigating the psychometric characteristics and clinical utility of the SOAPP in 397 patients, Akbik et al. (2006) found patients classified at high risk were significantly younger, with altered urine screening results (p<0.05) than low risk patients. The factor analysis also revealed the presence of 5 factors, called: 1) History of substance abuse; 2) Legal problems; 3) Craving medications; 4) Heavy smoking and 5) Mood swings. Moore et al. (2009), in a study to examine the efficacy of the SOAPP and other tools in predicting the risk of opioid misuse, found good sensitivity for the tool (0.72); combining the data from the SOAPP with those from a semi-structured clinical interview designed to investigate prior treatments used, the presence of emotional distress and prior substance abuse, the sensitivity increased to 0.90.

e2. *The Screener and Opioid Assessment for Patients with Pain – Revised* (SOAPP-R) is a 24-item version developed by Butler et al. (2008) in order to overcome some limitations of the original SOAPP. The new version, tested on a sample of 283 patients, proved to have good internal consistency (Cronbach's α = 0.88); the cut-off of 18 shows adequate sensitivity (0.81) and specificity (0.68). Patients with low SOAPP-R scores appear to be at less risk of developing a substance abuse disorder.

f.   The *Opioid Risk Tool* (ORT, Webster et al., 2005) is a self-administered tool developed to estimate the probability that the patient displays aberrant drug behaviours during long-term opioid treatment. The ORT consists of 5 items which investigate the following risk factors: family history of substance abuse (alcohol, drugs or prescribed medicines); personal history of substance abuse (alcohol, drugs or prescribed medicines); age (if between 16 and 45 years); history of childhood sexual abuse; presence of psychological distress (attention deficit disorder, obsessive-compulsive disorder, bipolar disorder, schizophrenia and depression). Each factor has a different weight in determining the potential risk of drug misuse, and so a specific numerical value is assigned to each, which also varies according to the sex of the respondent. There are three risk levels: scores from 0 to 3 are indicative of low risk; scores from 4 to 7 determine moderate risk; finally, scores of 8 or more are indicative of a high risk of misuse. This questionnaire was validated on 108 women and 77 men with chronic pain, followed for a period of 12 months from the initial appointment. 94% of the patients classified as low risk based on the total ORT score did not display aberrant drug behaviours in the year in which they were monitored, while 90.9% of the patients with scores of the cut-off value of 8 or more displayed aberrant drug behaviours.

g.   The *Addiction Behaviour Checklist* (ABC, Wu et al., 2006) consists of 20 items to be administered in the form of an interview. The items are grouped in two principal categories: 1) addicted behaviours noted during visit (e.g. "patient running out of medications early"; "receiving narcotics from other providers"); 2) addictive behaviours observed within the visit (e.g. "patient appearing sedated"; "patient expressing concern about the future availability of narcotics"). Finally, there is a further question that can be used if family members of the patient are present during the medical appointment ("significant others express concern over patient's use of analgesic"). The answer system is binary (yes/no): each affirmative answer is assigned a point and the total score can vary from 0 to 20. To investigate its psychometric characteristics, the ABC was administered to 136 patients with chronic pain prescribed long-term opioid treatment. The tool proved to have high inter-rater validity (0.94 – 0.95) and significant concurrent validity: a significant correlation (r=0.40; p< .01) was found between the ABC score and the Prescription Drug Use Questionnaire (PDUQ, Compton et al., 1998) score. A cut-off value of 3 on this tool is able to provide a good estimate of appropriate/inappropriate use that the patient will make of the drug. For scores of 3 or more, the authors suggest that the patient should be monitored frequently, including more frequent urine toxicology screening.

h.   The *Diagnosis Intractability Risk and Efficacy Score* (DIRE, Belgrade et al., 2006) is a tool that is compiled by a multidisciplinary team of physicians and psychologists. It consists of 4 scales: Diagnosis, Intractability, Risk (4 subcategories) Efficacy. Each class requires assessment on a 3 point scale, where a score of 1 corresponds to characteristics and behaviours that are indicative of a negative prognosis, and a score of 3 is indicative of suitability for treatment with opioids. The Diagnosis factor requires the clinician to determine the extent to which the patient's diagnosis is sufficiently compelling or advanced to warrant an aggressive pharmacological approach. The Intractability factor requires a determination of how many appropriate treatments the patient has undergone and how he or she is involved in the treatment, i.e. if they play a passive or an active role in managing their pain. The Risk factor was created to estimate the extent to which the patient would adhere to the instructions of the clinician during treatment. As stated above, it comprises four categories: Psychological health assesses the psychiatric and psychological status of the patient; Chemical health assesses the patient's relationship with substances with potential risk of abuse; Reliability assesses compliance with treatment in the past, whether or not the patient attends appointments and following the physician's recommendations fully; Social support assesses the patient's support network and his or her ability to function in life roles, such as work, school, parenting, etc. Efficacy assesses the analgesic effectiveness of opioids, based on physical functionality and patient's pain self-report. When efficacy cannot be assessed because the patient has not yet started to take opioids, or takes them in quantities that are too low (less than the equivalent of 30 mg/day of morphine) a score of 2 is attributed. All the scales and subscales of the Risk factor are firstly assessed individually and then added together to obtain the DIRE score. The total score can vary from a minimum of 7 to a maximum of 21; scores between 14 and 21 are indicative of a greater degree of patient compliance and, in general, greater treatment efficacy. The psychometric analyses of the original version, carried out on a group of 61 patients with chronic pain, shown an internal consistency alpha coefficient of 0.80 and an inter-rater validity of 0.95.

i.   The Drug Abuse Screening Test (DAST, Yudko et al., 2007) is a self-administered questionnaire consisting of 28 items with binary (yes/no) answers. Scores of 6 or more indicate the presence of substance dependence or abuse. In addition to the complete version of the questionnaire, which can be too time-consuming in some clinical contexts, there are various short versions of the DAST, based on 10 items instead of 28. The 28-item DAST has proved to have high test-retest reliability ($r = 0.85$) and good internal consistency (Cronbach's α 0.92-0.94). The tool has shown good sensitivity, between 81% and 96%, and good specificity (from 71% to 94%). One limitation of the tool is the fact that it is susceptible to falsification and may therefore not identify those people who, while abusing the drug, intentionally give false answers. Moreover, the tool is predictive of substance abuse but does not specifically examine the aberrant drug behaviours.

2.4.1 Ways of monitoring treatment

A number of different tools have been created for clinicians to monitor opioid treatment and as checklists for the systemic observation of aberrant drug behaviours. The tools most widely mentioned in the literature are described briefly below.

The *Prescription Opioid Therapy Questionnaire* (POTQ; Michna et al., 2004) is a tool with 11 items to which the clinician must answer yes or no to assess opioid misuse. The items reflect the behaviours suggested by Chabal et al. (1997) as indicative of substance abuse. These behaviours include multiple unauthorised dosage increases, episodes of lost or stolen prescriptions, frequent unplanned visits to the clinic or emergency room, excessive telephone calls and inflexibility about treatment options. Patients who were positively rated on two or more of the items met criteria for prescription opioid misuse.

The *Pain Assessment and Documentation Tool* (PADT; Passik et al., 2004; Passik et al., 2005) is a brief (takes between 10 to 20 minutes to complete) clinician-directed interview. The clinician asks the patients questions that are organized in four primary areas called the "Four A's" and are notably: Analgesia - focuses on pain intensity (numeric rating scales) and pain relief; Activities of Daily Living - focuses on whether the patient's functioning since the last assessment is better, same, or worse; Adverse Events - identifies whether the patient is experiencing side effects from current pain relievers, and if so, what they are; potentially Aberrant Drug-Related Behaviours - assesses 17 aberrant behaviours. The availability of this checklist is likely to improve the ability of clinicians to capture problematic behaviours and implement appropriate actions in response. In addition, there is a fifth section on "Assessment" which identifies a specific analgesic plan.

The *Current Opioid Misuse Measure* (COMM, Bultler at al., 2007) is a tool with 17 items, asking the patient how he or she currently uses pain medication. For each behaviour listed (e.g. "how often have you needed to take pain medications belonging to someone else?"), the patient must indicate the frequency of each behaviour on a 5 point Likert scale (0 = "never"; 4 = "very often"). The current 17-item version of COMM was created from the 40-item version produced from the concept mapping work carried out by 26 pain and addiction professionals. Validation of the tool was carried out on 227 patients with chronic pain. Scores of 9 or more (sensitivity=0.77; specificity=0.68) are considered to be indicative of high risk of drug abuse. The tool has excellent internal consistency (Cronbach's α= 0.86) and very good test-retest reliability one week after its first administration (r = 0.86).

As well as the tools mentioned above, urine drug screens and other laboratory tests can help the clinician to understand if the patient is using illegal substances or non-prescribed drugs. It is important to supplement the observation-based tools with laboratory tests. In fact, Katz et al. (2003) showed that even if a clinician has been very careful to detect aberrant drug behaviours, some signals may be missed: approximately 20% of patients considered compliant with the treatment prescribed by expert clinicians actually tested positive in urine toxicology screening. Urine screening is an economical and non-invasive monitoring strategy that enables most drugs to be identified between 1 and 3 days after they were taken (Heit & Gourley, 2004). In addition, urine screening may be very useful in preventing opioid abuse, detecting the presence of illegal substances, identifying those patients who are not taking the prescribed drugs, or those who are using non-prescribed opioids (Atluri & Sudarshan, 2003). However, the results of urine toxicology screening must be interpreted with caution, since they may not always be correct, and in some cases can produce false positives and false negatives. Moreover, some substances are not detected by standard urine screening, and so clinicians must result to more specific or costly urine tests (or to blood or hair analysis). For this reason the results of urine drug screen should be considered a further piece of the puzzle in assessing patients with problematic opioid use behaviours (Ballantyne, 2009).

2.5 The research

This section describes the preliminary results of a prospective longitudinal study to identify some procedures that allow the risk of opioid misuse to be determined in patients with chronic non-cancer pain. Specifically, the study examines the efficacy and clinical utility of the Pain Medication Questionnaire – PMQ (Adams et al. 2004) and the Diagnosis, Intractability, Risk and Efficacy – DIRE (Belgrade et al. 2006). The PMQ was selected because it is a self-administered scale that can easily be integrated into clinical-care routine, and the DIRE because it is an assessment tool used in a multidisciplinary setting that requires a medical and psychological assessment of the patient. In addition, both tools have been shown to possess characteristics that make them suitable for use in clinical practice: good psychometric properties in their original version, easy to complete, and sufficiently short to administer and score.

The specific aim of the study is to identify and examine the efficacy of a clinical protocol for the systematic assessment of patients who are candidates for starting opioid treatment. As a preliminary step, the predictive validity of the Italian versions of the PMQ and the DIRE was investigated: until now the Italian versions of these instrument are not available. Besides, the capacity of the two tools to predict opioid misuse was compared to the subjective estimate made by the physician based on his or her clinical experience. Furthermore, the presence of possible relationships between aberrant drug behaviours and the presence of risk factors for treatment compliance was examined, as was any use of illegal substances established by urine drug tests. Finally, the efficacy of the treatment was analysed the patient's perceived quality of life and pain experience after 2 and 4 months after the start of treatment.

2.5.1 Subjects

The preliminary data presented below refer to 25 patients treated in the Pain Relief and Palliative Care Unit. The inclusion criteria were: age between 18 and 70 years; presence of non-cancer pain for at least 6 months; pain intensity assessed on an 11 point Numerical Rating Scale of at least 4 in the last month; good knowledge/understanding of Italian; absence of cognitive deficit; use of fixed regime weak opioids insufficiently efficacious; other pharmacological and non-pharmacological treatments used for at least 3 months not sufficiently efficacious; no significant decrease in life expectancy; informed consent to participation in the study obtained.

	Descriptives (mean SD or % frequency)
Age	56.2 (10.6)
Sex	
- Women	17 (68.0%)
- Men	8 (32.0%)
Education (years)	
- 5	5 (20.0%)
- 8	10 (41%)
- 9-13	9 (35%)
- >13	1 (4%)
Marital status	
- Never married	2 (8%)
- Married	13 (52%)
- Divorced	3 (11%)
- Widowed	7 (27%)
Occupation	
- Employed	6 (24%)
- Housewife	7 (28%)
- Unemployed	1 (4%)
- Retired	11 (44%)
Type of pain	
- Nociceptive	10 (40%)
- Neuropathic	5 (20%)
- Mixed	10 (40%)
Duration of pain (months)	88.2 (57.7)

Table 4. Socio-demographic characteristics.

The socio-demographic and clinical characteristics of the group of subjects are represented in table 4. The mean age is 56.2 years (±10.6) and 68% are women. Most subjects were not working at the time of the study due to their pain condition. Regarding the characteristics of their pain symptoms, the most prevalent types were nociceptive (40%) or mixed (40%); the average duration of the pain condition was 88.2 months (±57.7). There were no statistically significant differences between men and women in any of the descriptive variables considered.

2.5.2 Instruments

The *Checklist for medical selection* is a tool constructed ad hoc that enabled physicians to collect information needed to check the suitability of the patient for inclusion in the study. It includes the collection of personal data (age, sex, nationality), clinical data (disorder causing the pain, characteristics of the pain, prior pharmacological and non-pharmacological treatments) and the assessment of pain intensity (in the last month) using the *11-point Numerical Rating Scale* (NRS-11). The doctor must also indicate the drug administration route (oral or transdermal) and the initial dosage.

The *11-point Numerical Rating Scale* (NRS-11) is a pain assessment scale in which the patient is asked to report the intensity of the pain, over a specific time interval, with a number from 0 to 10, where 0 indicates no pain and 10 the worst possible pain.

The risk opioid misuse was assessed using the Pain Medication Questionnaire- PMQ (Adams et al., 2004) and the Diagnosis Intractability Risk and Efficacy Score - DIRE; Belgrade et al. 2006): see § 2.4 for a detailed description of these tools. The Italian version of the tools elaborated for this study was authorised and approved by the original Authors.

The *Medical risk prediction* requires the physician to provide an estimate, based on his or her clinical experience, of the risk of opioid misuse, answering 3 questions on an 11 point numerical scale: compliance with medical treatment (0=no compliance; 10=maximum compliance), risk of abuse and/or underuse of the drug (0=no risk, 10=maximum risk) and expected efficacy of treatment (0=no efficacy, 10=maximum efficacy).

The *Medical control form* was designed to collect clinical information about the progress of the treatment, any side effects, and the intention to continue or suspend treatment. It contains also a list of aberrant drug behaviours, based on the reference literature; the physician must tick those behaviours displayed by the patient (e.g. The patient uses other opioids in addition to those prescribed, The patient displays little interest in managing himself and his rehabilitation).

Urine toxicology screening was performed with fast immunodosages that could be read visually, allowing the qualitative determination of the pharmacological substances and their metabolites present in the urine. For opiates, marijuana and buprenorfin, QuikStrip™ OneStep immunodosages were used; QuikPac II™ OneStep were used to detect the presence of amphetamines, metamphetamines and cocaine.

Regarding the psychological assessment the following tools were used.

The *Initial pain interview* is a semi−structured interview designed to reconstruct the clinical history of the pain, and its progress over time. The interview is used to gather a wide range of personal information (e.g. marital status, level of education, employment status, etc.) and other information about the pain and its interference in daily activities. The habits and behaviours that, based on the literature, are considered risk factors for aberrant opioid use were also investigated (smoking, alcohol consumption patterns, use of drugs, family history of alcohol and/or drug abuse, sexual abuse).

The *Visual Analogue Scale* (VAS) consists of a 10 cm long horizontal line, the start and end points of which are labelled "no pain" and "worst possible pain". The patient is asked to mark the precise points corresponding to his or her maximum, minimum and habitual pain in the last month.

The *Minnesota Multiphasic Personality Inventory II* (MMPI-2; Hataway e McKinley, 1989; Italian adaptation by Pancheri et al., 1996) is a self-administered questionnaire used to assess personality characteristics. It consists of 567 items to be answered "true" or "false". Scores are obtained referred to three control scales and ten clinical scales (Hypochondria, Depression, Hysteria, Psychopathic Deviate, Masculinity – Femininity, Paranoia, Psychasthenia, Schizophrenia, Hypomania and Social Introversion).

The *Beck Depression Inventory II* (BDI-II; Beck et al., 1996; Italian adaptation by Ghisi et al., 2006) is a 21-item self-administered questionnaire commonly used among chronic pain patients to determine their depressive reaction, assessing both the cognitive component (e.g. sadness, pessimism) and the somatic component (e.g. loss of appetite, sleep disorders).

The *State Trait Anxiety Inventory-Y* (STAI-Y, Spielberger,1983; Italian adaptation by Pedrabissi and Santinello, 1989) is a 40-item questionnaire that assesses the level of patient anxiety. Two scores can be obtained, referring to two subscales that assess state anxiety (i.e. the anxiety experienced by the patient at the time they complete the questionnaire) and trait anxiety (i.e. the anxiety that the patient habitually experiences).

The *Pain Related Self-Statement Scale* (PRSS; Flor and Turk, 1988; Italian adaptation by Ferrari et al., 2004) is a self-administered scale developed to assess the cognitions specifically triggered in the pain situation that might inhibit or promote coping responses. The tool consists of 18 items, from which two total scores can be obtained for the subscales called Catastrophizing and Coping.

The *Nottingham Health Profile* (NPH, Hunt et al., 1985; Italian adaptation by Bertin et al, 1992) was used to assess quality of life. It consists of 38 items covering 6 content areas: physical mobility, energy, sleep, pain, social isolation, emotional reactions. The scores are expressed on percentage scales and correspond to the level of compromise perceived by the subject in the quality of life area considered.

The *Multidimensional Pain Inventory* (MPI, Kerns et al., 1985; Italian adaptation by Ferrari et al., 2000) is a 61-item self-administered questionnaire that allow a multidimensional assessment of the pain experience. The tool is divided into 3 parts: the first focuses on assessing the intensity of the pain, its interference in the life of the patient, the patient's perceived control of the pain and of events in his or her life (it consists of the following subscales: pain severity, interference, life-control, affective distress and support). The second part investigates the patient's perception of the responses of his or her significant others to his or her pain communications (negative/solicitous and distracting responses). The third part examines the frequency with which the patient carries out common daily activities (household chores, outdoor work, distant activities, social activities and general activity).

Finally, the *McGill Pain Questionnaire* (MPQ, Melzack, 1983; Italian adaptation by Maiani and Sanavio, 1985) is a tool consisting of a list of 78 adjectives related to pain grouped into 20 subclasses of homogeneous content; within each subgroup the descriptors are arranged in order of increasing intensity. The subject is invited to choose the adjective that best describes his or her pain in each category. The tool allows the pain to be assessed as an experience with three major dimensions: sensory-discriminative, motivational-affective and cognitive-evaluative.

2.5.3 Procedure

The study is observational prospective and longitudinal; patient selection, data collection and the subsequent follow-ups took place from December 2009 to March 2011 in the Pain Relief and Palliative Care Unit of Vicenza hospital. The study consisted of the following assessment phases: patient selection, collection of pre-treatment data, 2 and 4 month follow-ups (figure 3).

The specialist physician selected patients according to the personal and clinical criteria indicated above, as well as by using the numerical scale to assess pain intensity. Patients who were candidates for opioid treatment were asked to undergo psycho-clinical assessment in accordance with the multidisciplinary care diagnostic protocol, for patients with chronic non-cancer pain referred for opioid treatment at our Centre.

Pre-treatment data were collected in the two week period following selection. It consisted of the compilation of the questionnaire to determine the risk of opioid misuse (PMQ) by the patient, and the compilation of the DIRE by the team of pain specialists. Questionnaires to assess the intensity and experience of pain (VAS, MPI, MPQ, PRSS) and affective/emotional state (STAI-Y, BDI-II), quality of life (NHP) and personality characteristics (MMPI-2) were also administered. Medical and psychological follow-ups were scheduled 2 and 4 months after the start of treatment. At 2 months, medical data such as the presence of any side effects, changes in dosage, presence of aberrant drug behaviours and any intention to stop treatment were collected for treatment monitoring. The PMQ was administered again, to assess its reliability over time, and the questionnaires assessing quality of life and pain experience (VAS, MPI and NHP) were also administered. The same medical and psychological data were collected at 4 months, apart from the PMQ. At both follow-up appointment urine drug test was proposed. The study protocol was approved by the competent Ethics Committee.

PATIENT SELECTION	PRE-TREATMENT	2 MONTH FOLLOW-UP	4 MONTH FOLLOW-UP
• Checklist for medical selection • Intensity of pain in the last month ≥4/10 (NRS)	*Medical assessment* • Medical risk prediction *Psychological assessment* • Risk of opioid misuse (PMQ) • Initial pain interview • Pain intensity (VAS) • Personality characteristics (MMPI-II) • Affective-emotional state (STAI-Y,BDI-2) • Pain experience and coping strategies (MPI,MPQ,PRSS) • Quality of life (NHP) *Team assessment* • Risk of opioid misuse (DIRE)	*Medical assessment* • Medical control form • Urine drug tests	*Medical assessment* • Medical control form • Urine drug tests *Psychological assessment* • Pain intensity (VAS) • Experience of pain (MPI) • Quality of life (NHP)

Fig. 3. Study procedures

2.5.4 Statistical analysis

Continuous variables are expressed with mean, standard deviation, minimum and maximum and centiles into which the variables fall, when possible. Discrete and nominal variables are reported in frequency tables with the related percentages. To examine the differences between continuous variables, Student's parametric t test was used, with Chi squared for the comparison of frequency distributions.

The reliability of the PMQ was assessed using test-retest, and Cronbach's α, while the internal consistency of the DIRE was determined from Cronbach's α.

Correspondence Analysis was used to examine the relationship between the PMQ and DIRE scores obtained by the patients in the pre-treatment phase and the number of aberrant drug behaviours detected in the patients at the medical follow-ups recorded in the "Medical control form", the duration of treatment and the presence of the drug in the urine. Analysis of variance and correlational analysis with Spearman's non-parametric coefficient were used to analyse the relationship between the PMQ scores and the DIRE and the clinical variables related to pain, psychological function and quality of life.

2.5.5 Results

All the patients reported continuous pain; table 5 shows the mean values for pain intensity (assessed using the VAS) and the data on pharmacological treatment in the three assessment phases. No significant gender differences were found in maximum, minimum or habitual pain intensity. However, there was a statistically significant reduction in maximum and minimum pain intensity from the pre-treatment to the 2 month follow-up ($F_{1,24}$= 4.64; $F_{1,24}$= 6.75 respectively; both for $p<0.05$); from pre-treatment to the 4 month follow-up the only difference was in maximum VAS ($F_{1,24}$= 8.21; $p<0.01$). This variation was not influenced by the active substance administration route.

Analysing the type of pharmacological treatment, it may be noted that at both the start of the pharmacological treatment and at the subsequent follow-ups, the most frequently administered active substance was oxycodone. The administration route during the data collection phases remained primarily oral. The drug dosages were transformed into equivalent mg of morphine, and classified as mild/average/high based on the indications supplied by Bruera et al. (1995). Regarding the dosage, it showed a tendency to increase at the 4 month follow-up.

Approximately half (46%) of the patients reported the presence of at least one side effect at the follow-ups; the most frequently reported side effects were sleepiness (29%), constipation (29%) and nausea (21%). The drug administration route did not appear to have any effect on the number and type of side effects reported by the patients.

With respect to the psychological indicators investigated in the pre-treatment assessment, it was found that, based on the personality profile obtained with the MMPI-2, 56.2% of women and 33.3% of men had clinically significant scores in at least one of the clinical scales with psychopathological content (Paranoia, Schizofrenia, Hypomania). As for the affective-emotional variables, the mean total score at BDI-II in the initial treatment phase was 24.6 (SD= 13.40) in women and 18.2 (SD= 9.94) in men; the level of depression was clinically significant (scores higher than 95th percentile) in 61% of women and 50% of men. Considering trait anxiety, the mean score was 52.7 (SD= 11.97) in women and 46.2 (SD= 7.22) in men, with 27.7% clinically significant levels of anxiety only in women (scores higher than 95th percentile). Regarding PRSS, the subjects reported a mean score of 3.20 (range 0-5, SD= 1.15) on the Catastrophizing scale and 2.76 on the Coping scale (range 0-5, SD= 0.88).

	Initial treatment	2 month follow-up	4 month follow-up
	Mean (SD)	Mean (SD)	Mean (SD)
Pain intensity	Mean (SD)	Mean (SD)	Mean (SD)
- maximum VAS	90.2 (12.9)	80.6 (16.4)	78.7 (28.3)
- minimum VAS	33.1 (22.4)	24.0 (18.7)	31.8 (19.6)
- habitual VAS	55.5 (20.6)	52.6 (13.8)	56.1 (24.5)
	Frequency (%)	Frequency (%)	Frequency (%)
Drug active substance			
- Oxycodone	12 (48%)	12 (48%)	15 (60%)
- Fentanyl	10 (40%)	6 (24%)	5 (20%)
- Hydromorphone	3 (12%)	4 (16%)	5 (20%)
- Buprenorphine	-	3 (12%)	-
Route of administration			
- Oral	15 (60%)	16 (64%)	20 (80%)
- Transdermal	10 (40%)	9 (36%)	5 (20%)
Dosage (mg morphine)	Frequency (%)	Frequency (%)	Frequency (%)
- Mild (<60 mg)	24 (96%)	11 (44%)	6 (24%)
- Average (60-300mg)	1 (4%)	14 (56%)	11 (44%)
- High (>300 mg)	-	-	8 (32%)

Table 5. Pain intensity, active medication taken, administration route and dosage in initial treatment and in subsequent follow-ups.

In the description of the pain characteristics at the MPQ, higher scores emerged in the evaluative and affective -evaluative dimensions (means 0.87 and 0.73, respectively) , while the lower scores referred to the affective and mixed-sensory dimensions (means 0.4 and 0.52, respectively).

In the MPI the subjects reported high mean on "Pain severity" (mean: 4.6; SD= 0.9), "Interference" (mean: 4.3; SD= 1.1) and "Affective distress" (mean: 3.6; SD= 1.1) in the pre-treatment assessment. Quality of life, measured using the NHP, appears more compromised in the following areas: "Emotional reactions" (mean: 80; SD= 56), "Pain" (mean: 77; SD= 26.2) and "Energy" (mean: 64; SD= 40). There were no statistically significant variations in the mean scores at the start of treatment and at the subsequent follow-ups for either the MPI or the NHP.

As for the tools to assess the risk of opioid misuse, the mean score at the PMQ was 24.59 (SD=9.43); there were no significant gender differences in the PMQ scores. Figure 4 shows the three different levels of the PMQ scores that, according to the cut-offs established by Dowling et al. (2007), identify a low/moderate or high risk of drug misuse. Overall, 36% of the subjects were found to be at high risk of misuse, 20% at moderate risk, and the remaining 44% at low risk. The distribution in the three risk levels between men and women was comparable.

The group was subsequently divided into patients with high PMQ scores (H-PMQ; n=9) and patients with low PMQ scores (L-PMQ; n=11) in order to analyse the presence of any significant differences in the psychological variables considered in the study. The patients with H-PMQ had a mean score of 3.78 on the Catastrophizing scale of the PRSS, statistically higher than that of the L-PMQ patients (mean 2.61) (t=-3.16; p<0.01); while on the Coping scale the H-PMQ subjects had mean scores that were significantly lower than those of the L-PMQ group (t=-2.18; p<0.05). Further statistical differences were found for the "HS" scale

(Hypocondria) of the MMPI-2, in which the H-PMQ subjects had scores that were significantly higher than the L-PMQ subjects (means 21 and 16.5 respectively, t=23.60; p<0.05) and for the total depression score in the BDI-II (H-PMQ mean =27.36; L-PMQ mean =17.88; t=26.18, p<0.05).

As for the predictive validity of the tool, a highly significant correlation was found between the total PMQ score (high risk of opioid misuse) and the number of aberrant drug-related behaviours noted by the physician at the 4 month follow-up (r=0.95; p<0.01). Significant correlations were also found between the PMQ score and the "HS" (Hypochondria) scale of the MMPI-2 (r=0.49; p<0.01), the total score in the BDI-II (r=0.43; p<0.05), the trait anxiety score of the STAI-Y (r=0.38; p<0.05) and the "emotional reaction" scale of the NHP (r=0.39; p<0.05).

The mean time required by the patient to complete the tool was 12'02" (SD=6.35; range: 4-30). Finally, analysis of internal consistency produced an alpha coefficient of 0.82, indicating that the tool has excellent internal coherence; the test-retest reliability at 2 months was very high (r= 0.76; p<0.001).

In the DIRE, the mean score assigned by the multidisciplinary team was 15.35; in this case too there were no significant differences in the mean scores of men and women. Figure 5 shows the percentage of patients suitable or not suitable for treatment based on DIRE total Score according to the cut-offs established by Belgrade et al. (2006). Most women (81.2%) and men (87.5%) were found suitable to start chronic opioid treatment according to the DIRE score.

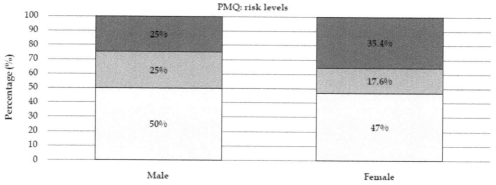

Fig. 4. Percentage of patients with low/moderate/high risk level for opioid misuse, based on PMQ scores.

The total DIRE score was not found to be significantly correlated with the number of aberrant drug behaviours recorded by the physician at 2 and 4 months; however, a significant negative correlation (r=0.83; p<0.05) was found between the scores in the "Risk" category of the DIRE (psychological risk, chemical health, reliability, social support) and the number of aberrant drug behaviours recorded by the physician at the 4 month follow-up.

The total DIRE score correlates negatively with the total BDI-II score (r=0.46, p<0.01) and with many of the MMPI-2 scales, and specifically: "PD" (Psychopathic Deviate) (r= 0.44; p<0.05), "PA" (Paranoia) (r= 0.40; p<0.05), "D" (Depression) (r= 039; p<005); "FAM" (Family Problems) (r= 044; p<005), "WRK" (Work Interference) (r= 040; p<005) and "TRT"(Negative Treatment Indicators) (r= 0.39; p<0.05).

The mean time required by the multidisciplinary team to complete the tool was 7'23" (SD=3.38; range: 1-16). The internal consistency of the Italian version of the tool was 0.48, which is very low; the item that contributed least to the internal consistency of the DIRE was Diagnosis (α if item deleted=0.51).

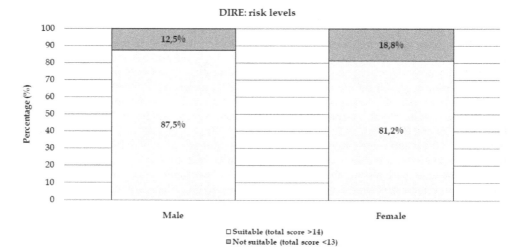

Fig. 5. Percentage of patients suitable or not suitable for treatment based on DIRE total Score.

As for the concurrent validity of the two tools, there were no significant correlations between the total scores of the PMQ and the DIRE. However, there was a moderate negative correlation ($r=0.36$; $p< 0.05$) between high total PMQ scores (high risk of opioid misuse) and low scores in the Risk category of the DIRE.

Both the PMQ and the DIRE proved to be more effective than the Medical risk prediction in estimating the risk of drug misuse: the subjective estimate of the physician based on his or her clinical experience does not in fact correlate with the aberrant drug behaviours displayed by the patient at 2 and 4 months.

In the urine toxicology screening, only one patient tested negative for the active principle at the two month follow-up, while all the patients were positive for the drug used at the four month follow-up. None of the patients tested positive for illegal substances.

In relation to aberrant drug behaviours, most of the subjects (71%) displayed no aberrant drug behaviour at the two month follow-up; there was a potential misuse indicator in 19%, and the remaining 10% displayed three or more. At the 4 month follow-up, 22% of the patients displayed three or more aberrant drug behaviours while no indicators of misuse were found in 56% of the subjects.

Regarding other factors that according to the literature might be predictive for improper use of opioids, none of the patients reported that they abused alcohol or narcotic substances at assessment; 4.9% reported a personal history of alcohol abuse and 5.4% stated that they had abused illegal substances in the past. 7.3% of the subjects had a family history of alcohol abuse and 2.4% had a family history of the use of narcotic substances. None of the patients reported that they had suffered sexual abuse in childhood or adolescence, 17.1% of the patients had a prior psychiatric diagnosis and 9.8% of the subjects were being treated by a psychiatrist at the time of the evaluation.

2.5.6 Discussion

The main purpose of this study was to identify clinical procedures that allow to estimate the risk of opioid misuse in patients with chronic non-cancer pain treated as outpatients in a pain relief centre. With this aim, two tools were selected and adapted in Italian – the Pain Medication Questionnaire (PMQ) and the Diagnosis, Intractability, Risk and Efficacy Score (DIRE). These tools examine the perspectives of the patient and the multispecialist team, respectively.

The preliminary results reported above show that the PMQ has a good capacity to predict the risk of drug misuse by the patient. A strong correlation was found between high PMQ scores and the number of aberrant drug behaviours reported by the physician 4 months after the start of the study.

From the PMQ scores, 36% of the subjects were found to be at high risk of misuse, 20% at moderate risk, and the remaining 44% at low risk. High PMQ scores (high risk of misuse) were found to be associated with higher levels of anxiety, depression and persistent body-related worries. Furthermore, those patients classified as high risk of misuse, based on the cut-offs suggested by Dowling et al. (2007), were found to be significantly more depressed, and with a greater tendency to somatise their emotional distress than those classified as low risk. High risk patients were also found to be less active in managing their pain condition, and to have a greater propensity to produce pessimistic and catastrophic thoughts about their pain symptoms. The association that emerged, between high PMQ scores and the presence of symptoms of depression, appears to be in line with the findings of Holmes et al. (2006) in their work assessing the long-term utility of the PMQ in 271 subjects. In this study the low risk patients had mean BDI scores that were significantly lower than those of the high risk of misuse group.

Furthermore, based on the initial results, the PMQ has demonstrated adequate internal consistency and good reliability over time. This suggests that the items composing it measure a single construct, and that the tool provides a reliable estimate of the risk of medication misuse. In addition, completing the PMQ requires just over ten minutes of the patient's time, and this makes it easy to incorporate into clinical practice.

To summarise, the tool seems to possess a good predictive capacity in relation to the use that the patient will make of the drug, and his or her compliance with treatment. The total score on the questionnaire, and the stratification of risk based on the cut-offs suggested by the authors therefore appear to be reliable indicators that the clinician can use to plan regular treatment monitoring. The strong association between high PMQ scores and the presence of symptoms of depression, tendency to somatisation and catastrophization, suggest that pharmacological treatment with opioids needs to be combined with psychological treatment to reduce the affective and emotional distress and modify the patient's dysfunctional convictions and behaviours in relation to use of the drug.

As for the Italian version DIRE, the preliminary results show that the total score for risk of drug misuse is a poor predictor with limited psychometric quality. The Risk category, which specifically assesses psychosocial aspects such as psychological adaptation, substance abuse, reliability in complying with previous treatments and perceived social support in life context, is an exception to this. The tool in fact has low internal consistency, which improves slightly when the Diagnosis factor is removed. This means that the items of which the tool is composed are very heterogeneous, and that the tool probably has a multifactorial structure. Our finding does not agree with the results reported by Belgrade et al. (2006) in the original validation study, in which the DIRE displayed a very high internal consistency. The total score of the DIRE - Italian version - is not at present predictive of the number of aberrant drug behaviours detected by the physician at the follow-ups. This seems to be in line with the work of Moore et al. (2007), who found that the DIRE had low sensitivity (0.17) in predicting aberrant drug behaviours. The authors suggest that the DIRE is more than simply an addiction risk tool and some of its items may not to be appropriate to predict drug misuse. However, as mentioned above, the score of the Risk category was found to be predictive of the number of aberrant drug behaviours at 4- months follow-up. This result is coherent with the findings of many studies on opioid abuse risk factors, which found that the factors considered to be most predictive of opioid abuse are the presence of psychiatric disorders (Compton et al., 1998; Sullivan et al., 2006) and a personal and/or family history of substance abuse or drug abuse (Dunbar & Katz, 1996; Schieffer et al., 2005). Our data indicate that a low score (not suitable for opioid treatment) is associated with depressive symptoms, the presence of paranoid personality traits and family and work difficulties. Completing the DIRE requires a few minutes of the team's time, but this must be preceded by an in-depth psychological assessment of the patient to determine if psychiatric disorders and past abuse, or current alcohol or substance abuse, are present.

The two tools selected do not appear to be correlated; instead, it is clear that there is an association between high PMQ scores (high risk of misuse) and low scores in the DIRE Risk category.

The prediction made by the physician based on his or her clinical experience was not found to be valid in estimating the risk of opioid misuse. This result highlights the need to use tools specifically created to assess the risk of opioid addiction in the chronic pain patient; clinical experience can be used to understand and contextualize the results obtained from these scales, but seems to be insufficient on its own.

So far as the experience of pain and the indicators of psychophysical function are concerned, the use of opioid drugs proved efficacious in reducing the maximum and minimum intensity of the perceived pain 2 months after the start of the treatment. A parallel improvement in the quality of life of the patients was not recorded by the questionnaire used in this study. This result seems to be in line with the data in the literature: despite ongoing research and the growing use of opioids in clinical practice, the effect of this treatment on the quality of life of the patient remains a subject of debate (Dillie et al., 2008). The reduction in pain, unaccompanied by an improvement in physical function and quality of life, indicates that these patients need psychological support, to examine their life habits, coping strategies and any secondary gain that might interfere with recovery of a state of psychophysical well-being. Quality of life is in fact a wide ranging concept, influenced by perception of one's health in a biopsychosocial sense, level of independence, social relationships and interaction with one's own specific environmental context in a complex way (Apolone et al., 1997).

As for the psychological variables considered in the study, half of the men and 60% of the women reported clinically significant levels of depression; and almost 30% of the women displayed high levels of anxiety. These data are in line with the findings of many authors, that clinically significant levels of depression and anxiety are very frequent in patients with chronic pain (Banks & Kerns, 1996; Boersma & Linton, 2006; Dersh et al., 2006; Gatchel, 2005; Vlayen & Linton, 2000). In addition, there was a high incidence of alterations in patients' personality profiles: over half of the women and approximately one third of the men reported high scores in at least one of the clinical content scales of the MMPI-2. This result too seems coherent with the reports in the literature, that the presence of psychiatric and personality disorders is more frequent in these patients (Banta-Green et al., 2009a; Haller & Acosta; 2010), and therefore it is advisable to involve a psychotherapist or psychiatrist in the treatment process (Chou, 2009; Chou et al, 2009a; Chou et al, 2009b; Chou et al, 2009c; Trescot et al., 2006; Trescot at al., 2008).

The analyses carried out to date have shown that only one patient in twenty five did not test positive to the prescribed drug; and no patients tested positive for illegal substances in the urine toxicology screening. These data seem very different to those of other studies, which found the prevalence of abuse of illegal substances in patients being treated with opioid to be 16% (Machikanti et al., 2006), 20% (Heit & Gourlay, 2004) or 40.3% (Ives et al., 2006). The preliminary results seem to suggest that in our context the more frequent problem may be the underuse of opioid analgesics rather than their compulsive use and abuse: this interpretation is supported by the difficulty, frequently expressed by our patient, in accepting these drugs for fear of dependence, loss of mental lucidity or being socially stigmatised as drug addicted. A further important objective of the management of patients who are candidates for opioid treatment in a multidisciplinary setting is thus to assess their convictions about the use of these drugs and their expectations of treatment, so as to be able to modify any dysfunctional beliefs and unrealistic hopes for the outcome of treatment.

The limitations of this study are primarily the small number of subjects examined and the differing distribution of men and women. In addition, the limited number of patients did not allow us to examine the effect of other variables that, based on the reference literature, can constitute risk factors for opioid addiction, such as a personal or family history of alcohol and/or substance abuse, or episodes of sexual abuse in childhood or adolescence.

Despite these limits, the high degree of correlation between risk of misuse and the psychological aspects supports the view that an in-depth assessment of the affective-emotional, cognitive and behavioural variables of the patient is crucial. So future research may be focused on understanding which psychological variables are most connected to the risk of opioid misuse (e.g. personality traits, anxiety, depression, etc.) so as to be able to develop tailored psychological interventions that maximise treatment efficacy, with positive outcomes for quality of life and overall well-being, as well.

Overall the results that have emerged so far highlight the need for a multidisciplinary assessment of patients who are candidates for opioid treatment so as to improve compliance and treatment benefits. The use of tools specifically designed to determine the risk of inappropriate use of the drug has proved to be more efficacious that the opinion expressed by the clinician based on his or her experience. The strong association between psychosocial distress and high risk of opioid misuse also suggests that pharmacological treatment should be combined with psychological interventions that can reduce the anxiety-depression symptoms and correct any irrational ideas about the use of these drugs. Furthermore, systemic monitoring of treatment and regular urine drug screen can contribute to improve adherence to treatment.

3. Conclusions

Chronic non-cancer pain remains a condition that affects a large number of people throughout the world, and is associated with significantly compromised quality of life. Although many pharmacological and non-pharmacological treatments have been proposed to manage chronic pain, the results have proved disappointing for a significant proportion of patients.

Opioid drugs seem promising for the management of chronic pain of medium-severe intensity, but many uncertainties remain about the long-term use of these drugs and the risk of dependence and abuse. In this respect, many guidelines and protocols with recommendations have been developed in recent years precisely to allow safer and more targeted use of opioid drugs in chronic non-cancer pain syndromes; these recommendations highlight, primarily, the importance of carrying out stratification of risk in the patient who is a candidate for pharmacological treatment with opioids. A number of standardised tools have been developed with the aim of identifying and objectively measuring the risk of abuse, dependence and aberrant drug behaviours.

This chapter has presented the preliminary results of a study that aims to analyse the clinical utility of the Italian adaptation of two tools for stratification of the risk: a self-administered patient questionnaire, the Pain Medication Questionnaire, and a team assessment tool, the Diagnosis Intractability Risk and Efficacy Score.

These tools have been used as part of a multidisciplinary medical and psychological assessment and treatment protocol; the data in the literature, confirmed in our study, clearly indicates that there is a frequent association between high risk of opioid misuse and the presence of psychological distress (Banta-Green et al., 2009a; Haller & Acosta; 2010). This emphasizes the importance of a physical, psychological and social assessment before starting treatment with opioids. In this respect, based on literature data and the preliminary results of the study described, we believe that an effective psychological assessment must consist of an initial clinical interview, specific tools to assess the risk of drug misuse, and questionnaires that investigate the patient's subjective experience of pain, perceived quality of life and personality characteristics. The interview, which may be more or less structured, is essential to understand the individual's experience of pain and its interference in the patient's family, professional, social and emotional life; it also allows the clinician to investigate behaviour habits related to opioid misuse (e.g. prior abuse of alcohol or illegal substances) and the presence of traumatic experiences such as sexual abuse in childhood or adolescence. During the interview the clinician may also identify any fears and worries about taking these drugs, the patient's expectations of the treatment and their reliability in following the indications of the therapist. Further areas of investigation concern the strategies that the patient uses to deal with the pain, and the possible presence of secondary gain that could compromise the efficacy of the treatment. Our results show that the indications provided by the specifically designed tools are more reliable than the clinical experience of the specialist physician in estimated aberrant drug behaviours. Investigation of the emotional-affective state of the patient, and his or her personality characteristics, always an important aspect of the multidimensional assessment of chronic pain, appears indispensable when long-term opioid therapy is initiated, since the presence of depression, anxiety or personality disorders has been found to be correlated with a greater risk of addiction. Pain coping strategies and any tendency to "catastrophize" must also be investigated using suitable questionnaires. Based on our experience, patients at greater risk of opioid misuse in fact seem to display a passive attitude to the management of their pain condition, and to have exaggeratedly pessimistic expectations of the progress of their symptoms. Finally, it is important to systematically assess the quality of life of these patients, as effective pain relief should always be accompanied by functional improvements in their physical, psychological and social area. The preliminary results of our study show that reduction in pain intensity of pain due to opioids does not seem to be accompanied by an improvement in physical and psychological functionality. This indicates that the patient needs to be monitored not only in medical term, but also from a psychological perspective, to be able to make cognitive, emotional and behavioural changes that can enhance and consolidate the efficacy of the treatment.

From our experience in the Italian context, the prevalence of addiction or misuse in patients with chronic pain in treatment with opioids appears to be low. The systematic assessment of risk using the tools created in recent years allows the clinician to overcome some biases, such as the overestimation of the risk of addiction, and hence avoid considering the entire population of chronic pain patients to be at risk of abuse.

The treatment of pain is a public health problem that is of such critical importance as to constitute an international imperative, as well as a fundamental human right (Brennan et al., 2007); opioid drugs appear as a potential resource to manage chronic pain efficaciously. However, their targeted use must be preceded by a suitable assessment of the patient by a multidisciplinary team that clarifies not only the causes of the pain, but also any risk factors or dysfunctional psychological aspects related to use of the drug, so as to increase the benefits of treatment and reduce the costs.

4. Acknowledgments

We would like to thank all the medical and nursing staff of the Pain and Palliative Care Unit from Vicenza Hospital for the precious contribution to the realization of this study.

5. References

Adams, L., Gatchel, R., Robinson, R., Polatin, P., Gajraj, N., Deschner, M. & Noe, C. (2004). Development of a self-report screening instrument for assessing potential opioid medication misuse in chronic pain patients. *Journal of Pain and Symptom Management*, Vol. 27, No. 5, (May), pp. 440-456.

Akbik, H., Butler, S., Budman, S., Fernandez, K. & Jamison R. (2006).Validation and clinical application of the Screener and Opioid Assessment for Patients with Pain (SOAPP). *Journal of Pain and Symptom Management*, Vol. 32, No. 3, (September), pp. 287-293.

American Society of Addiction Medicine (2001). *Definitions Related to the Use of Opioids for the Treatment of Pain: Consensus Statement of the American Academy of Pain Medicine, the American Pain Society, and the American Society of Addiction Medicine.* Last accessed June 2011, available from:
http://www.pcssmethadone.org/pcss/documents2/ASAM_DefinitionsRelated ToUseOpioidsPain.pdf.

Apolone, G., Ballatori, E., Mosconi, P. & Roila, F. (Ed. Pensiero Scientifico) (1997). *Misurare la qualità di vita in oncologia: aspetti di metodo ed applicativi.* Il Pensiero Scientifico Editore, Roma, Italy. ISBN: 8870027880.

Atluri, S. & Sudarshan, G. (2003). Evaluation of abnormal urine drug screens among patients with chronic non-malignant pain treated with opioids. *Pain Physician.* Vol. 6, No. 4, (October), pp. 407-409.

Back, S.E., Payne, R.A., Waldrop, A.E., Smith, A., Reeves, S. & Brady, K.T. (2009). Prescription opioid aberrant behaviors: a pilot study of sex differences. *Clinical Journal of Pain.* Vol. 25, No. 6, (July-August), pp: 477-484.

Bair, M.J., Robinson, R.L., Katon, W. & Kroenke, K. (2003). Depression and pain comorbidity: a literature review. *Archives of Internal Medicine.* Vol. 163, No. 20, (November), pp. 2433-2445.

Ballantyne, J. (2007). Opioid analgesia : perspectives on right use and utility. *Pain Physician*, Vol. 10, No. 3, (May), pp. 479-491.

Ballantyne, J.C. & Shin, N.S. (2008). Efficacy of opioids for chronic pain: a review of the evidence. *Clinical Journal of Pain, Vol.* 24, No. 6, (July-August), pp. 469-478.

Ballantyne, J.C. (2009). U.S. opioid risk management initiatives International Association for the Study of Pain (IASP), Vol. XVII, No. 6, (November). Last accessed June 2011, available from:
http://www.iasp-pain.org/AM/AMTemplate.cfm?Section=HOME,HOME,HOME,HOME&SECTION=HOME,HOME,HOME,HOME&TEMPLATE=/CM/ContentDisplay.cfm&CONTENTID=10419

Banks, S.M. & Kerns, R.D. (1996). Explaining high rates of depression in chronic pain: a diathesis-stress framework. *Psychological Bulletin.* Vol 119, No. 1, (January), pp. 95-110.

Banta-Green, C.J., Merrill, J.O., Doyle, S.R., Boudreau, D.M. & Calsyn, D.A. (2009a). Opioid use behaviors, mental health and pain development of a typology of chronic pain patients. *Drug and Alcohol Dependence.* Vol. 104, No. 1-2, (September), pp. 34-42.

Banta-Green, C.J., Merrill, J.O., Doyle, S.R., Boudreau, D.M. & Calsyn, D.A. (2009b). Measurement of opioid problems among chronic pain patients in a general medical population. *Drug and Alcohol Dependence.* Vol. 104, No. 1-2, (September), pp. 43-49.

Beck, A. T., Steer, R. A., & Brown, G. K. (1996). *Manual for the Beck Depression Inventory,* 2nd ed. San Antonio, TX: The Psychological Corporation.

Belgrade, M. J., Schamber, D. & Lindgren, B. R. (2006). The DIRE Score: predicting outcomes of opioid prescribing for chronic pain. *The Journal of Pain*, Vol. 7, No. 9, (September), pp. 671-681.

Bertin, G., Niero, M. & Porchia, S. (1992). L'adattamento del Nottingham health profile al contesto italiano. In *The european group for quality of life and health measurement*, European guide to the Nottingham Health Profile, Escubase, Montpellier.

Bhamb, B., Brown, D. Anderson, J., Balousek, S. & Fleming, M.F. (2006). Survey of select practice behaviors by primary care physicians on the use of opioids for chronic pain. *Current Medical Research & Opinion*, Vol. 22, No. 9, (September), pp. 1859-65.

Boersma, K. & Linton, S.J. (2006). Psychological processes underlying the development of a chronic pain problem: a prospective study of the relationship between profiles of psychological variables in the fear-avoidance model and disability. *The Clinical Journal of Pain.* Vol. 22, No. 2, (February), pp. 160-166.

Bonica, J.J. (1991) History of pain concepts and pain therapy. *The Mount Sinai Journal of Medicine*, Vol. 53, No. 3, (May), pp. 191-202.

Bonica, J.J. (Ed. Delphino). (1992). *Il Dolore: Diagnosi, prognosi e terapia.* Antonio Deplhino, ISBN 978-887-2870-48-8, Roma, Italia.

Breivik, H., Collett, B., Ventafridda, V., Cohen, R. & Gallacher, D. (2006). Survey of chronic pain in Europe: prevalence, impact on daily life, and treatment. *European Journal of Pain.* Vol. 10, No. 4, (May), pp. 287-333.

Brennan, F., Carr, D.B. & Cousins, M. (2007). Pain management: a fundamental human right. *Anesthesia & Analgesia.* Vol. 105, No. 1, (July), pp. 205-221.

Brown, R.L. & Rounds, L.A. (1995). Conjoint screening questionnaires for alcohol and other drug abuse: criterion validity in a primary care practice. *Wisconsin Medical Journal.* Vol. 94, No. 3, pp.135-140.

Bruera, E., Schoeller,T., Wenk, R., MacEachern, T., Marcelino, S., Hanson, J. & Suarez-Almazor, M. (1995). A prospective multicenter assessment of the Edmonton staging system for cancer pain. *Journal of Pain and Symptom Management.* Vol. 10, No. 5, (July), pp. 348-355.

Buelow, A.K., Haggard, R. & Gatchel, R.J. (2009). Additional validation of the pain medication questionnaire in a heterogeneous sample of chronic pain patients. *Pain Practice.* Vol. 9, No. 6, (November-December), pp. 428-434.

Butler, S.F., Budman, S.H., Fernandez, K. & Jamison, R.N. (2004). Validation of a screener and opioid assessment measure for patients with chronic pain. *Pain.* Vol. 112, No. 1-2, (November), pp. 65-75.

Butler, S.F., Budman, S.H., Fernandez, K.C., Houle, B., Benoit, C., Katz, N. & Jamison, R.N. (2007). Development and validation of the Current Opioid Misuse Measure. *Pain.* Vol. 130, No. 1-2, (July), pp. 144-156.

Butler, S.F., Fernandez, K., Benoit, C., Budman, S.H. & Jamison, R.N. (2008). Validation of the revised Screener and Opioid Assessment for Patients with Pain (SOAPP-R). *The Journal of Pain.* Vol. 9, No. 4, (April), pp. 360-372.

Caudill-Slosberg, M.A., Schwartz, L.M. & Woloshin, S. (2004). Office visits and analgesic prescriptions for musculoskeletal pain in US: 1980 vs 2000. *Pain,* Vol. 109, No. 3, (June), pp. 514-19.

Centers for Disease Control and Prevention (2007). National and state medical expenditures and lost earnings attributable to arthritis and other rheumatic conditions - United States, 2003. *Morbidity and Mortality Weekly Report.* Vol. 56, No. 1, (January), pp. 4-7.

Chabal, C., Erjavec, M.K., Jacobson, L., Mariano, A. & Chaney, E. (1997). Prescription opiate abuse in chronic pain patients: clinical criteria, incidence, and predictors. *The Clinical Journal of Pain.* Vol. 13, No. 2, (June), pp. 150-155.

Chou, R. (2009). 2009 clinical guidelines from the American Pain Society and the American Academy of Pain Medicine on the use of chronic opioid therapy in chronic noncancer pain. What are the key messages for clinical practice?. *Polskie Archiwem Medycyny Wewnętrznej,* Vol. 119, No. 7-8, (July-August), pp. 469-477.

Chou, R., Ballantyne, J.C., Fanciullo, G.J., Fine, P.G. & Miaskowski, C. (2009c). Research gaps on use of opioids for chronic noncancer pain: findings from a review of the evidence for an American Pain Society and American Academy of Pain Medicine clinical practice guideline. *The Journal of Pain,* Vol. 10, No. 2, (February), pp. 147-159.

Chou, R., Fanciullo, G.J., Fine, P.G., Adler, J.A., Ballantyne, J.C., Davies, P., Donovan, M.I., Fishbain, D.A., Foley, K.M., Fudin, J., Gilson, A.M., Kelter, A., Mauskop, A., O'Connor, P.G., Passik, S.D., Pasternak, G.W., Portenoy, R.K., Rich, B.A., Roberts, R.G., Todd, K.H. & Miaskowski C. (2009a). American Pain Society-American Academy of Pain Medicine Opioids Guidelines Panel. Clinical guidelines for the use of chronic opioid therapy in chronic noncancer pain. *The Journal of Pain,* Vol. 10, No. 2, (February), pp.113-130.

Chou, R., Fanciullo, G.J., Fine, P.G., Miaskowski, C., Passik, S.D. & Portenoy, R.K. (2009b). Opioids for chronic noncancer pain: prediction and identification of aberrant drug-related behaviors: a review of the evidence for an American Pain Society and American Academy of Pain Medicine clinical practice guideline. *The Journal of Pain,* Vol. 10, No. 2, (February), pp. 131-146.

Collett, B.J. (1998). Opioid tolerance: the clinical perspective. *British Journal of Anaesthesia.* Vol. 81, No. 1, (July), pp. 58-68.

Compton, P., Darakjian, J. & Miotto, K. (1998). Screening for addiction in patients with chronic pain and problematic substance use: evaluation of a pilot assessment tool. *Journal of Pain and Symptom Management,* Vol. 16, No. 6, (December), pp. 355-363.

Compton, P.A., Wu, S.M., Schieffer, B., Pham, Q. & Naliboff, B.D. (2008). Introduction of a self-report version of the Prescription Drug Use Questionnaire and relationship to medication agreement noncompliance. *Journal of Pain and Symptom Management.* Vol. 36, No. 4, (October), pp. 383-395.

Dersh, J., Gatchel, R.J., Mayer, T., Polatin, P. & Temple, O.R. (2006). Prevalence of psychiatric disorders in patients with chronic disabling occupational spinal disorders. *Spine.* Vol. 1, No. 31, (May), pp. 1156-1162.

Dersh, J., Gatchel, R.J., Polatin, P. & Mayer, T. (2002). Prevalence of psychiatric disorders in patients with chronic work-related musculoskeletal pain disability. *Journal of Occupational and Environmental Medicine.* Vol. 44, No. 5, (May), pp. 459-468.

Dews, T.E., Mekhail, N. (2004). Safe use of opioids in chronic noncancer pain. *Cleveland Clinic Journal of Medicine.* Vol. 71, No. 11, (November), pp. 897-904.

Dillie, K.S., Fleming, M.F., Mundt, M.P. & French, M.T. (2008). Quality of life associated with daily opioid therapy in a primary care chronic pain sample. *Journal of the American Board of Family Medicine.* Vol. 21, No. 2, (March-April), pp.108-17.

Dowling, L.S., Gatchel, R.J., Adams, L.L., Stowell, A.W. & Bernstein D. (2007). An evaluation of the predictive validity of the Pain Medication Questionnaire with an heterogeneous group of patients with chronic pain. *Journal of Opioid Management,* Vol 3, No. 5, (September-October), pp. 257-266.

Dunbar, S.A. & Katz, N.P. (1996). Chronic opioid therapy for nonmalignant pain in patients with a history of substance abuse: report of 20 cases. *Journal of Pain and Symptom Management.* Vol. 11, No. 3, (March), pp. 163-171.

Edlund, M.J., Steffick, D., Hudson, T., Harris, K.M. & Sullivan, M. (2007). Risk factors for clinically recognized opioid abuse and dependence among veterans using opioids for chronic non-cancer pain. *Pain.* Vol. 129, No. 3, (June), pp. 355-362.

Elliott, A.M., Smith, B.H., Hannaford, P.C., Smith, W.C. & Chambers, W.A. (2002). The course of chronic pain in the community: results of a 4-year follow-up study. *Pain.* Vol. 99, No. 1-2, (September), pp. 299-307.

Ferrari, R., Fipaldini, E. & Birbaumer, N. (2004). La valutazione del controllo percepito sul dolore: la versione italiana del Pain Related self-Statement Scale e del Pain Related Control Scale. *Giornale Italiano di Psicologia.* Vol. 1, No. 1, (March), pp. 187-208. ISSN : 0390-5349.

Ferrari, R., Novara, C., Sanavio, E. & Zerbini, F. (2000). Internal structure and validity of the Multidimensional Pain Inventory, italian language version. *Pain Medicine.* Vol. 1, No. 2, (June), pp. 123-30.

Fishbain, D.A. (1999). Approaches to treatment decisions for psychiatric comorbidity in the management of the chronic pain patient. *The Medical Clinics of North America.* Vol. 83, No. 3, (May), pp. 737-760.

Fleming, M.F., Balousek, S.L., Klessig, C.L., Mundt, M.P. & Brown, D.D. (2007). Substance use disorders in a primary care sample receiving daily opioid therapy. *Journal of Pain,* Vol. 8, No. 7, (July), pp. 573-582.

Flor, H., Turk, D.C. (1988). Chronic back pain and rheumatoid arthritis: predicting pain and disability from cognitive variables. *Journal of Behavioral Medicine.* Vol. 11, No. 3, (June), pp. 251-265.

Friedman, R., Li, V. & Mehrotra, D. (2003). Treating pain patients at risk: evaluation of a screening tool in opioid-treated pain patients with and without addiction. *Pain Medicine.* Vol. 4, No. 2, (June), pp. 182-185.

Garcia, J. & Altman, R.D. (1997). Chronic pain states: pathophysiology and medical therapy. *Seminars in Arthritis and Rheumatism,* Vol. 27, No. 1, (August), pp. 1–16.

Gatchel, R.J. (Ed. American Psychological Association) (2005). *Clinical essentials of pain management.* APA Press. Washington DC. ISBN: 1591471532

Ghisi, M., Flebus, G.B., Montano, A., Sanavio, E. & Sica, C. (Ed. Giunti Organizzazioni Speciali) (2006). *Beck Depression Inventory – second edition. Adattamento italiano: manuale.* Giunti O.S., pp. 1-79, Firenze, Italy.

Gureje, O., Von Korff, M., Simon, G.E. & Gater, R. (1998). Persistent pain and well-being: A World Health Organization study in primary care. *The Journal of the American Medical Association.* Vol. 280, No. 2, (July), pp. 147-151.

Haller, D.L. & Acosta, M.C. (2010). Characteristics of pain patients with opioid-use disorder. *Psychosomatics.* Vol. 51, No. 3, (May), pp. 257-66.

Hathaway, S.R. & McKinley, J.C. (1989). *MMPI-2: Manual for administration and scoring,* University of Minnesota Press, Minneapolis, MN

Heit, H.A. & Gourlay, D.L. (2004). Urine drug testing in pain medicine. *Journal of Pain and Symptom Management.* Vol., 27, No. 3, (March), pp. 260-267.

Højsted, J. & Sjøgren, P. (2007). Addiction to opioids in chronic pain patients: A literature review. *European Journal of Pain,* Vol. 11, No. 5, (July), pp. 490- 518.

Holmes, C.P., Gatchel, R.J., Adams, L.L., Stowell, A.W., Hatten, A., Noe, C. & Lou, L. (2006). An opioid screening instrument: long-term evaluation of the utility of the Pain Medication Questionnaire. *Pain Practice.* Vol. 6, No. 2, (June), pp. 74-88.

Hunt, S. M., McEwan, J. & McKenna, S. P. (1985). Measuring health status: a new tool for clinicians and epidemiologists. *Journal of the Royal College of General Practitioner.* Vol. 35, No. 273, (April), pp. 185-188.

Ives, T.J., Chelminski, P.R., Hammett-Stabler, C.A., Malone, R.M., Perhac, J.S., Potisek, N.M., Shilliday, B.B., DeWalt, D.A. & Pignone, M.P. (2006). Predictors of opioid misuse in patients with chronic pain: a prospective cohort study. *BMC Health Services Research.* Vol. 4, No. 6, (April), pp: 6:46.

Kalso, E., Allan, L., Dellemijn, P.L., Faura, C.C., Ilias, W.K., Jensen, T.S., Perrot, S., Plaghki, L.H. & Zenz, M. (2003). Recommendations for using opioids in chronic non-cancer pain. *European Journal of Pain,* Vol 7, No. 5, pp. 381-6.

Katz, N.P., Sherburne, S., Beach, M., Rose, R.J., Vielguth, J., Bradley, J. & Fanciullo, G.J. (2003). Behavioral monitoring and urine toxicology testing in patients receiving long-term opioid therapy. *Anesthesia and Analgesia.* Vol. 97, No. 4, (October), pp. 1097-1102.

Kerns, R.D., Turk, D.C. & Rudy, T.E. (1985). The West Haven-Yale Multidimensional Pain Inventory (WHYMPI). *Pain.* Vol. 23, No. 4, (December), pp. 345-356.

Linton, S.J., Hellsing, A.L. & Hallden, K. (1998). A population based study of spinal pain among 35-45-year old individuals. *Spine.* Vol. 23, No. 13, (July), pp. 1457-1463.

Loeser, J.D. & Melzack, R. (1999). Pain: an overview. *Lancet,* Vol. 8, No. 352, (May), pp. 1607-1609.

Loeser, J.D. (2000). Pain and suffering. *The Clinical Journal of Pain,* Vol. 16, No. 2, (June), pp. 2-6.

Luo, X., Pietrobon, R., Sun, S.X., Liu, G.G. & Hey, L. (2004). Estimates and patterns of direct health care expenditures among individuals with back pain in the United States. *Spine.* Vol. 29, No. 1, (January), pp. 79-86.

Maiani, G. & Sanavio, E. (1985). Semantics of pain in Italy: the Italian version of the McGill Pain Questionnaire. *Pain.* Vol. 22, No. 4, (August), pp. 399-405.

Manchikanti, L., Benyamin, R., Datta, S., Vallejo, R. & Smith, H. (2010). Opioids in chronic noncancer pain. *Expert Review of Neurotherapeutics.* Vol. 10, No. 5, (May), pp. 775-789, ISSN 1473-7175.

Manchikanti, L., Cash, K.A., Damron, K.S., Manchukonda, R., Pampati, V. & McManus, C.D. (2006). Controlled substance abuse and illicit drug use in chronic pain patients: an evaluation of multiple variables. *Pain Physician*. Vol. 9, No. 3, (July), pp: 215-225.

Manchikanti, L., Manchukonda, R., Pampati, V. & Damron, K.S. (2005). Evaluation of abuse of prescription and illicit drugs in chronic pain patients receiving short-acting (hydrocodone) or long-acting (methadone) opioids. *Pain Physician*. Vol. 8, No. 3, (July), pp. 257-261.

Manchikanti, L., Pampati, V., Damron, K.S., Fellows, B., Barnhill, R.C. & Beyer, C.D. (2001). Prevalence of opioid abuse in interventional pain medicine practice settings: a randomized clinical evaluation. *Pain Physician*. Vol. 4, No. 4, (October), pp. 358-365, ISSN 1533-3159.

Maniadakis, N. & Gray, A. (2000). The economic burden of back pain in the UK. *Pain*. Vol. 84, No. 1, (January), pp. 95-103.

Mannion, R.J. & Woolf, C.J. (2000) Pain mechanisms and management: a central perspective. *Clinical Journal of Pain*, Vol. 16 Supplement, pp. 144-156.

Melzack R. (Raven Press) (1983). *The McGill Pain Questionnaire*. In: Pain Measurement and Assessment. Raven Press, pp. 41-48, New York, USA.

Merskey, H. & Bogduk, N. (Ed.s Merskey & Bogduk) (1994). *Classification of Chronic Pain: descriptions of chronic pain syndromes and definitions of pain terms, II edition*. IASP press, Seattle, USA, ISBN 978-0931092053

Merskey, H. (1986a). Classification of chronic pain. Descriptions of chronic pain syndromes and definitions of pain terms. Prepared by the International Association for the Study of Pain, Subcommittee on Taxonomy. *Pain*, Suppl. 3, pp. 1-226

Merskey, H. (1986b). Variable meanings for the definitions of disease. *Journal of Medicine and Philosophy*, Vol. 11, No. 3, (August), pp. 215-232.

Michna, E., Ross, E.L., Hynes, W.L., Nedeljkovic, S.S., Soumekh, S., Janfaza, D., Palombi, D. & Jamison, R.N. (2004). Predicting aberrant drug behavior in patients treated for chronic pain: importance of abuse history. *Journal of Pain and Symptom Management*. Vol. 28, No. 3, (September), pp. 250-258.

Moore, T.M., Jones, T., Browder, J.H., Daffron, S. & Passik, S.D. (2009). A comparison of common screening methods for predicting aberrant drug-related behavior among patients receiving opioids for chronic pain management. *Pain Medicine*. Vol. 10, No. 8, (November), pp. 1426-1433.

Noble, M., Treadwell, J.R., Tregear, S.J., Coates, V.H., Wiffen, P.J., Akafomo, C. & Schoelles, K.M. (2010). Long-term opioid management for chronic noncancer pain. *Cochrane Database of Systematic Reviews*. Vol. 20, No. 1, (January), pp. 214-228.

Office of Applied Studies, Substance Abuse and Mental Health Services Administration (SAMHSA). (2009). *Trends in Nonmedical Use of Prescription Pain Relievers: 2002 to 2007*. Last accessed June 2011, Available from: http://oas.samhsa.gov/2k9/painRelievers/nonmedicalTrends.pdf.

Office of Applied Studies, Substance Abuse and Mental Health Services Administration (SAMHSA). (2008). *Results from the 2007 National Survey on Drug Use and Health: National findings*. Last accessed June 2011, Available from: http://oas.samhsa.gov/p0000016.htm.

Pancheri, P., Sirigatti, S., & Biondi, M. (1996). *Adaptation of the MMPI-2 in Italy*. In J. N. Butcher (Ed.), International adaptations of the MMPI-2: Research and clinical applications (pp. 416-441). Minneapolis, MN: University of Minnesota Press.

Passik, S.D. (2009). Issues in long-term opioid therapy: unmet needs, risks, and solutions. *Mayo Clinic Proceedings*. Vol. 84, No. 7, (July), pp. 593-601

Passik, S.D., Kirsh, K,L,, Whitcomb, L., Portenoy, R.K., Katz, N.P., Kleinman, L., Dodd, S.L. & Schein, J.R. (2004). A new tool to assess and document pain outcomes in chronic pain patients receiving opioid therapy. *Clinical Therapeutics*. Vol. 26, No. 4, (April), pp. 552-561.

Passik, S.D., Kirsh, K.L., Donaghy, K.B. & Portenoy, R.K. (2006). Pain and aberrant drug-related behaviours in medically ill patients with and without histories of substance abuse. *The Clinical Journal of Pain*. Vol. 22, No. 2, (February), pp. 173-181.

Passik, S.D., Kirsh, K.L., Whitcomb, L., Schein, J.R., Kaplan, M.A., Dodd, S.L., Kleinman, L., Katz, N.P. & Portenoy, R.K. (2005). Monitoring outcomes during long-term opioid therapy for noncancer pain: results with the Pain Assessment and Documentation Tool. *Journal of Opioid Management*. Vol. 1, No. 5, (November-December), pp. 257-266.

Pedrabissi, L. & Santinello, M. (Ed. Giunti Organizzazioni Speciali) (1996). STAI, State-Trait Anxiety Inventory, Forma Y: Manuale. Giunti OS, Firenze, Italy.

Portenoy, R.K. (1996) Opioid therapy for chronic nonmalignant pain: a review of the critical issues. *Journal of Pain and Symptom Management*. Vol. 11, No. 4, (April), pp. 203-217.

Portenoy, R.K. (2000). Current pharmacotherapy of chronic pain. *Journal of Pain and Symptom Management*. Vol. 19, No. 1 Suppl., (January), pp. 16-20.

Portenoy, R.K. (2004) Appropriate use of opioids for persistent non-cancer pain. *Lancet*. Vol. 364, No. 9436, (August-September), pp. 739-740.

Rosenblum, A., Marsch, L.A., Joseph, H. & Portenoy R.K. (2008). Opioids and the treatment of chronic pain: controversies, current status, and future directions. *Experimental and Clinical Psychopharmacology*.Vol. 16, No. 5, (October), pp. 405–416.

Savage S.R. (1993). Addiction in the treatment of pain: significance, recognition, and management. *Journal of Pain Symptom Management*. Vol. 8, No. 5, (July), pp. 265-278.

Savage S.R. (2002). Assessment for addiction in pain-treatment settings. *Clinical Journal of Pain*. Vol. 18, No. 4 Suppl, (July-August), pp: 28-38.

Schieffer, B.M., Pham, Q., Labus, J., Baria, A., Van Vort, W., Davis, P., Davis, F. & Naliboff, B.D. (2005). Pain medication beliefs and medication misuse in chronic pain. *The Journal of Pain*. Vol. 6, No. 9, (September), pp. 620-629.

Spielberger, C.D (Ed. Mind Garden) (1983). *State-Trait Anxiety Inventory for adults*. Mind Garden, Palo Alto, CA, USA.

Sullivan, M.D., Edlund, M.J., Zhang, L., Unützer, J. & Wells, K.B. (2006). Association between mental health disorders, problem drug use, and regular prescription opioid use. *Archives of Internal Medicine*. Vol. 166, No. 19, (October), pp. 2087-2093.

Trescot, A.M., Boswell, M.V., Atluri, S.L., Hansen, H.C., Deer, T.R., Abdi, S., Jasper, J.F., Singh, V., Jordan, A.E., Johnson, B.W., Cicala, R.S., Dunbar, E.E., Helm, S., Varley, K.G., Suchdev, P.K., Swicegood, J.R., Calodney, A.K., Ogoke, B.A., Minore, W.S. & Manchikanti, L. (2006). Opioid guidelines in the management of chronic non-cancer pain. *Pain Physician*, Vol. 9, No. 1, (January), pp. 1-39.

Trescot, A.M., Helm, S., Hansen, H., Benyamin, R., Glaser, S.E., Adlaka, R., Patel, S. & Manchikanti, L. (2008). Opioids in the management of chronic non-cancer pain: an update of American Society of the Interventional Pain Physicians (ASIPP) guidelines. *Pain Physician*, Vol. 11, No. 2 Suppl., (March), pp. 5-62.

Turk, D. & Okifuji, A. (2002). Psychological factors in chronic pain: evolution and revolution. *Journal of Consulting and Clinical Psychology*. Vol. 70, No. 3, (June), pp. 678-690.

van Leeuwen, M.T., Blyth, F.M., March, L.M., Nicholas, M.K. & Cousins, M.J. (2006). Chronic pain and reduced work effectiveness: the hidden cost to Australian employers. *European Journal of Pain*. Vol. 10, No. 2 (February), pp. 161-66.

Verhaak, P.F., Kerssens, J.J., Dekker, J., Sorbi, M.J. & Bensing, J.M (1998). Prevalence of chronic benign pain disorder among adults: a review of the literature. *Pain*. Vol. 77, No. 3, (September), pp. 231-239.

Vlaeyen, J.W. & Linton, S.J. (2000). Fear-avoidance and its consequences in chronic musculoskeletal pain: a state of the art. *Pain*. Vol. 85, No. 3, (April), pp. 317-332.

Wasan, A.D., Butler, S.F., Budman, S.H., Benoit, C., Fernandez, K. & Jamison, R.N. (2007). Psychiatric history and psychologic adjustment as risk factors for aberrant drug-related behaviour among patients with chronic pain. *Clinical Journal of Pain*. Vol. 23, No. 4, (May), pp. 307-315.

Webster, L. R. & Webster, R. M. (2005). Predicting aberrant behaviors in opioid-treated patients: preliminary validation of the Opioid Risk Tool. *Pain Medicine*, Vol. 6, No. 6, (November-December), pp. 432-442.

White, W., Ernest Kurtz, M.A., & Acker, C. (2001a). *Combined Addiction Disease Chronologies*. Last accessed June 2011, available from: http://silkworth.net/kurtz/Kurtz-1864-1879-OCR.pdf.

White, W., Ernest Kurtz, M.A., & Acker, C. (2001b). *Combined Addiction Disease Chronologies*. Last accessed June 2011, available from: http://silkworth.net/kurtz/Kurtz-1900-1919-OCR.pdf.

Winkelmann, A., Perrot, S., Schaefer, C., Ryan, K., Chandran, A., Sadosky, A. & Zlateva, G. (2011). Impact of fibromyalgia severity on health economic costs: results from a European cross-sectional study. *Applied Health Economics and Health Policy*. Vol. 9, No. 2, (March), pp. 125-136.

World Health Organization (1990). Cancer pain relief and palliative care: report of a WHO expert committee. *Technical Report Series 804*. Geneva, Switzerland.

World Health Organization (1998). The use of essential drugs: report of a WHO Expert Committee. *Technical Report Series No. 882*, Geneva, Switzerland.

World Health Organization (1986). Cancer pain relief, Geneva, Switzerland.

World Health Organization. (2002). Achieving balance in national opioids control policy: guidelines for assessment. Geneva, Switzerland.

Wu, S., Compton, P., Bolus, R., Schieffer, B., Pham, Q., Baria, A., Van Vort, W., Davis, F., Shekelle, P. & Naliboff, B. (2006). The Addiction Behaviors Checklist: validation of a new clinician based measure of inappropriate opioid use in chronic pain. *Journal of Pain and Symptom Management*, Vol. 32, No. 4, (October), pp. 342-351.

Yelin, E., Cisternas, M.G., Pasta, D.J., Trupin, L., Murphy, L. & Helmick, C.G. (2004). Medical care expenditures and earnings losses of persons with arthritis and other rheumatic conditions in the United States in 1997: total and incremental estimates. *Arthritis and Rheumatisms*. Vol. 50, No. 7, (July), pp. 2317-2326.

Yudko, E., Lozhkina, O. & Fouts, A. (2007). A comprehensive review of the psychometric properties of the Drug Abuse Screening Test. *Journal of Substance Abuse Treatment*. Vol. 32, No. 2, (March), pp. 189-198.

4

The Role of Peripheral Nerve Blocks in the Interdisciplinary Care of Children with Chronic Pain: A Case Series and Review of the Literature

Gillian R. Lauder[1] and Nicholas West[2]
[1]Department of Anesthesia, British Columbia Children's Hospital (BCCH),
[2]Pediatric Anesthesia Research Team, University of British Columbia (UBC),
Canada

1. Introduction

Chronic pain of childhood is an extremely complex condition which can lead to damaging effects on physical and social wellbeing. Some children with severe chronic pain embark on a downward spiral of decreased physical, psychological and social functioning. This includes loss of mobility and inability to participate in physical and sporting activities, poor sleep, difficulty concentrating on school work, school absenteeism, social isolation and family stress. As chronic pain persists the child can experience increased pain intensity, distress, anxiety and depression. When enmeshed in this disordered lifestyle the child and their family require coordinated integrated care. The interdisciplinary team management approach, based on pharmacology, physiotherapy and psychology, is now well established to be the standard of care for children with chronic pain. Treatment goals are targeted to individual children after careful consideration of the history and examination. In appropriately selected children peripheral nerve blocks can provide immediate and effective pain relief. This chapter will present a referenced review of the literature on interdisciplinary paediatric chronic pain management whilst highlighting the role of peripheral nerve blocks. The case histories of eight paediatric patients with chronic pain who gained significant relief from peripheral nerve blocks will be presented.

The International Association for the Study of Pain (IASP) defines pain as "an unpleasant sensory or emotional experience associated with actual or potential tissue damage, or described in terms of such damage" (1986). One defining characteristic of pain is its duration. Acute pain is relatively short-term pain that typically lasts until the underlying cause has been identified and treated. On the other hand, chronic pain is understood to mean prolonged pain or "pain that extends beyond the expected period of healing" (Turk & Okifuji, 2001) and while defined time frames that determine a diagnosis of chronic pain vary, the definition adopted by most studies, including those cited here, is pain lasting longer than three months.

Chronic pain can have its roots in one or a combination of types of pain mechanism. Types of pain include nociceptive, inflammatory, neuropathic or psychogenic pain (DSM-IV "Pain Disorder"). Extreme caution is required before labelling a patient with a diagnosis of psychogenic pain, functional pain or somatisation disorder as the true prevalence of these conditions is extremely low. Most patients with chronic pain will have psychosocial elements to their suffering, but this does not mean that the pain is "psychogenic".

Nociceptive pain is felt in response to noxious stimuli, such as the trauma associated with injury, oncological and other disease processes as well as following surgery. This pain functions as a protective and interpretable symptom: 'it hurts here' means 'here is the damage' and can be a straightforward guide to what needs to be treated or allowed to heal. *Inflammatory pain* occurs as a result of inflammatory mediators in many disease processes or associated with healing following acute trauma or surgery. If either nociceptive or inflammatory pains are left unrecognised or undertreated they can lead to ongoing and then chronic pain. *Neuropathic pain* signifies some dysfunction in the nervous system itself and is a major cause of chronic suffering, occurring in about 6-7% of the population (Vinik, 2010).

Neuropathic pain may derive from some identifiable damage to the nerves, resulting from a disease process, inflammation or accidental damage during trauma or surgery, or may result from a failure of integration and function of the peripheral and central nervous systems. Many conditions previously labelled as functional pain are now known to have peripheral and central nervous elements, which would re-class them as neuropathic pain. Complex regional pain syndrome (CRPS) is an immuno-neurological disorder (Fechir et al, 2008). It may be associated with no nerve lesion (type I) or may be related to some identifiable nerve lesion (type II). Chronic conditions like functional abdominal pain syndrome (FAPS) and CRPS have been under-recognised by physicians, but are experienced by a significant number of adolescents (Clouse et al, 2006; Kachko et al, 2008). In summary, a combination of pain mechanisms may be involved in the development of chronic pain conditions.

1.1 The epidemiology of paediatric chronic pain

The epidemiology of chronic pain in children is less well understood than it is in adults, but some useful studies have been published in the last decade that help us to understand the overall scale of the problem and to elicit some socio-demographic particulars of the affected population. A survey of over 5,000 children aged 0 – 18 years in the Netherlands reported that 25% had experienced some form of chronic or recurrent pain (Perquin et al, 2000). A Spanish study, of 561 schoolchildren aged 8 – 16 years, reported an incidence of 37%, but concluded that only 5% suffer moderate or severe chronic pain (Huguet & Miró, 2008). In a Canadian study of 495 schoolchildren aged 9 - 13, more than half reported having experienced at least one recurrent pain, typically characterised as a headache, stomach pain or 'growing pain'. Although 46% reported a 'long-lasting' pain, the researchers judged that in many cases this represented a recurrent pain condition; nonetheless, 6% of children were classified as having possible, probable or definite chronic pain (van Dijk et al, 2006).

While these studies highlight the methodological difficulties in distinguishing acute, recurrent and chronic pain from children's responses to questionnaire and interview questions, these statistics clearly also demonstrate that childhood chronic pain is a significant problem: slightly more than one child in every twenty is a chronic pain sufferer; that is, at least one child in every average-sized classroom in every school. Perquin et al (2000) conclude that childhood chronic pain is 'a common experience' and that the incidence of severe chronic pain amongst adolescents should provoke both concern and further research from the healthcare community.

The Role of Peripheral Nerve Blocks in the Interdisciplinary Care of Children with Chronic Pain: A Case Series and Review of the Literature

103

Previous pain experiences, cognitive, emotional and behavioural factors, family background, environment, peer group and culture have an influence on the impact, perception and biopsychosocial outcomes of chronic pain. Children living in lower educated, lower income families have been found to be at a greater risk of suffering recurrent pain, which is consistent with adult studies (Grøholt et al, 2003). Children suffering chronic pain themselves are quite likely to be living with another chronic pain sufferer, whether parent or sibling, and further investigation suggests that pre-existing chronic pain in the family environment is a predictor of both physical and psychological effects on the child (Lynch et al, 2006). Ethnicity and area of residence also appear to affect prevalence rates. For example, in Canada, the incidence of chronic pain is higher among Aboriginal people and, for males, is higher in rural areas (Ramage-Morin & Gilmour, 2010). There may also be cultural differences in the perception and reporting of pain (Mailis-Gagnon et al, 2007).

While chronic pain is clearly not confined to the developed world, most published studies provide figures for European or North American children, which may not be generalisable to different environments. A US study found that 13% of 12-13 year-olds and 17% of 15-16 year-olds experience abdominal pain every week (Hyams et al, 1996), while Dutta et al (1999) reported a considerably higher incidence (74%) in India. However, with gastrointestinal infections more widespread than the inflammatory bowel disease seen in developing countries, these figures probably represent the outcome of different disease processes (Ganesh et al, 2010). Abu-Saad Huijer (2010) considers the effects of war and traumatic events. Despite an absence of research in this area, he argues that chronic pain has been linked with post-traumatic stress disorders and that, as a consequence, we may expect to see a different profile of chronic pain among children affected by armed conflict.

In developed countries, headache, abdominal and musculoskeletal pain form the primary foci of chronic and recurrent pain among the paediatric population. In their study of Canadian 9-13 year olds, van Dijk et al (2006) received reports of recurrent headaches (32%), growing pains (21%), stomach pains (19%) and muscle aches (2%). Perquin et al (2000) had published similar findings from their survey of Dutch schoolchildren, in which they also analysed reports of pain at multiple locations. They found that the single location pain was most often reported. The combination of headache and abdominal pain was the most commonly reported multiple pain, found in 25% of all children. This greater than one pain profile was significantly more prevalent in adolescent girls.

Recent figures from a Statistics Canada health report identify chronic pain among 2.4% of males and 5.9% of females aged 12 to 17 years (Ramage-Morin & Gilmour, 2010). It has been reported that girls are as much as three times more likely to report chronic pain than boys (Martin et al, 2007). Perquin et al (2000) also showed a significant increase in the prevalence of chronic pain in girls. These girls were aged between 12 and 14 which may well be linked with the onset of menstruation. In general, abdominal pain is significantly more likely to be reported by girls and limb pain (or growing pains/muscle aches) is significantly more likely to be reported by boys (Perquin et al, 2000; van Dijk et al, 2006). A review on gender and pain suggests potential mechanisms within social and psychological processes, such as coping processes and catastrophising, are likely to contribute to the repeatedly observed sex differences in pain (Fillingim et al, 2009).

Aetiology and predisposition to chronic pain in children is largely unknown and depends on the type of pain. Factors associated with the development of chronic pain include surgery, trauma, emotional distress and chronic disease. In many cases, a definitive aetiology is difficult to establish. Even chronic post-surgical pain (CPSP) can be difficult to diagnose and consequently remains under-recognised. However, it represents a significant clinical problem. A 2006 review suggests that CPSP occurs after 10-50% of operations and results in severe chronic pain in 2-10% of these patients (Kehlet et al, 2006). This may, in fact, represent a significant portion of chronic pain sufferers. A UK study found that 22.5% of chronic pain patients developed their condition after surgery (Crombie et al, 1998). CPSP will often be neuropathic, resulting from nerve damage during surgery, though it could also be an ongoing inflammatory/nociceptive mechanism. The incidence of CPSP in the adult population is found to depend on a number of perioperative factors which include: genetic predisposition, degree of pre-operative anxiety, depression, pre-operative pain status, the surgical pain model, surgical technique, length of surgery and the quality of acute postoperative pain management (Kehlet et al, 2006; Macrae, 2008). The probability of an adult developing chronic pain after mastectomy or hernia surgery is decreased with increased age (Poleshuck et al, 2006; Poobalan et al, 2003). How this relationship to age translates to children and adolescents is not known as there is no published literature on CPSP in children. Six out of the eight paediatric cases presented in this chapter developed chronic pain following surgery.

Untangling factors to establish clear causality for the development of paediatric chronic pain is a challenge. Whether initiated by surgery or injury or other cause, it is a complex multi-factorial process. Understanding this mechanism requires not only a search for a cause, but also a clearer understanding of the effects of chronic pain. It is established that some paediatric chronic pain conditions have been under-diagnosed. Better recognition and early treatment of these conditions requires that healthcare providers understand the effects of chronic pain on a child and their family.

1.2 The impact of chronic pain on children and their families
Childhood chronic pain has a negative impact on physical, psychological and social function. It can prevent a child participating in sporting activities and other forms of exercise. It can cause sleep disruption and fatigue. It can contribute to depression and anxiety. It can affect school work through fatigue, poor memory and concentration and result in reduced school attendance. Friendships and family relationships are disrupted which may lead to varying degrees of social isolation. An Australian study of 207 children and adolescents attending a paediatric pain management clinic found that 95% had missed school, 90% had been unable to participate in some sporting activity and 71% had suffered some sleep disruption (Chalkiadis, 2001). Roth-Isigkeit et al (2005) found that 30-40% of children/adolescents with pain reported effects of their pain on school attendance, hobbies, social contacts, appetite, sleep, as well as increased utilization of health services because of their pain. An understanding of the range and interaction of all these different effects is crucial to the effective recognition and treatment of chronic pain in children.

These impacts on daily living can be bundled into the notion of Health-Related Quality of Life (HRQoL), which may be defined as *"an individual's subjective assessment of his or her functioning and emotional state"* (Gold et al, 2009) and can be used for comparative purposes. One such measurement instrument is the Pediatric Quality of Life Inventory (PedsQL), which contains items relating specifically to both physical and psychosocial function (the latter comprising emotional, social and school function) and can be completed by self-report or parent-proxy (Varni et al, 2001). Using this instrument, a US study of 100 patients, aged

The Role of Peripheral Nerve Blocks in the Interdisciplinary Care of Children with Chronic Pain: A Case Series and Review of the Literature

105

2–21 years, attending a chronic pain clinic found that the HRQoL scores of these patients were not only considerably lower than scores obtained from normal healthy children, but were significantly lower than scores observed in children with rheumatological or cancer disease (Vetter, 2008). Another US study found that the mean PedsQL score for a cohort of 69 children and adolescents (aged 8 – 18 years) seeking outpatient pain management services, fell below the 'at-risk cut-off score' for all dimensions except social functioning, suggesting that the majority of these children were experiencing significant disruption in their day-to-day lives. The message from these studies is clear: the effects of chronic pain on a child's quality of life are wide-ranging and profound.

School functioning has received perhaps the most attention (Palermo, 2000). It demonstrates the most marked detriment of all the psychosocial dimensions of the PedsQL scale (Vetter, 2008; Gold et al, 2009) and clearly illustrates the complex effects of chronic pain on quality of life. A child with chronic pain may experience a range of problems which impact on their schooling: fatigue and/or poor sleep profile prevents early morning waking; pain inhibits physical ability to get to school, to sit in a classroom for long periods or to participate in physical activities; fear of pain by accidentally being knocked during recess times inhibits social interaction and imparts a sense of isolation, difference and not being involved with peers; poor memory and concentration affects schoolwork; as school work becomes missed or incomplete these unfinished projects become a barrier to return to school if workload is not controlled; and the school may represent an environment where their pain condition is not properly understood or tolerated.

For all these reasons school absences are common. In a survey of adolescent chronic pain sufferers aged 12-17 in Boston USA, 44% missed more than one-quarter of school days and 20% had missed more than half (Logan et al, 2008). Of course, schools typically offer only a limited degree of health-related support. In the Boston study, two-thirds of participants had received some form of accommodation from their school, such as being sent to the nurse's office, being sent home in pain, reduction in workload, extension on an assignment, and so on. Nonetheless, 44.3% of parents reported their child's grades had suffered (Logan et al, 2008) and missing school can clearly have negative consequences that extend beyond academic performance to a child's physical, emotional and social development. Six of the eight cases presented in this chapter had missed significant amounts of school.

Assessing the impact of chronic pain on a child's life is an important but problematic task. There are a number of reasons for this difficulty.

Firstly, the specific effects of chronic pain are not easily isolated from one another. For example, fatigue may be a mediating factor between pain and school functioning (Gold et al, 2009). Anxiety also plays a complex role in moderating the relationship between pain and function. Tsao et al (2007) studied anxiety sensitivity, or the fear of anxiety sensations, in 87 children aged 10-18 presenting at a US chronic pain clinic. Anxiety sensitivity was found to be linked with academic and/or social limitations, where those limitations arose from emotional rather than physical difficulties. Greater anxiety sensitivity was associated with lower self-esteem and perceived general and mental health, and with more behavioural problems and family disruption, but did not appear to affect physical functioning (Tsao et al, 2007). In a similar study of 222 adolescents aged 11 to 19 years attending two chronic pain clinics in the UK, Cohen et al (2010) found that in children with low anxiety, level of pain was a good predictor of physical and social function, but that high levels of anxiety prompted poorer function regardless of the level of pain.

Secondly, the impact of chronic pain on health and quality of life often extends beyond any immediate effects. For example, more than 50% of adolescents with chronic pain report some symptoms of insomnia (compared with less than 20% of healthy adolescents), and while these may initially be related directly to the experience of pain, behavioural patterns can transform this disruption into a primary sleep disorder (Palermo et al, 2010). Furthermore, chronic pain in childhood appears to increase the risk of developing further chronic conditions in adulthood. Adults, who have suffered recurrent headaches as children, are at an increased risk not only of headaches, but other physical and psychiatric symptoms (Fearon & Hotopf, 2001). Similarly, a longitudinal cohort study of paediatric FAPS patients, aged 6 to 18 at enrolment, found that, 15 years later, those with unresolved FAPS experienced higher levels of non-abdominal chronic pain (including migraine, tension-type headaches, and pelvic, back and limb pain) than those with resolved FAPS or normal controls (Walker et al, 2010).

Thirdly, the effects of chronic pain are felt not just by the child, but become a burden for the whole family. The child may no longer participate in shared physical activities, limiting family excursions and fun. Relationships with parents, siblings and other family members are put under strain resulting in anxiety and depression (Eccleston et al, 2004). A number of studies report associations between family functioning and the level of a child's pain-related disability, generally finding that the worse the disability, the greater the family dysfunction (Lewandowski et al, 2010). While it is difficult to interpret the causal relationship underpinning this association with confidence, it is likely that causation runs in both directions: a child's chronic pain has an adverse effect on family life; family problems make it more difficult for the child to cope and so worsen the experience of pain. The impact of chronic pain on the family matches the adverse impact experienced by families caring for children at home with severe cerebral palsy or birth defects (Vetter, 2008).

Daily care arrangements for the child/adolescent with chronic pain require additional support, which may cost money or require a parent to give up a job. The direct and indirect costs of caring for a child with chronic pain have been estimated. A UK study calculated, from a sample of 52 families, that the total annual cost, to a family living with a child in chronic pain, was as much as £14,160 or, approximately, $25,000 (Sleed et al, 2005). This figure included direct healthcare costs for the child and other family members and indirect costs such as loss of earnings, adaptations to housing, over-the-counter medications and care assistance. This is a potentially ruinous sum for low-income families.

Fourthly, physical and social effects of chronic pain carry another associated economic burden, which may be less easily identified and difficult to quantify. Diminished school function and educational achievement will have potential long-term career and economic cost for both the child and for society.

Finally, the immediate effects of chronic pain have the potential to feed back negatively on the physical and psychosocial health of children and their families. This further reduces their capacity to cope. Unremitting pain can cause sleep disruption and fatigue. Missing school leads to social isolation. The extra burden of stress and financial hardship on families makes them less able to provide the required care. The physical, psychological and social effects of chronic pain can lead the child and their family into a downward spiral, from which it is difficult to emerge without inter-disciplinary support. It is crucial that physicians not only identify the wider psychosocial effects of chronic pain, but recognise that these effects are contributory factors which play an important role in the ongoing pain and functioning of their patient (Jensen, 2011). With the goal of optimal patient care in mind, a clinician should consider including interventions that address these factors in their treatment strategies for children with chronic pain.

1.3 Interdisciplinary team management of children with chronic pain

Management of children and adolescents with severe suffering and extensive pain-related disability as a result of chronic pain requires an interdisciplinary approach (Eccleston et al, 2003). This includes the treatment modalities of pharmacology, physiotherapy and psychology running in parallel or, more importantly, enmeshed with one another. How these elements are balanced is dependant on each individual child and takes into consideration the type and duration of pain, as well as the impact of pain on particular biopsychosocial aspects of the child's life.

1.3.1 Pharmacology

The pharmacological approach to management of a child with chronic pain requires consideration of the type of pain, the impact of the pain on the child's biopsychosocial functions and the potential side effects of the medications. Medications need to be individualised to each child and continually re-assessed for efficacy and side effects. If medications are having no impact at therapeutic dosage they need to be discontinued and the child re-evaluated for consideration of other appropriate agents. Close liaison with psychiatry is advised prior to and following up on prescription of mood stabilising medications. It is important to emphasise that pharmacological interventions are only one part of an interdisciplinary approach to improve function in children/adolescents with chronic pain. Table 1 provides a summary of the medications that may be considered in the pharmacological treatment of paediatric chronic pain.

Drug	Dose	Comments
Acetamin-ophen	**>3 months of age to adolescents:** 10-15 mg/kg/dose PO Q4H PRN (max 75 mg/kg/day)	Central analgesic action via cannabinoid or prostaglandin mechanism Hepatotoxic in acute overdose or with chronic long term use; risk factors for toxicity include fever, prolonged fasting (>48 hrs), concomitant interacting drugs, obesity, poorly controlled diabetes, liver disease, viral infections and malnutrition Doses apply to normal healthy children (i.e. no hepatic or renal compromise)
Ibuprofen	5-10 mg/kg/dose PO Q6-8H (max 40 mg/kg/day)	Non steroidal anti-inflammatory agent; should not be used concomitantly with other NSAIDs Use caution in patients with aspirin hypersensitivity, hepatic or renal insufficiency Administer with food or milk to lessen GI upset; contraindicated with active GI bleeding and ulcer disease
Naprosyn	**Children >2 years:** 5-7 mg/kg/dose PO/PR Q8-12H	Non steroidal anti-inflammatory agent; should not be used concomitantly with other NSAIDs Contraindicated with active GI bleeding and ulcer disease; administer with food or milk to avoid GI upset; common GI side effects include abdominal pain, appetite loss, stomatitis or constipation May cause photosensitive vesicular rash (pseudoporphyria)

Drug	Dose	Comments
Tramadol (Ultram, Ralivia)	**Immediate-release form: Children:** 1-2 mg/kg Q4-6H PRN (max: 400 mg/day or 8 mg/kg/day) **Adolescents:** 50-100 mg Q4-6H PRN (max: 400 mg/day) **Extended-release form: Adolescents:** Initial: 100 mg PO daily; titrate by 100 mg increments every 2-3 days PRN (max: 300 mg/day).	An opioid analgesic with norepinephrine and serotonin effects Side effects include nausea and vomiting; tolerability is improved by gradual dose titration. Caution in renal and/or hepatic impairment Tramadol is metabolized to active form (i.e. a prodrug) Inter-individual pharmacogenomic variations affect efficacy Serotonin syndrome reported with concurrent use of serotonergic drugs Seizures reported with concurrent TCAs, SSRIs, and opioids or with conditions that lower seizure threshold Withdrawal symptoms may develop if abruptly discontinued; do not suddenly stop long-term treatment; wean dose by 25% per week Extended release product given ONCE daily.
Topical Lidocaine	Topical: 5% under occlusive dressing for 12 hours (once per day)	Blockade of upregulated sodium channel receptors in injured nerves. Useful for very localised pain Minimal side effects (mild skin reactions)
Amitriptyline	Initial: 0.1 mg/kg/dose PO HS; increase as needed and tolerated over 2-3 wks to 0.5-2 mg/kg/dose HS	Tricyclic antidepressant agent (TCA) used in low dose for chronic neuropathic pain; prevents the re-uptake of serotonin and norepinephrine. Pretreatment ECG required to exclude arrhythmia potential. Drug interactions via cytochrome p450 system; contraindicated if MAO inhibitors used within 14 days; tricyclics have limited efficacy for treatment of depression in children and adolescents Side effects include: sedation, confusion, weakness, fatigue, tremor, sweating, headache, anticholinergic effects, cardiovascular effects (including orthostatic hypotension, tachycardia, prolonged QTc and arrhythmias at higher plasma levels), decreased seizure threshold. Sedative side effect used to help with improved sleep profile If one TCA not helpful due to intolerable side effects try another with a different SE profile before abandoning this modality of pharmacological therapy (Nortriptyline is less sedating, doxepin less anticholinergic). Analgesic effect may not occur for 2 weeks from commencement. A withdrawal syndrome is documented for Tricyclics (flu-like symptoms, dizziness, mood changes). Assess patient carefully and limit prescribed quantities to minimum effective dose; do not suddenly stop long-term treatment; wean dose by 25% per week.
Gabapentin	**Children:** titrate to effect over a few days, starting at 2 mg/kg once or twice daily, then increase to TID dosing to a maximum of 35 mg/kg/24hr (max 3600 mg/day)	Calcium channel α 2-δ ligand; calcium channel blocker when neuron hyperexcited Analgesic, anticonvulsant, anxiolytic, and sleep-modulating activities. Side effects may include somnolence, ataxia, fatigue and behaviour change. Gradual dose increase helps to minimize sedation; increased

The Role of Peripheral Nerve Blocks in the Interdisciplinary Care of Children with Chronic Pain: A Case Series and Review of the Literature

109

Drug	Dose	Comments
		oral doses are associated with decreased bioavailability; do not administer with antacids; primarily excreted unchanged in the urine, therefore need to adjust dose in renal impairment Maximum dose often not be needed for maximum effect; do not suddenly stop long-term treatment; wean dose by 25% per week.
Pregabalin	**Children > 10 years:** Initial: 25 mg PO daily Titrate upward to effect to 2.5 mg/kg PO BID or max 300 mg/day	Calcium channel α 2-δ ligand; calcium channel blocker when neuron hyperexcited. Similar in mechanism to gabapentin Side effects may include somnolence, ataxia, fatigue and behaviour change. Gradual dose increase helps to minimize sedation; increased oral doses are associated with increased bioavailability; do not administer with antacids; primarily excreted unchanged in the urine, therefore need to adjust dose in renal impairment. Maximum dose often not be needed for maximum effect; do not suddenly stop long-term treatment; wean dose by 25% per week.
Opioids	For dosing of different agents see Compendium of Pharmaceuticals and Specialties	mu-opioid agonist Additive sedative effects with other medications and/or alcohol Side effects include sedation, nausea, vomiting, constipation, pruritis, tolerance dependance opioid induced hyperalgesia, addiction Long-term use rarely indicated in children; addiction potential should be assessed prior to commencement of opioids; opioid prescription should follow national guidelines for safe practice
Venlafaxine	**Initial Dose:** 37.5 – 75 mg PO Once DAILY **Increment:** 37.5-75 mg every 4-7 days **Usual Dose Range:** 75-225 mg/day	Serotonin/norepinephrine reuptake inhibitor (SNRI) Effective in the treatment of Depression, Generalized Anxiety Disorder, Social Anxiety Disorder, Panic Disorder. Also used to treat ADHD, Post-Traumatic Stress Disorder and Obsessive-Compulsive Disorder. Side effects include: headache, nausea, increased heart rate and blood pressure (more prominent at higher doses), anorexia/weight loss, drowsiness, dizziness, dry mouth, sweating, tremor and impaired sexual function (adolescents/adults). Administer with food or milk to decrease GI upset; full beneficial effects may not be seen until 4 weeks of therapy completed. ***Warnings issued by Health Canada regarding use of antidepressants in pediatric patients.***
Clonidine	1-4 micrograms/kg/dose PO Q4-6H	An alpha adrenergic receptor antagonist; metabolism is hepatic and renal (roughly 50:50); drug interactions with beta blockers, tricyclic anti-depressants Sedative, anxiolytic and analgesic effects; a useful adjunct used to minimise other analgesic drug doses such as opioids Side effects include sedation, dry mouth, hypotension Do not suddenly stop long-term treatment; wean dose by 25% per week to prevent rebound hypertension

Table 1. Modalities of medications that may be considered in outpatient paediatric chronic pain management

1.3.2 Physiotherapy

Chronic pain sufferers often experience some level of physical incapacity and many adopt activity patterns that can make their pain worse, such as alternating episodes of over-activity and under-activity (Birkholtz et al, 2004). Physiotherapy plays an important role in the interdisciplinary treatment of chronic pain in children and adolescents. Eccleston & Eccleston (2004) divide it into the following four components:

- *Exercise* – this is used to increase aerobic endurance, flexibility, strength and overall fitness, which all have potential benefits for pain reduction;
- *Education* – this helps the patient relate their pain to their anatomy, physiology and activity levels and to address issues such as fear of movement and the potential for re-injury;
- *Behavioural management* – this may involve physical retraining and activity pacing, aiming for a gradual increase in the range and extent of movement, including a steady return to any activities abandoned since the onset of pain (see also Harding et al, 1998);
- *Performance assessment* – there is a clear link between reduced pain and improved physical function; the physiotherapist is well-placed to assess treatment progress.

Other reports of physiotherapy interventions in the treatment of chronic pain stress the importance of the interdisciplinary approach. For example, a combination of physical therapy and CBT has been shown to be effective in treating CRPS in children (Lee et al, 2002). Harding et al (1998) also highlight the need to integrate behavioural and cognitive components in activity training to minimise distress and unhelpful beliefs.

1.3.3 Psychology

There are a number of psychological factors, which are directly involved in the perception, reporting and self-management of pain. These include fear, vigilance to the feeling and threat of pain, catastrophising, avoidance of pain-inducing activity, sadness, depression, anger and self-denigration. Psychological factors are also important in coping mechanisms, taking action, and being able to predict or make sense of pain and its consequences (Eccleston, 2001). Psychologists provide continual education/reassurance on the pathophysiology of the chronic pain condition and teach mind-body techniques like breathing, muscle relaxation exercises, self-hypnosis, imagery, and cognitive strategies. These techniques help reduce the impact of pain on daily living and mood.

Cognitive behaviour therapy (CBT) is central to the notion of interdisciplinary care. CBT refers to an *"integration of treatments aimed at reducing or extinguishing the influence of the factors that maintain patients' maladaptive behaviours, beliefs and patterns of thought... and is delivered by a team of pain therapists, including anaesthetists, clinical psychologists and physiotherapists"* (Eccleston, 2001). Interdisciplinary CBT programmes aimed at adolescents with chronic musculoskeletal pain have been found to improve physical function, reduce emotional distress, increase attendance at school and reduce medicine consumption (Eccleston et al, 2003; de Blécourt et al, 2008). Furthermore, there is evidence to suggest that an interdisciplinary framework is beneficial for the family members involved. Schurman & Friesen (2010) report that an 'integrative care' approach in a paediatric Abdominal Pain Clinic (that is, service delivered by a gastroenterologist and a psychologist) was acceptable to families, produced higher satisfaction scores and, crucially, improved receptivity to treatment recommendations.

Relaxation strategies and plans to improve sleep hygiene are a vital part of the psychologist's role. When schooling has been impacted by pain, the psychologist helps teachers become more aware of the condition and its impact on schoolwork. The psychologist helps to negotiate or advocate for any accommodations needed in order to help the child succeed at school. Psychologists help the child and their family identify and resolve stresses such as anxiety or depression that could be preventing return to function.

A Cochrane Review determined that there is strong evidence for psychological therapies being effective in the treatment of headaches in children and some evidence for their efficacy in the treatment of musculoskeletal and recurrent abdominal pain (Eccleston et al, 2009). Psychological interventions are often, and ideally, delivered as part of an interdisciplinary approach and consequently there are few randomized-controlled-trial (RCT) studies providing definite evidence for individual therapies (McGrath & Holahan, 2003). Nonetheless, psychological techniques are a vital component of the interdisciplinary approach and experienced therapists will select particular techniques according to the needs of the individual patient.

1.3.4 Interventional therapies

Interventional procedures offered at Canadian paediatric *multidisciplinary pain treatment facilities* (MPTFs) include continuous epidural infusions, single epidural injections, facet injections, stellate ganglion nerve blocks, peripheral nerve blocks, trigger point injections, sympathetic blocks with local anaesthetic, Botox injections, intravenous regional anaesthesia, paravertebral nerve blocks and radiofrequency lesioning (Peng et al, 2007). Nerve blocks are used widely among Canadian anaesthesiologists who specifically practice chronic pain management: of those, 84% perform nerve blocks, compared with 60% who use pharmacotherapy, and a majority of them estimated that more than 40% of their patients require some form of nerve block as part of their treatment programme (Peng & Castano, 2005).

However, there is very little evidence to demonstrate that interventions benefit a patient more than would be seen from a placebo response. The literature is comprised of case reports and small case series, along with a few randomized, placebo-controlled trials (RCTs). For example, therapeutic lumbar facet joint nerve blocks can provide effective pain relief and functional improvement (Manchikanti et al, 2010). However, epidural corticosteroid injections for sciatica appear to offer only transient benefit (Arden et al, 2005). Results of RCTs are not always consistent, however. For example, one RCT has shown that radiofrequency lesioning of the dorsal root ganglion for treatment of chronic lumbosacral radicular pain appears not to be more effective than control treatment with local anaesthetic (Geurts et al, 2003); on the the other hand, another RCT has shown that it is both safe and effective (Simopoulos et al, 2008). For some techniques, such as myofascial trigger point injections, it has not even been possible to establish a consensus on methods for diagnosis or treatment (Tough et al, 2007). Furthermore, any RCTs that have been done mainly comprise adult studies. The evidence of efficacy in children/adolescents is even more limited and more research is required. There are also rare but significant iatrogenic risks associated with some of these interventions. Injection therapies for lower back pain carry the risk of paraspinal, spinal end epidural abscesses or meningitis (Gaul et al, 2005).

Despite this negative portrayal of interventional medicine for chronic pain "absence of evidence is not evidence of absence" (Altman & Bland, 1995) and there are many pain physicians and patients, including those in this case series, who have derived enormous benefit from interventional treatments.

2. Case reports

The cases are described below and summarised in table 2.

No	Gender	Age	Weight	Site of pain	Duration (months)	Diagnosis	Block(s) performed
1	Male	16	60kg	Chest	5	Intercostal neuralgia related to Nuss bar	Intercostal nerve blocks (1 diagnostic and 3 therapeutic)
2	Male	14	56kg	Abdomen	9	Abdominal wall pain	Bilateral rectus abdominis sheath blocks (diagnostic and therapeutic)
3	Male	18	60kg	Groin	12	Ilioinguinal neuralgia following hydrocele repair	Ilioinguinal nerve blocks (1 diagnostic and 3 therapeutic)
4	Male	15	66kg	Abdomen	3	Neuropathic pain, *not* incisional hernia	Intercostal nerve block; rectus sheath block.
5	Male	9	25kg	Groin	4	Genitofemoral or ilioinguinal neuralgia following orchidopexy	Rectus abdominis sheath block
6	Female	15	45kg	Rib	8	Intercostal neuralgia, post-surgery	intercostal nerve blocks (diagnostic and therapeutic)
7	Female	9	33kg	Abdomen	2	Abdominal wall pain following laparascopic appendectomy	Bilateral rectus abdominis sheath blocks (diagnostic and therapeutic)
8	Female	17	66kg	Rib	7	Intercostal neuralgia	Intercostal nerve blocks (diagnostic and therapeutic)

Table 2. Summary of cases

2.1 Case 1: A 16-year-old adolescent with chest pain related to a Nuss bar

A 60kg 16-year-old male presented with a 5 month history of right sided chest wall pain. He had undergone a Nuss procedure for cosmetic repair of pectus excavatum one year prior to presentation and had received satisfactory acute pain management with epidural analgesia. He was referred to the Pain Service by his surgeon. His pain was precipitated by a sudden lateral movement, but aggravated by activity, laughter and bending down. The pain was described as "shooting". The pain was not relieved by ibuprofen and/or acetaminophen.

This young man, an active kick-boxer, was extremely fit and well. However, his pain was so unremitting that he had to stop all sporting activities and was completely sedentary. His sleep was not disrupted, nor was his school attendance or academic performance. However, he was very frustrated that his pain prevented him pursuing his kick-boxing and his ability to perform simple physical tasks. He was able to maintain friendships, but could not engage in some of the more physical social activities.

On examination, his pain was found to radiate laterally from the site of his Nuss bar on the right side, in one dermatomal level at the level of the 7th rib from midaxillary line to sternum. There was no pain on palpation or deep inspiration/expiration. There was no numbness, allodynia or skin changes. Palpation of the thoracic spines, costochondral junctions, and left side of chest were unremarkable and pain free. His chest X-ray (CXR) revealed that his Nuss bar had not moved, with no bony reaction or wire migration. The CXR was otherwise normal. The presumed diagnosis was intercostal neuralgia.

A diagnostic intercostal nerve block was performed, which provided effective short-term symptomatic relief so a follow-up therapeutic block was done 10 days later. For the therapeutic block, 5mls of 0.25% bupivicaine with 1/200,000 epinephrine and 10mg triamcinolone was injected at four sites: at the affected rib, one above, one below and at the right sided Nuss bar insertion scar site. This provided complete pain relief to allow the patient to return to his previous physical activities.

He required repeat therapeutic blocks at 3 months and 1 year from the initial block for resurgence of pain, but had no further pain up to and after the removal of the Nuss bar.

2.2 Case 2: A 14-year-old male with abdominal pain

A 56kg 14-year-old male presented with a 9 month history of abdominal pain. There was no apparent precipitating event. He was referred to the Pain Service after multiple referrals and investigations had excluded a remedial cause for his pain but drawn a blank on a diagnosis. The pain was described as a dull, aching pain, present all the time, but worse with exercise and on palpation. There was no pattern to his pain or any relation to his diet. There were no other symptoms related to the abdominal system. The pain was not relieved by ibuprofen, acetaminophen or homeopathic remedies.

This young man had been extremely fit and well. However his pain was such that he had to stop all his sporting activities, experienced difficulty getting to sleep, was depressed and grumpy with his family and had been absent from school for the preceding 6 months.

On examination, his abdomen was slim and soft, with normal bowel sounds, no masses and no organomegaly. There was tenderness in the midline above the umbilicus, which was worse on abdominal wall tensing (Carnett's test positive). The presumed diagnosis was chronic abdominal wall pain.

A diagnostic bilateral rectus sheath block was performed above the umbilicus under ultrasound control which provided effective short-term symptomatic relief so a follow-up therapeutic block was done two weeks later. For the therapeutic block 10mls of 0.25% bupivicaine with 1/200,000 epinephrine and 20mg triamcinolone was injected at each site. He did not require repeat therapeutic blocks.

Two weeks after his therapeutic block, he slowly returned to his normal activity levels, sleeping and eating patterns and resumed his previous happy demeanour. The following term, he returned to school and reported no subsequent absences.

2.3 Case 3: An 18-year-old with groin pain after hydrocele repair

A 60kg 18-year-old male presented with a 1 year history of a shooting pain in his groin, which was present all the time and radiated down the medial aspect of his thigh to his knee. There was no apparent precipitating event; however, he was a competitive fencer and had undergone a left hydrocele repair 6 months prior to the onset of pain. The pain was worse in morning, walking up stairs and mobilizing from lying down. He had episodes of severe pain 2-3 times per day, which lasted several hours.

He was referred to the Pain Service after multiple referrals and investigations had excluded a remedial cause for his pain, but drawn a blank on a diagnosis. The pain was not relieved by acetaminophen.

This young man had been extremely fit and well. However his pain was such that his appetite was reduced, he was losing weight and he had to stop all his physical activities to the point that his future competitive aspirations were severely compromised. He continued to attend school, but was under pressure to compete in the fencing team. His mood during this period was described as 'testy'.

On examination, he had pain on palpation of the hydrocele repair scar, but no pain on palpation underneath inguinal ligament. He had a full range of non-painful movements of his lumbar spine, hips and knees with normal bulk, tone & power in his lower limbs, and brisk but equal knee and ankle jerk reflexes. He exhibited a downgoing plantar reflex and bilateral abdominal reflexes. His abdomen was slim and soft, with normal bowel sounds, no masses and no organomegaly. There was no apparent numbness to light touch of his scar or thigh and no allodynia, skin or hair changes. There was no pain to palpation in his scrotum or penis. The presumed diagnosis was ilioinguinal neuralgia.

A diagnostic ilioinguinal nerve block was performing under ultrasound control which provided effective short-term symptomatic relief so a follow-up therapeutic block was done one week later. For the therapeutic block 20mls of 0.25% bupivacaine with 1/200,000 epinephrine and 20mg triamcinolone was injected between the internal oblique and transverse abdominis muscles; some was also injected under the scar site from his hydrocele repair. This provided complete pain relief.

His mood and eating pattern improved within the first month, but he did require repeat therapeutic blocks at 5 months and 11 months following the initial block. These provided good pain relief to allow the patient to make a graded return to competitive fencing.

2.4 Case 4: A 15-year-old male with a suspected incisional hernia

A 66kg 15-year-old male presented with a 3 month history of left upper quadrant pain associated with a bulge just lateral & inferior to the incision from a congenital diaphragmatic hernia repair when he was 14 months old. The pain was described as a burning, stabbing sensation. He exhibited no symptoms related to the respiratory, cardiovascular or abdominal systems.

He had been extremely fit and well. However his pain was such that he could not stand up straight, suffered pain with all activity and was unable to sleep soundly because he could not get comfortable. He had completely lost his appetite and had lost 10kg in weight. He became depressed and ceased to interact with friends. His suffering affected his family deeply: his parents' relationship suffered, his sister became depressed. He could not sit or concentrate and consequently missed 5 months of school.

An upper gastrointestinal endoscopy was normal. Surgical repair of the suspected incisional hernia revealed no hernia of the abdominal wall. Pain occurred in the immediate postoperative period. This pain did not respond to simple analgesics or hydromorphone. He was referred to the Pain Service and a diagnosis of neuropathic pain was made.

Intercostal nerve blocks were administered to the left sided 9th, 10th, and 11th ribs. This provided effective short-term symptomatic relief, so a follow-up therapeutic block was done a week later. For the therapeutic block, 5ml of 0.25% bupivacaine with 1/200,000 epinephrine & 10mg triamcinolone was injected at the same 3 intercostal spaces; in addition, the same amount was administered as a left rectus sheath block under ultrasound control, adjacent to the site of surgery. On awakening, the patient reported that his pain had gone.

This treatment provided immediate pain relief, which allowed the patient to return to his normal self. His appetite returned the next day. Within a few days, he was laughing again and was sleeping normally. Within 2 months he had started gym. He quickly caught up with most of his schoolwork and was now motivated to do additional study during the summer vacation. He resumed contact with friends and his family were able to return to normal. He did not require repeat therapeutic blocks.

2.5 Case 5: A 9-year-old with post-orchidopexy pain

A 25kg 9-year-old male presented with a 4 month history of left sided groin pain. He had been experiencing this pain for three years on and off, but it had been worse since his orchidopexy surgery 4 months prior to the consultation. He was referred to the Pain Service by his surgeon.

He continued to attend school, but had to visit the nurse twice a day and lie down to recover his strength. Often the school requested that he be collected and taken home early. He found it difficult to engage in physical or social activities and had to give up Tae Kwon Do. He was often woken with pain and cramps and cried as a result of his pain.

The pain was described as "stabbing". It was not relieved by ibuprofen and/or acetaminophen. On examination, there was no numbness, allodynia or skin changes and Carnett's test was positive. The presumed diagnosis was genitofemoral or ilioinguinal neuralgia.

A diagnostic rectus abdominis sheath block was performed, under ultrasound control: 15ml 0.25% bupivicaine, 1/200,000 epinephrine was injected into the rectus sheath and between the transverse abdominis and internal oblique; 10ml was injected at his flank at the anterior superior iliac spine; and some was injected at his orchidopexy scar site. On awakening, the patient reported the pain was gone.

A therapeutic block was not done in this case. He was able to resume a normal sleeping pattern within 2 weeks, was much happier and once again able to spend time with friends. He made a gradual return to Tae Kwon Do and normal schooling with no absences.

2.6 Case 6: A 15-year-old female with chest pain following removal of exostosis

A 45 kg 15-year-old female presented at the Complex Pain Clinic with post-surgical chest pain. Successful removal of an exostosis from her right rib cage was followed by the gradual emergence of a new, sharp pain, which was present every day. It worsened during the day and with sitting or physical activity.

It was 8 months since her surgery. She had missed some school, had stopped gymnastics classes and soccer training completely and had to limit her social activities. She was grumpy with friends and family. Physiotherapy had not helped, but ketorolac (10mg twice a day as needed), psychology, TENS and laser therapy were judged to have provided some benefit.

She was examined by the interdisciplinary team. Physical examination revealed that her pain was localised to the right anterolateral aspect of her 10th rib, close to the exostosis excision; there was no associated numbness, no allodynia and no skin colour change. The physiotherapist noted that her right waist crease and elevated iliac crest suggested a protective response, but that she had a full range of motion in spine and extremities. The psychologist determined that she was not overly anxious or depressed, despite some ongoing family conflicts. A preliminary diagnosis of intercostal neuralgia was made.

A diagnostic intercostal nerve block was performed. This provided effective short-term symptomatic relief so a follow-up therapeutic block was done 3 weeks later. The therapeutic block comprised: 5ml 0.25% bupivicaine with 1/200,000 epinephrine & 2mg/ml triamcinolone injected at 3 sites above & below the affected rib; and 4ml 0.25% bupivicaine with 1/200,000 epinephrine & 1mg/ml triamcinolone injected under the scar site.

Though she did not return to gymnastics, her tiredness was resolved and she was able to begin soccer refereeing a week later. She was more energetic, happier and able to spend time with friends again. Her concentration and focus improved which enabled her to achieve better grades at school.

2.7 Case 7: A 9-year-old female with persistent pain following appendectomy

A 33kg 9-year-old female presented with right-sided abdominal pain, which had begun 3 days after a laparoscopic appendectomy two months previously. The pain, present all the time, but varying in intensity, was described as 'stabbing'. It was worse with activity and at the end of the day.

She had experienced disturbed sleep and was often woken by pain. She had only attended school for only three or four days since her surgery and was completely unable to attend her rhythmic gymnastics classes. Her appetite was reduced and her pain was worse after eating. She became anxious and this period of uncertainty was a tremendously stressful time for her whole family. Tramadol, ibuprofen and acetaminophen had not helped her pain.

A physical examination revealed a positive Carnett's test and normal bowel sounds. Her femoral pulses were present and equal. There was no lymphadenopathy in the inguinal region or neck and no organomegaly. There was no allodynia, no numbness and no skin colour change at the site of her pain. Pain was increased by squatting, walking, use of upper extremities and right leg raises. Right hip flexor function and ability to do sit-ups were limited by pain. She was diagnosed with abdominal wall pain secondary to surgery for laparoscopic appendectomy.

A diagnostic abdominal wall block was performed, which provided effective short-term symptomatic relief so a follow-up therapeutic block was performed two weeks later. The therapeutic block was administered on the right side using ultrasound control, with a 22-gauge IV cannula. A total of 10ml 0.25% bupivicaine with 2mg/ml triamcinolone was injected: 4ml into rectus sheath and 6ml between the transverse abdominus and internal oblique muscles.

On awakening she reported her right side was numb. She experienced an achy bruising pain for 36 hours, which settled down. She was soon able to return to normal sleeping, eating and activity levels. She returned to gymnastics within 3 weeks and was back to her previous level of activity within 2 months. She was significantly happier and quickly re-established her relationships with friends. She returned to school within 2 weeks and was back to a full timetable within a month.

2.8 Case 8: A 17-year-old female with rib pain

A 66kg 17-year-old female presented with a 6 month history of right-sided lower rib pain. It may have been caused by an injury incurred playing volleyball. She described it as a 'stabbing', burning pain that sometimes radiated to the back or the epigastrum. She had no pain-free days. The pain was worse at night, with deep-breathing and with sitting for long periods of time.

She experienced considerable difficulty maintaining a normal sleep balance: she had trouble getting to sleep and was woken at least once a night in pain, often for long periods. As a consequence, she was often very fatigued, which she felt made her pain worse. She had a reduced appetite in the morning and had stopped all sporting activities. She showed some signs of depression and isolated herself from friends and family. She struggled to concentrate and missed approximately 40% of school.

The Role of Peripheral Nerve Blocks in the Interdisciplinary Care of Children with Chronic Pain: A Case Series and Review of the Literature

117

A variety of therapies had been tried, including psychology, physiotherapy, acupuncture, TENS and two sessions with a chiropractor, but these had afforded only partial pain relief. Acetaminophen and non-steroidal anti-inflammatory agents were not effective. She obtained some relief from morphine, consuming up to 50mg each day. The presumed diagnosis was intercostal neuralgia.

A diagnostic intercostal nerve block was performed, which provided effective short term symptomatic relief so a follow-up therapeutic block was done three weeks later. For the therapeutic block, a total of 12ml 0.25% bupivicaine with 1/200,000 epinephrine was injected at 3 sites; one above & below and at the site of the affected rib on the right side.

This treatment allowed her to make a gradual return to normal. She began exercising again after 2 weeks, started sleeping deeper and longer and was generally in much better mood. She was able to sit and concentrate once again and resumed social activities with friends.

3. Discussion

3.1 Diagnosis and selection criteria for the use of peripheral nerve blocks

The cases described in this chapter demonstrate that, in properly selected children and adolescents, a peripheral nerve block can be an extremely beneficial component of interdisciplinary care. The case histories demonstrate the effective use of targeted nerve blocks for specific pain conditions such as ilioinguinal block for ilioinguinal neuralgia. The children and adolescents affected are often extremely physically active prior to the first reports of pain. They are usually previously fit and well with no previous pain or medical problems. There is typically an inciting event. The pain is characteristically neuropathic in description with sharp shooting elements and allodynia. The pain distribution is often dermatomal but not necessarily associated with numbness. The pain is not responsive or resolved with simple medications. The impact of the pain is considerable in its effects on physical function, schooling, mood and family dynamics.

3.2 Effective techniques in the use of peripheral nerve blocks

Peripheral nerve blockade in paediatric chronic pain has previously been described specifically for chronic abdominal wall pain (Skinner & Lauder, 2007). Due to the lack of evidence to guide therapy, the following recommendations are the opinion of the author (GL). Peripheral nerve blocks are done under sedation or general anesthesia to minimise further stress and pain to children and adolescents. Strict sterile procedure is followed. Plain local anaesthetic is used for the initial block to ensure that the diagnosis is correct prior to installation of steroids. Peripheral nerve blocks are done whenever possible under ultrasound control to maximise the chance of an effective block by ensuring the local anaesthetic is deposited in the correct plane or near the correct nerve. A diagnostic peripheral nerve block is considered to have worked if the local anaesthetic provided numbness in the dermatomal region to be blocked and also resulted in a clinically significant reduction in pain (>50% reduction). A therapeutic block is only performed after a positive diagnostic block. To achieve a therapeutic peripheral nerve block the same block is performed under ultrasound control with local anaesthetic and steroid (1-2mg/ml of trimcinolone to a maximum dose of 40mg). Peripheral nerve blocks are only offered if children and adolescents are willing to participate in the whole team approach with adherence to paced activity and integration with psychology. The duration of effect of a therapeutic block is extremely varied and may be related to time from diagnosis as well as to the degree in which paced return to activity is adhered to following successful block. Subsequent therapeutic blocks tend to last longer than the previous.

3.2.1 Pharmacology
The steroid element of the therapeutic peripheral nerve block is considered to either reduce inflammation or result in thinning of the connective tissue around painful nerves (Suleiman & Johnston, 2001). There is no consensus on the correct dose of steroid that should be used for peripheral nerve blocks in children. Steroids have local and systemic side effects. The local effect of fascial thinning may have detrimental effects with repeat injections (Suleiman & Johnston, 2001). Side effects of ongoing or chronic systemic steroids include carbohydrate intolerance, hypothalamic-pituitary-adrenal suppression, growth failure (Hochberg, 2002) and others such as immunosuppression, cataracts, pseudomotor cerebri, pancreatitis steroid psychosis, and steroid myopathy (Rimsza, 1978). The incidence of major systemic side effects to infrequent intermittent steroid injections is not known.

3.3 The mechanism and effects of the treatment
The specific effects of peripheral nerve blocks rely on the action of pharmacological agents such as local anaesthetics and triamcinolone. However, broader elements of care are also significant. In the context of an ongoing treatment regime, it is particularly important to consider the psychosocial dynamics of the diagnosis and treatment processes, including development of trust in the healthcare team and springboard effects from the realization of interim treatment goals. It is presumed that the combination of these effects creates/initiates a break or change in the pain cycle and reverses the changes that occurred within the peripheral and central nervous system to cause chronic pain.

3.3.1 Nonspecific treatment effects
We may like to think that when a patient gets better, it is the direct and intentional result of medical intervention, but it may not be quite so straightforward. Jamison (2011) identifies three mechanisms, which may contribute to any improvement in a patient's pain or functioning – (i) the specific or intended effects of any treatment, (ii) natural history and (iii) nonspecific effects of treatment – and there may be some interaction between these elements. Nonspecific treatment effects are the outcomes of patient encounters with healthcare providers. These include attention, stimulation of the desire to get better, reduced anxiety, increased understanding, trust, hope, optimism and improved ability to cope (Jamison, 2011). One important nonspecific treatment effect with children and adolescents is for others, including healthcare providers, to believe that they have pain. These non-specific treatment effects represent a complex array of psychosocial variables that, when utilized correctly, can bestow huge benefit to the patient's sense of wellbeing and outcomes.
The team's attention to the broader effects of pain on daily functioning and quality of life is crucial. What does the child's pain mean to them? What does it mean to their family? What are the patient goals of therapy and are they achievable? As discussed, psychosocial effects of pain such as sadness, frustration, anxiety or depression can become contributory factors to the continuation or worsening of pain in a vicious circle that is hard to escape without effective support. If they remain unrecognized and untreated, these factors may hinder the progress of any management plan.
It has been established that the style of communication adopted by a physician can have a dramatic effect on patient patient's health outcomes (Di Blasi et al, 2001; Griffin et al, 2004;

Verheul et al, 2010). Meaningful two-way communication between healthcare provider and patient is crucial. However, a patient-centred dialogue may depend on circumstances, as physicians appear to adopt a more patient-centred style of communication with patients who participate actively in the discussion (Cegala & Post, 2009). In paediatric care, the communication is, typically, three-way between provider, patient and parent or caregiver which makes adopting a patient-centred approach will often be more challenging. Effective communication, in this context, means using appropriate terminology and actively listening to both patient and parent as well as giving attention to their body language. Factors which have to be considered include: identifying patient and parental expectations, i.e. goal directed therapy; devoting enough time to acquire the whole pain-related history; interpreting non-responsiveness; identifying hidden messages conveyed in what's being said and not said; understanding family beliefs, hopes and fears; asking potentially embarrassing questions separately and in confidence; conveying empathy; introducing appropriate humour into the dialogue; conveying expertise and credibility in pain management; establishing trust; not causing more pain on examination; providing an agreed workable goal-directed and achievable management plan.

3.3.2 Placebo response to peripheral nerve block intervention

Without the evidence of a randomized double blind placebo controlled trial, it is not easy to stipulate that the interventional blocks are the overriding therapeutic modality in this case series. Many would argue that this represents a placebo response. A placebo response refers to the psychobiological response seen after administration of a placebo (a non therapeutic modality) in an individual or groups of patients. Placebo treatments have known effects on the endogenous pharmacology, cognitive and conditioning systems in humans (Fields & Levine, 1981; de la Fuente-Fernandez et al, 2001; Meissner et al, 2007; Wager et al, 2007; Benedetti, 2008; Scott et al, 2008; Eippert et al, 2009; Finniss et al, 2009).

Expectations have the strongest evidence for contributing to the placebo response, especially placebo analgesia. Within the neuro-pharmacological aspect of an analgesic placebo response, there is evidence for the role of endogenous endorphins as some placebo analgesic responses are reversed with naloxone. The respiratory centres, serotonin secretion, hormone secretion, immune responses and heart function are also involved in the biological response to placebo analgesic treatments (Finniss et al, 2009).

Whatever the mechanism of therapeutic benefit, placebo responses are potentially embedded in every intervention for pain relief (Robinson, 2009). The key message from our case series is that plain local anaesthetic nerve block provided only temporary relief for 7 out of 8 cases. Only when local anaesthetic and steroid was used, in conjunction with their ongoing interdisciplinary care, did these children and adolescents turn their lives around to their pre-pain level of functioning. If only a placebo response, it would be expected to last 1-3 months only. Only 2 of the cases required repeat therapeutic blocks which were performed greater than three months after the initial therapeutic block. This all points to a mainly therapeutic effect, but would have to be supported by a properly conducted study.

4. Conclusion

Chronic pain of childhood is an extremely complex condition which can have devastating effects on physical, psychological and social functioning. The interdisciplinary team management approach, based on pharmacology, physiotherapy and psychology, is the standard of care for children with severe or ongoing chronic pain. However, in a small proportion of appropriately selected children peripheral nerve blocks can provide immediate, effective and long-term pain relief. The case histories outlined in this chapter demonstrate the enormous impact that pain can have on a child, their functioning and their families. The significant relief received from peripheral nerve blockade indicates that this is a modality that must be considered when the history and examination findings match those presented. However, formal studies are required to definitively evaluate the effectiveness of the peripheral nerve block intervention.

5. Acknowledgement

The authors would like to thank UBC's *Pediatric Anesthesia Research Team* and the children and adolescents reported in this chapter for allowing us to detail their pain journey.

6. References

Abu-Saad Huijer, H. (2010) 'Chronic pain in children and adolscents: a review', *Lebanese Medical Journal*, Vol. 58, No. 2, pp. 105-10, ISSN 0023-9852

Altman, D. & Bland, J. (1995) 'Statistics notes: Absence of evidence is not evidence of absence', *British Medical Journal*, Vol. 311, No. 7003, p.485, ISSN 0007-1447

Arden, N., Price, C., Reading, I., Stubbing, J., Hazelgrove, J., Dunne, C., Michel, M., Rogers, P. & Cooper, C. (2005) 'A multicentre randomized controlled trial of epidural corticosteroid injections for sciatica: the WEST study', *Rheumatology* , Vol. 44, No. 11, pp. 1399-406, ISSN 1462-0324

Benedetti F. (2008) 'Mechanisms of placebo and placebo-related effects across diseases and treatments', *Annual Review of Pharmacology and Toxicology*, Vol. 48, pp. 33–60, ISSN 0362-1642

Birkholtz, M., Aylwin, L. & Harman, R. (2004) 'Activity pacing in chronic pain management: one aim, but which method? Part one: introduction and literature review', *British Journal of Occupational Therapy*, Vol. 67, No. 10, pp. 447-452, ISSN 0308-0226

Cegala, D. & Post, D. (2009) 'The impact of patients' participation on physicians' patient-centered communication', *Patient Education and Counseling*, Vol. 77, No. 2, pp. 202-8, ISSN 0738-3991

Chalkiadis, G. (2001) 'Management of chronic pain in children', *The Medical journal of Australia*, Vol. 175, No. 9, pp. 476-9, ISSN 0025-729X

Clouse, R., Mayer, E., Aziz, Q., Drossman, D., Dumitrascu, D., Mönnikes, H. & Naliboff, B. (2006) 'Functional abdominal pain syndrome', *Gastroenterology*, Vol. 130, No. 5, pp. 1492-7, ISSN 0016-5085

Cohen, L., Vowles, K. & Eccleston, C. (2010) 'The impact of adolescent chronic pain on functioning: disentangling the complex role of anxiety', *The Journal of Pain*, Vol. 11, No. 11, pp. 1039-46, ISSN 1526-5900

Crombie, I., Davies, H. & Macrae, W. (1998) 'Cut and thrust: antecedent surgery and trauma among patients attending a chronic pain clinic ', *Pain*, Vol. 76, No. 1-2, pp. 167-71, ISSN 0304-3959

de Blécourt, A., Schiphorst Preuper, H., Van Der Schans, C., Groothoff, J., Reneman, M. (2008) 'Preliminary evaluation of a multidisciplinary pain management program for children and adolescents with chronic musculoskeletal pain', *Disability and Rehabilitation*, Vol. 30, No. 1, pp. 13-20, ISSN 0963-8288

The Role of Peripheral Nerve Blocks in the Interdisciplinary Care of Children with Chronic Pain: A Case Series and Review of the Literature

121

de la Fuente-Fernandez, R., Ruth, T., Sossi, V., Schulzer, M., Calne, D. & Stoessl, A. (2001) 'Expectation and dopamine release: mechanism of the placebo effect in Parkinson's disease', *Science*, Vol. 293, No. 5532, pp.1164-6, ISSN 0036-8075

Di Blasi, Z., Harkness, E., Ernst, E. Georgiou, A. & Kleijnen, J. (2001) 'Influence of context on health outcomes: a systematic review', *The Lancet*, Vol. 357, No. 9258, pp. 757-62, ISSN 0140-6736

Dutta, S., Mehta, M. & Verma, I. (1999) 'Recurrent abdominal pain in Indian children and its relation with school and family environment', *Indian Pediatrics*, Vol. 36, No. 9, pp. 917-20, ISSN 0019-6061

Eccleston, C. (2001) 'Role of psychology in pain management', *British Journal of Anaesthesia*, Vol. 87, No. 1, pp. 144-52, ISSN 0007-0912

Eccleston, C., Malleson, P., Clinch, J., Connell, H. & Sourbut, C. (2003) 'Chronic pain in adolescents: evaluation of a programme of interdisciplinary cognitive behaviour therapy', *Archives of Disease in Childhood*, Vol. 88, No. 10, pp. 881–885, ISSN 0003-9888

Eccleston, C., Crombez, G., Scotford, A., Clinch, J. & Connell, H. (2004) 'Adolescent chronic pain: patterns and predictors of emotional distress in adolescents with chronic pain and their parents', *Pain*, Vol. 108, No. 3, pp. 221-229, ISSN 0304-3959

Eccleston, Z. & Eccleston, C. (2004) 'Interdisciplinary management of adolescent chronic pain: developing the role of physiotherapy', *Physiotherapy*, Vol. 90, No. 2, pp. 77-81, ISSN 0031-9406

Eccleston, C., Palermo, T., Williams, A., Lewandowski, A. & Morley, S. (2009) 'Psychological therapies for the management of chronic and recurrent pain in children and adolescents', *The Cochrane Database of Systematic Reviews*, Vol. 15, No. 2, CD003968, ISSN 1469-493X

Eippert, F., Bingel, U., Schoell, E., Yacubian, J., Klinger, R., Lorenz, J. & Büchel, C. (2009) 'Activation of the opioidergic descending pain control system underlies placebo analgesia', *Neuron*, Vol. 63, No. 4, pp. 533-43, ISSN 0896-6273

Fearon, P. & Hotopf, M. (2001) 'Relation between headache in childhood and physical and psychiatric symptoms in adulthood: national birth cohort study', *British Medical Journal*, Vol. 322, pp. 1145, ISSN 0959-8138

Fechir, M., Geber, C. & Birklein, F. (2008) 'Evolving understandings about complex regional pain syndrome and its treatment', *Current Pain and Headache Reports*, Vol. 12, No. 3, pp. 186-191, ISSN 1531-3433

Fields, H. & Levine, J. (1981) 'Biology of placebo analgesia', *The American Journal of Medicine*, Vol. 70, No. 4, pp. 745-6, ISSN 0002-9343

Fillingim, R., King, C., Ribeiro-Dasilva, M., Rahim-Williams, B. & Riley 3rd, J. (2009) 'Sex, gender, and pain: a review of recent clinical and experimental findings', *The Journal of Pain*, Vol. 10, No. 5, pp. 447-485, ISSN 1526-5900

Finniss, D., Nicholas, M. & Benedetti, F. (2009) 'Placebo analgesia - understanding the mechanisms and implications for clinical practice', *Reviews in Pain*, Vol. 3, No. 2, pp. 15-19

Ganesh, R., Arvind Kumar, R., Suresh, N. & Sathiyasekeran, M. (2010) 'Chronic abdominal pain in children', *The National Medical Journal of India*, Vol. 23, No. 2, pp. 94-9, ISSN 0970-258X

Gaul, C., Neundörfer, B. & Winterholler, M. (2005) 'Iatrogenic (para-) spinal abscesses and meningitis following injection therapy for low back pain', Pain, Vol. 116, No. 3, pp. 407-10, ISSN 0304-3959

Geurts, J., van Wijk, R., Wynne, H., Hammink, E., Buskens, E., Lousberg, R., Knape, J. & Groen, G. (2003) 'Radiofrequency lesioning of dorsal root ganglia for chronic lumbosacral radicular pain: a randomised, double-blind, controlled trial', *The Lancet*, Vol. 361, No. 9351, pp. 21-6, ISSN 0140-6736

Gold, J., Mahrer, N., Yee, J. & Palermo, T. (2009) 'Pain, fatigue and health-related quality of life in children and adolescents with chronic pain', *The Clinical Journal of Pain*, Vol. 25, No. 5, pp. 407-412, ISSN 0749-8047

Griffin, S. , Kinmonth, A., Veltman, M., Gillard, S., Grant, J. & Stewart, M. (2004) 'Effect on health-related outcomes of interventions to alter the interaction between patients and practitioners: a systematic review of trials', *Annals of Family Medicine*, Vol. 2, No. 6, pp. 595-608, ISSN 1544-1709

Grøholt, E., Stigum, H., Nordhagen, R. & Köhler, L. (2003) 'Recurrent pain in children, socio-economic factors and accumulation in families', *European Journal of Epidemiology*, Vol. 18, No. 10, pp. 965-75, ISSN 0393-2990

Harding, V. & Williams, A. (1998) 'Activities training: Integrating behavioural and cognitive methods with physiotherapy in pain management', *Journal of Occupational Rehabilitation*, Vol. 8, No. 1, pp. 47-60, ISSN 1053-0487

Hochberg, Z. (2002) 'Mechanisms of steroid impairment of growth', *Hormone Research*, Vol. 58, Suppl. 1, pp. 33–38, ISSN 0301-0163

Huguet, A. & Miró, J. (2008) 'The severity of chronic pediatric pain: an epidemiological study', *The Journal of Pain*, Vol. 9, No. 3, pp. 226-36, ISSN 1526-5900

Hyams, J., Burke, G., Davis, P., Rzepski, B. & Andrulonis, P. (1996) 'Abdominal pain and irritable bowel syndrome in adolescents: a community-based study', *The Journal of Pediatrics*, Vol. 129, No. 2, pp. 220-6, ISSN 0022-3476

International Association for the Study of Pain (1986) 'Pain terms: a current list with definitions and notes on usage', *Pain*, Vol. 24, Supplement 1, pp. S215-21, ISSN 0167-6482

Jamison, R. (2011) 'Nonspecific treatment effects in pain medicine', *Pain Clinical Updates*, Vol. 19, No. 2, pp. 1-7, ISSN 1083-0707

Jensen, M. (2011) 'Psychosocial approaches to pain management: an organisational framework', *Pain*, Vol. 152, No. 4, pp. 717-725, ISSN 0304-3959

Kachko, L., Efrat, R., Ben Ami, S., Mukamel, M. & Katz, J. (2008) 'Complex regional pain syndromes in children and adolescents', *Pediatrics International*, Vol. 50, No. 4, pp. 523-7, ISSN 1328-8067

Kehlet, H., Jensen, T. & Woolf C. (2006) 'Persistent postsurgical pain: risk factors and prevention', Lancet. 2006, Vol. 367, No. 9522, pp. 1618-25, ISSN 0140-6736

Lee, B., Scharff, L., Sethna, N., McCarthy, C., Scott-Sutherland, J., Shea, A., Sullivan, P., Meier, P., Zurakowski, D., Masek, B. & Berde, C. (2002) 'Physical therapy and cognitive behavioural treatment for complex regional pain syndromes', *Journal of Pediatrics*, Vol. 141, No. 1, pp. 135-40, ISSN 0022-3476

Lewandowski, A., Palermo, T., Stinson, J., Handley, S. & Chambers, C. (2010) 'Systematic review of family functioning in families of children and adolescents with chronic pain', *The Journal of Pain*, Vol. 11, No. 11, pp. 1027-38, ISSN 1526-5900

Logan, D., Simons, L., Stein, M. & Chastain, L. (2008) 'School impairment in adolescents with chronic pain', *The Journal of Pain*, Vol. 9, No. 5, pp. 407-416, ISSN 1526-5900

Lynch, A., Kashikar-Zuck, S., Goldschneider, K. & Jones, B. (2006) 'Psychosocial risks for disability in children with chronic back pain', *The Journal of Pain*, Vol . 7, No. 4, pp. 244-51, ISSN 1526-5900

Macrae, W. (2008) 'Chronic post-surgical pain: 10 years on', *British Journal of Anaesthesia*, Vol. 101, No. 1, pp. 77-86, ISSN 0007-0912

Mailis-Gagnon, A., Yegneswaran, B., Nicholson, K., Lakha, S., Papagapiou, M., Steiman, A., Ng, D., Cohodarevic, T., Umana, M. & Zurowski, M. (2007) 'Ethnocultural and sex characteristics of patients attending a tertiary care pain clinic in Toronto, Ontario', *Pain Research & Management*, Vol. 12, No. 2, pp. 100-6, ISSN 1203-6765

Manchikanti, L., Singh, V., Falco, F., Cash, K. & Pampati, V. (2010) 'Evaluation of lumbar facet joint nerve blocks in managing chronic low back pain: a randomized, double-blind, controlled trial with a 2-year follow-up', *International Journal of Medical Sciences*, Vol. 7, No. 3, pp. 124-35, ISSN 1449-1907

Martin, A., McGrath, P., Brown, S. & Katz, J. (2007) 'Children with chronic pain: impact of sex and age on long-term outcomes', *Pain*, Vol. 128, No. 1-2, pp. 13-9, ISSN 0304-3959

McGrath, P. & Holahan, A-L. (2003) 'Psychological Interventions with children and adolescents: evidence for their effectiveness in treating chronic pain', *Seminars in Pain Medicine*, Vol. 1, No. 2, pp. 99-109, ISSN 1537-5897

Meissner, K., Distel, H. & Mitzdorf, U. (2007) 'Evidence for placebo effects on physical but not on biochemical outcome parameters: a review of clinical trials', *BMC Medicine*, Vol. 5, No. 3, ISSN 1741-7015

Palermo, T. (2000) 'Impact of recurrent and chronic pain on child and family daily functioning: a critical review of the literature', *Developmental and Behavioral Pediatrics*, Vol. 21, No. 1, pp. 58-69, ISSN 0196-206X

Peng, P. & Castano, E. (2005) 'Survey of chronic pain practice by anaesthesiologists in Canada', *Canadian Journal of Anesthesia*, Vol. 52, No. 4, pp. 383-9, ISSN 0832-610X

Peng, P., Stinson, J., Choiniere, M. & Dion, D. (2007) 'Dedicated multidisciplinary pain management centres for children in Canada: the current status', *Canadian Journal of Anesthesia*, Vol. 54, No. 12, pp. 985-91, ISSN 0832-610X

Perquin, C., Hazebroek-Kampschreur, A., Hunfeld, J., Bohnen, A., van Suijlekom-Smit, L., Passchier, J. & van der Wouden, J. (2000) 'Pain in children and adolescents: a common experience', *Pain*, Vol. 87, No. 1, pp. 51-8, ISSN 0304-3959

Poleshuck, E., Katz, J., Andrus, C., Hogan, L., Jung, B., Kulick, D. & Dworkin, R. (2006) 'Risk factors for chronic pain following breast cancer surgery: a prospective study', *The Journal of Pain*, Vol. 7, No. 9, pp. 626-34, ISSN 1526-5900.

Poobalan, A., Bruce, J., Smith, W., King, P., Krukowski, Z., Chambers, W. (2003) 'A review of chronic pain after inguinal herniorrhaphy', The Clinical Journal of Pain, Vol. 19, No. 1, pp. 48-54, ISSN 0749-8047

Ramage-Morin, P. & Gilmour H. (2010) 'Chronic pain at ages 12 to 44', *Health reports / Statistics Canada* , Vol. 21, No. 4, pp 53-61, ISSN 0840-6529

Rimsza, M. (1978) 'Complications of corticosteroid therapy', *American Journal of Diseases of Children*, Vol. 132, No. 8, pp. 806–810, ISSN 0002-922X

Robinson, M. (2009) 'Placebo analgesia: Widening the scope of measured influences', *Pain*, Vol. 144, No. 1-2, pp. 5-6, ISSN 0304-3959

Roth-Isigkeit, A., Thyen, U,. Stöven, H., Schwarzenberger, J. & Schmucker, P. (2005) 'Pain among children and adolescents: restrictions in daily living and triggering factors', *Pediatrics*, Vol. 115, No. 2, pp. 152-62, ISSN 0031-4005

Schurman, J. & Friesen, C. (2010) 'Integrative treatment approaches: family satisfaction with a multidisciplinary paediatric Abdominal Pain Clinic', *International Journal of Integrated Care*, Vol. 10, July-Sept2010, pp. 1-9, ISSN 1568-4156

Scott, D., Stohler, C., Egnatuk, C., Wang, H., Koeppe, R. & Zubieta, J. (2008) 'Placebo and nocebo effects are defined by opposite opioid and dopaminergic responses', *Archives of General Psychiatry*, Vol. 65, No. 2, pp. 220–31, ISSN 0003-990X

Simopoulos, T., Kraemer, J., Nagda, J., Aner, M. & Bajwa, Z. (2008) 'Response to pulsed and continuous radiofrequency lesioning of the dorsal root ganglion and segmental nerves in patients with chronic lumbar radicular pain', *Pain Physician*, Vol. 11, No. 2, pp. 137-44, ISSN 1533-3159

Skinner, A. & Lauder, G. (2007) 'Rectus sheath block: successful use in the chronic pain management of pediatric abdominal wall pain', *Paediatric Anaesthesia*, Vol. 17, No. 12, pp. 1203-11, ISSN 1155-5645

Sleed, M., Eccleston, C., Beecham, J., Knapp, M. & Jordan, A. (2005) 'The economic impact of chronic pain in adolescence: Methodological considerations and a preliminary costs-of-illness study', *Pain*, Vol. 119, pp. 183-190, ISSN 0304-3959

Suleiman, S. & Johnston, D. (2001) 'The Abdominal Wall: An Over- looked Source of Pain', *American Family Physician*, Vol. 64, No. 3, pp. 431–438, ISSN 0002-838X

Tough, E., White, A., Richards, S. & Campbell, J. (2007) 'Variability of criteria used to diagnose myofascial trigger point pain syndrome--evidence from a review of the literature', *The Clincal Journal of Pain*, Vol. 23, No. 3, pp. 278-86, ISSN 0749-8047

Tsao, J., Meldrum, M., Kim, S. & Zeltzer, L. (2007) 'Anxiety sensitivity and health-related quality of life in children with chronic pain', *The Journal of Pain*, Vol. 8, No. 10, pp. 814-23, ISSN 1526-5900

Turk, D. & Okifuji, A. (2001). 'Pain terms and taxonomies' In: *Bonica's Management of Pain*, Loeser, D. (ed.), 3rd edn., pp. 18–25, Lippincott Williams & Wilkins, ISBN 0683304623

van Dijk, A., McGrath, P., Pickett, W. & VanDenKerkhof, E. (2006) 'Pain prevalence in nine- to 13-year-old schoolchildren', *Pain Research & Management*, Vol. 11, No. 4, pp.234-40, ISSN 1203-6765

Varni, J., Seid, M. & Kurtin, P. (2001) 'PedsQL 4.0: reliability and validity of the Pediatric Quality of Life Inventory version 4.0 generic core scales in healthy and patient populations', *Medical Care*, Vol. 39, No. 8, pp. 800-12, ISSN 0025-7079

Verheul, W., Sanders, A. & Bensing, J. (2010) 'The effects of physicians' affect-oriented communication style and raising expectations on analogue patients' anxiety, affect and expectancies', *Patient Education and Counseling*, Vol. 80, No. 3, pp. 300-6, ISSN 0738-3991

Vetter, T. (2008) 'A clinical profile of a cohort of patients referred to an anesthesiology-based pediatric chronic pain medicine program', *Anesthesia and Analgesia*, Vol. 106, No. 3, pp. 786-94, ISSN 0003-2999

Vinik, A. (2010) 'The approach to the management of the patient with neuropathic pain', *The Journal of Clinical Endocrinology and Metabolism*, Vol. 95, No. 11, pp. 4802-11, ISSN 0021-972X

Wager, T., Scott, D. & Zubieta, J-K. (2007) 'Placebo effects on human μ-opioid activity during pain', *Proceedings of the National Academy of Sciences of the USA*, Vol. 104, No. 26, pp.11056-61, ISSN 0027-8424

Walker, L., Dengler-Crish, C., Rippel, S. & Bruehl, S. (2010) 'Functional abdominal pain in childhood and adolescence increases risk for chronic pain in adulthood', *Pain*, Vol. 150, No. 3, pp. 568-72, ISSN 0304-3959

5

Psychological Strategies in Pain Management: Optimizing Procedures in Clinics

FuZhou Wang
Department of Anesthesiology and Critical Care Medicine,
The Affiliated Nanjing Maternity and Child Health Care Hospital,
Nanjing Medical University, Nanjing,
China

1. Introduction

Pain is the most awful sensory suffering that makes people exhausted. Although pain itself possesses protective role in keeping patients from further injury, it is still obliged to be treated for its negative effect on patients' physiological and psychological well-beings. Great progress has been made in our understanding of the therapeutic strategies with different agents and techniques on pain in the past decades, but the analgesic result is not as effective as we desired specifically when the acute process tends to be chronic (Li et al., 2011). As one of the important parts of somatosensory system, pain nets closely with spiritual and psychological feelings, which often results in analgesic failure when conventional pharmacological methods and means are used, and also raises questions on how to alleviate pain through psychotherapeutics (Manchikanti et al., 2011). Given the big difference in methods of psychological interventions and the association with the changing therapeutic context, the analgesic efficacy of psychosocial support fluctuates. Therefore, standardizing and optimizing the psychotherapeutic strategies in clinical practice would make it more effective in relieving pain. Here we review and prospect the psychological management of pain, and then give a recommendation of the therapeutic flow of the standardized optimal procedures.

2. Origins of psychological analgesia

Two hundreds years ago, the word "placebo" was defined by Robert Hooper in his dictionary to a more modern medical meaning as "any medicine adapted more to please than benefit the patient" (Hooper, 1811). In fact, this is the original description of psychological intervention in the field of medicine of which the meaning is broadened further during the following years. However, placebo therapies were becoming popular until the past century. To date, placebo medicine generally means (i) containing pharmacologically inactive ingredients, and (ii) the contents have pharmacological activity. The effect of placebo is mainly dependent on the psychological state of patients, therapeutic context and physicians' console. In contrast to placebo, nocebo was adapted to describe the negative effect (i.e. unpleasant consequence) occurs in expectation of a harmful occurrence when an inert substance was used. In pain medicine, both placebo and nocebo are also two majorities that can be used in psychological intervention. Therefore, psychological placebo (positive) or psychological nocebo (negative) are derived from the traditional conceptions of placebo or nocebo. Although the key patterns of psychological therapy is on the basis of the linguistic console from physicians or investigators, psychological analgesia with series of strategies of psychology is the result of the above-mentioned placebo or nocebo.

3. Mechanisms of psychological analgesia

Psychological analgesia is a broad concept that includes all aspects referring to the psychological intervention. Hypnosis, music therapy, preoperative education, and linguistic suggestion all belong to psychological approaches in pain control (Hobson et al., 2006; Patterson et al., 2010; Sen et al., 2010; Wang et al., 2008). Whatever psychological methods used in analgesia, common neurophysiological mechanisms exist and different models explain its function.

Functional magnetic resonance imaging (fMRI) verified an increase in neural activity during placebo associated psychological stimulation that is related to two major pain modulation mechanisms (Craggs et al., 2008): i) affective regulation which includes activation of the rostral anterior cingulate cortex, bilateral amygdala, and medial prefrontal cortex; and ii) higher cognitive regulation during which the posterior cingulate, pre-cuneus, rostral anterior cingulate cortex, perihippocampal gyrus, and the temporal lobes are activated. As the "gate theory" described that afferent inhibition blocks ascending signals from the periphery, psychological stimuli at the early period produce analgesic effect through a self-reinforcing feedback mechanism (Vase et al., 2005).

Several models give an in-depth understanding of the psychological stimulation associated analgesia. Conditioning, expectancy, motivation, and emotion are four psychological mediators involving in the process of analgesia. Conditioning model says that the interventional effect presented when the individual without knowing the stimulation would be and this process would not produce cognition (Williams & Rhudy, 2007). In this model, the perception of pain after psychological treatment largely depends on the learning history of the individual which determines the response variability under different context. The psychological conditioning as well as the verbal suggestion can turn tactile stimuli into pain and low-intensity pain into high-intensity pain. For this, the direct evidence was the conditioned pain reduction could be absolutely removed when the psychological stimuli were explained (Montgomery & Kirsch, 1997). Originally, conditioning is the primary response to psychological analgesia. Following conditioning, expectancy of the psychological stimuli to produce an effective analgesia takes place. Once the patients expect to have an improvement in pain management, the effect of psychological analgesia would play its role. Due to anxiety and fear to pain, patients generally want to have rapid and effective methods that can relieve their pain (Cornally & McCarthy, 2011; den Hollander et al., 2010; Kennedy et al., 2011), which consequently leads to an expectancy of their pain therapies. Under this condition, physicians' attitude and enthusiasm takes an important part in whether or not the psychological analgesia comes into play (Weintraub, 2005). Give patients the hope to conquer pain accompanying with a warmth care, the expected effect of psychological analgesia would be maximized. After expectancy, motivation of analgesia is another aspect in determining the effect of psychological interventions. If the patient desires for a relief of pain, the real analgesic role of psychological stimuli would be magnitude (Radat & Koleck, 2011). The motivation itself whether or not could predict the psychological effect on one type of pain needs to be explored at length, and could it be effective for different types of pain is also yet to be guaranteed. A body of literature has confirmed the role of emotions in pain perception and alleviation. Anxiety and stress are two main factors of emotion-associated psychological mediator. It is believed that anxiety is the cause of increased levels of pain, and reduction in anxiety produces analgesia (Luciano et al., 2011). Stress sometimes is related with increased levels of pain, but in some contexts, stress can produce analgesia (Donello et al., 2011; Wang et al., 2008). Therefore, the purpose of psychological suggestion in pain control is to alleviate patients' anxiety and stress, which in turn produces a feedback analgesia effect.

As described in the general model of the placebo-associated psychological analgesia, three consecutive stages exist when psychological treatment was given: the induction, psychophysiological mediation, and actualization (Goffaux et al., 2010). In the induction stage, three aspects compose the major contents including the introduction or initiation (therapeutic message; method of administration; follow-up and booster sessions; assessment of side effects), idiosyncratic variables (beliefs and values; personal history; innate predisposition) and therapeutic context (treatment objectives; therapeutic alliance; sociocultural factors). In the second stage, psychophysiological mediation composes of psychological and biological mechanisms. Psychological mechanisms include above-mentioned conditioning, expectancy, motivation, and emotion, and the biological mechanisms include neurochemical mediators (endorphins, dopamine, and other neurotransmitters/neuromodulators) and neurophysiology (activation of central modulatory mechanisms including descending inhibitory circuits). In the actualization stage, three main aspects exist including subjective experience (pain, emotions, quality of life, satisfaction, and related relief), behavioral markers (amount of analgesics consumed and overt pain behaviors), and physiological markers (physiological nociceptive activity, objective clinical indicators). As thus, when a psychological intervention is given, these three stages would be experienced. However, in consideration of the multiple phases of these stages, the actual effect of psychological analgesia may be variable in different individuals under different circumstances.

4. Efficacy of psychological analgesia

The analgesic effect of psychological approaches depends on types of pain, individual status, caregivers' attitude and contextual frame, which finally determines the efficacy of psychological analgesia. For postoperative pain, preoperative hypnosis could accelerate wound healing and alleviate pain intensity after mammoplasty (Ginandes et al., 2003), and reduce post-surgical pain and distress in patients undergone excisional breast biopsy (Schnur et al., 2008). However, in other surgical contexts, psychological interventions did not produce detectable difference compared with the control: relaxation training for spinal surgeries could not reduce postoperative pain (Gavin et al., 2006), and intraoperative music therapy also could not produce analgesia in Cesarean patients (Reza et al., 2007). Contrary to this, postoperative music can alleviate the pain and reduce the need for analgesics in patients who undergone Cesarean section (Ebneshahidi & Mohseni, 2008). Besides, in cardiac surgeries, music therapy produced effective role in alleviating anxiety and pain (Sendelbach et al., 2006). These different even controversial results raise questions on the real analgesia efficacy of psychological interventions. In fact, difference in interventional methods, types of surgeries, and professionals of investigators may all contribute to the changeable results of psychological analgesia. An attractive study performed to observe the influence of linguistic suggestion on postoperative pain management after abdominal surgeries, and found that negative words from nursing professionals results in therapeutic failure of patient-controlled analgesia, and suggested that a trusting psychological relationship between medical caregivers and patients should be established (Wang et al., 2008). Therefore, it is necessary to seek a standardized effective psychological method that can be employed at any time to alleviate pain and pain-associated psychological contributors.

Chronic pain, due to its multi-original property and hypo-responsiveness to traditional analgesics, is a complex pathological condition that needs to be cared with specific concentration. How to predict psychological problems in patients with chronic pain and then to take steps to overcome them plays pivotal role in alleviating this kind of pain. Modified Somatic Perception, Zung Questionnaires and Catastrophizing Scale are major means in predicting possible psychological factors in patients with chronic pain (Mannion et al., 1996; Meyer et al., 2008). These tools can help to identify psychological problems at early period that is crucial for understanding the development of acute pain into chronic and also possibly preventing its chronicity. Several studies considered psychological factors are contributors to patients' chronicity, but others did not find such a relationship (Roth et al., 2011a; Roth et al., 2011b; Roth et al., 2011c; Wallin et al., 2011; Xu et al., 2011). Various results in different studies questioned the real analgesic effect of psychological approaches in chronic pain management. Also, seek an optimized psychological procedure in chronic pain management is necessary for pain physicians.

5. Optimizing psychological analgesic procedure

Difference in methods of psychological interventions makes it difficult to reach a standardized uniform procedure that could be used for each individual at different pathological conditions. No matter what kind of methods employed, following four aspects are constant and also can be the interventional entry points: types of pain, individual expectancy status, therapeutic context, and professional level of physicians. Therefore, standardized psychological approach in analgesia should be based on these four factors. Besides, an optimized interventional flow of psychological analgesia from induction to performance to completion also will be standardized.

How to standardize the types of pain is so difficult because of its property of multiple originalities plus difference in its duration, intensity and responsiveness to pharmacological analgesics. To have a clear description and avoid an extra complexity of the standardization of the psychological procedure in the types of pain, here two major types of pain, acute and chronic, are discussed. First, acute pain is relatively easier to treat and generally resulted from traceable causes. So herein the acute pain is standardized on the basis of postoperative pain: surgical procedures → tissue injury → afferent fibers activation → dorsal root ganglion → spinal cord dorsal horn → ascending modulatory tracts → hypothalamus → cerebral cortex. However, chronic pain is refractory to pharmacological treatments and without assured causes. Here the standardization is based on chronic low back pain: regional chronic injury → persistent activation of peripheral fibers → spinal sensitization → reduction in pain threshold → activation of multiple brain regions. Although acute pain and chronic pain have different transduction pathways, they finally reach brain and then the perception is occur. This is the basis of the standardization when it is treated with psychological approaches.

Individual expectancy status is the second factor that needs to be standardized. Every one expects to have an effective method that can conquer the pain because of the unpleasant experience. Once a patient has such a hope, the psychological analgesia would play its role. However the psychological complexity makes people doubt the real efficacy of the analgesia. Therefore, give a timely psychological intervention along with patients' expectancy is the best way for analgesia through matching their different time windows. Under this condition, careful assessment of patients' psychological status with proper means would give physicians more information on what, how and when a psychological stimulation could be employed. In fact, psychological intervention if given appropriately at this moment exactly fills patients' psychological gap. If want take effective steps to control the pain, time communication with patients is the guarantee. So, the following flow is recommended: talk to confirm the expectancy → predisposition for psychological intervention → psychological preparation → increase confidence of conquering.

Therapeutic context is the environment where the patients go and seek for pain management. Whether clinics could provide proper and humanistic care or not determines the final conclusion of psychological analgesia. Due to big difference in the contextual background, it is hard to standardize the consulting environment. Here just give a proposal that should at least be followed when administering psychological interventions for pain control: i) avoiding negative stimuli; ii) establishing a warm setting; iii) patient-centered communication; iv) one-stop services. A trusting relationship between medical environment and patients could pave the way to a successful analgesia with psychological approaches.

Professional level of physician is the "software" that needs to be updated step by step and improved gradually with practice. Of course, personal morality is another crucial part that can give patients the "be-taken-seriously" feeling. Further, if the physician trained in psychological treatment, such professional knowledge in psychology would make the psychological analgesia more effective, and would produce the best efficacy in alleviating pain. This section, in fact, is the easiest one that can be improved after training and practice. Following is the suggestion on how to get better results in psychological analgesia: i) take patients' claim into heart; ii) build friend relationship with patients; iii) serve with the best professional knowledge; iv) psycho-language communication; v) unchangeable attitude and performance.

The changing window of man's mind is wide, and it is so easy to change when each above-mentioned part cannot satisfy the expectancy. Besides, the prone-to-be-broken psychological state would be shattered by improper intervention. Therefore, patients with different types of pain have various expectancy of analgesia that needs to be treated with optimal psychological procedures even at different clinics.

When performing psychological analgesia, following three-step procedure should be referred to. First step, induction: i) communicate without hint of psychological intervention; ii) confirm patient's psychological state; iii) predict patient's expectancy; iv) increase confidence that is bound to succeed. After this, the next step should be followed without interruption, i.e. performance: i) select a relatively quiet environment; ii) build a kind talking ambient; iii) give personalized linguistic intervention; iv) choose an interesting topic; v) talk without constraint; vi) observe psychological change during talking; vii) fine regulation in communication strategies. Following these procedures, the whole process of psychological intervention needs to be finalized, namely completion: i) conclude what have been talked; ii) thank patient's patience; iii) assess pain intensity with appropriate tools. Application of psychological linguistic suggestion should not be similar for one person at different visits, and the communicating environment should be changed time after time. The schematic flow of psychological intervention is presented in the Figure 1.

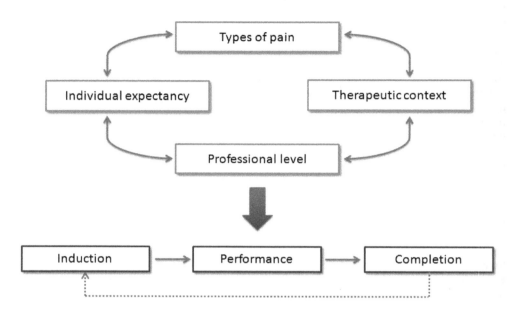

Fig. 1. Schematic flow of psychological analgesia.

6. Concluding remarks

Psychological activity is a complex emotional response that can be influenced by many factors. Psychological analgesia itself, however, is so complex that its efficacy is uncertain for different types of pain at different conditions. Therefore, how to select interventional methods and how to perform them for different patients with various psychological states is a thorny problem. Although here the optimized procedure of psychological analgesia is presented, it is necessary to be changed for different patients under different contextual conditions. Also this recommendation should favor the improvement of psychological intervention in pain management in future work.

7. References

Cornally, N. & McCarthy, G. (2011) Help-seeking behaviour for the treatment of chronic pain. *Br J Community Nurs* 16(2): 90-98.

Craggs, J.G.; Price, D.D.; Perlstein, W.M.; Verne, G.N. & Robinson, M.E. (2008) The dynamic mechanisms of placebo induced analgesia: Evidence of sustained and transient regional involvement. *Pain* 139(3): 660-669.

den Hollander, M.; de Jong, J.R.; Volders, S.; Goossens, M.E.; Smeets, R.J. & Vlaeyen, J.W. (2010) Fear reduction in patients with chronic pain: a learning theory perspective. *Expert Rev Neurother* 10(11): 1733-1745.

Donello, J.E.; Guan, Y.; Tian, M.; Cheevers, C.V.; Alcantara, M.; Cabrera, S.; Raja, S.N. & Gil, D.W. (2011) A peripheral adrenoceptor-mediated sympathetic mechanism can transform stress-induced analgesia into hyperalgesia. *Anesthesiology* 114(6): 1403-1416.

Ebneshahidi, A. & Mohseni, M. (2008) The effect of patient-selected music on early postoperative pain, anxiety, and hemodynamic profile in cesarean section surgery. *J Altern Complement Med* 14(7): 827-831.

Gavin, M.; Litt, M.; Khan, A.; Onyiuke, H. & Kozol, R. (2006) A prospective, randomized trial of cognitive intervention for postoperative pain. *Am Surg* 72(5): 414-418.

Ginandes, C.; Brooks, P.; Sando, W.; Jones, C. & Aker, J. (2003) Can medical hypnosis accelerate post-surgical wound healing? Results of a clinical trial. *Am J Clin Hypn* 45(4): 333-351.

Goffaux, P.; Léonard, G.; Marchand, S. & Rainville, P. (2010) Placebo analgesia. In: Beaulieu, P., Lussier, D., Porreca, F., Dickenson, A.H. (eds). *Pharmacology of Pain*. IASP Press, Seattle, pp. 451-473.

Hobson, J.A.; Slade, P.; Wrench, I.J. & Power, L. (2006) Preoperative anxiety and postoperative satisfaction in women undergoing elective caesarean section. *Int J Obstet Anesth* 15(1): 18-23.

Hooper, R. (1811) Quincy's Lexicon-Medicum. *A New Medical Dictionary*. London.

Kennedy, C.E.; Moore, P.J.; Peterson, R.A.; Katzman, M.A.; Vermani, M. & Charmak, W.D. (2011) What makes people anxious about pain? How personality and perception combine to determine pain anxiety responses in clinical and non-clinical populations. *Anxiety Stress Coping* 24(2): 179-200.

Li, A.; Montaño, Z.; Chen, V.J. & Gold, J.I. (2011) Virtual reality and pain management: current trends and future directions. *Pain Manag* 1(2): 147-157.

Luciano, J.V.; Martínez, N.; Peñarrubia-María, M.T.; Fernández-Vergel, R.; García-Campayo, J.; Verduras, C.; Blanco, M.E.; Jiménez, M.; Ruiz, J.M.; López del Hoyo, Y.; Serrano-Blanco, A. & FibroQoL Study Group. (2011) Effectiveness of a psychoeducational treatment program implemented in general practice for fibromyalgia patients: a randomized controlled trial. *Clin J Pain* 27(5): 383-391.

Manchikanti, L.; Giordano, J.; Fellows, B. & Hirsch, J.A. (2011) Placebo and nocebo in interventional pain management: a friend or a foe-or simply foes? *Pain Physician* 14(2): E157-E175.

Mannion, A.F.; Dolan, P. & Adams, M.A. (1996) Psychological questionnaires: do "abnormal" scores precede or follow first-time low back pain? *Spine (Phila Pa 1976)* 21(22): 2603-2611.

Meyer, K.; Sprott, H. & Mannion, A.F. (2008) Cross-cultural adaptation, reliability, and validity of the German version of the Pain Catastrophizing Scale. *J Psychosom Res* 64(5): 469-478.

Montgomery, G.H. & Kirsch, I. (1997) Classical conditioning and the placebo effect. *Pain* 72(1-2): 107-113.

Patterson, D.R.; Jensen, M.P.; Wiechman, S.A. & Sharar, S.R. (2010) Virtual reality hypnosis for pain associated with recovery from physical trauma. *Int J Clin Exp Hypn* 58(3): 288-300.

Radat, F. & Koleck, M. (2011) Pain and depression: Cognitive and behavioural mediators of a frequent association. *Encephale* 37(3): 172-179.

Reza, N.; Ali, S.M.; Saeed, K.; Abul-Qasim, A. & Reza, T.H. (2007) The impact of music on postoperative pain and anxiety following cesarean section. *Middle East J Anesthesiol* 19(3): 573-586.

Roth, R.S.; Punch, M. & Bachman, J.E. (2011a) Psychological Factors in Chronic Pelvic Pain due to Endometriosis: A Comparative Study. *Gynecol Obstet Invest* In press.

Roth, R.S.; Punch, M.R. & Bachman, J.E. (2011b) Patient beliefs about pain diagnosis in chronic pelvic pain: relation to pain experience, mood and disability. *J Reprod Med* 56(3-4): 123-129.

Roth, R.S.; Punch, M.R. & Bachman, J.E. (2011c) Psychological factors and chronic pelvic pain in women: a comparative study with women with chronic migraine headaches. *Health Care Women Int* 32(8): 746-761.

Schnur, J.B.; Bovbjerg, D.H.; David, D.; Tatrow, K.; Goldfarb, A.B.; Silverstein, J.H.; Weltz, C.R. & Montgomery, G.H. (2008) Hypnosis decreases presurgical distress in excisional breast biopsy patients. *Anesth Analg* 106(2): 440-444.

Sen, H.; Yanarateş, O.; Sızlan, A.; Kılıç, E.; Ozkan, S. & Dağlı, G. (2010) The efficiency and duration of the analgesic effects of musical therapy on postoperative pain. *Agri* 22(4): 145-150.

Sendelbach, S.E.; Halm, M.A.; Doran, K.A.; Miller, E.H. & Gaillard, P. (2006) Effects of music therapy on physiological and psychological outcomes for patients undergoing cardiac surgery. *J Cardiovasc Nurs* 21(3): 194-200.

Vase, L.; Robinson, M.E.; Verne, G.N. & Price, D.D. (2005) Increased placebo analgesia over time in irritable bowel syndrome (IBS) patients is associated with desire and expectation but not endogenous opioid mechanisms. *Pain* 115(3): 338-347.

Wallin, M.; Liedberg, G.; Börsbo, B. & Gerdle, B. (2011) Thermal detection and pain thresholds but not pressure pain thresholds are correlated with psychological factors in women with chronic whiplash-associated pain. *Clin J Pain* In press.

Wang, F.; Shen, X.; Xu, S.; Liu, Y.; Ma, L.; Zhao, Q.; Fu, D.; Pan, Q.; Feng, S. & Li, X. (2008) Negative words on surgical wards result in therapeutic failure of patient-controlled analgesia and further release of cortisol after abdominal surgeries. *Minerva Anestesiol* 74(7-8): 353-365.

Weintraub, M.I. (2003) Complementary and alternative methods of treatment of neck pain. *Phys Med Rehabil Clin N Am* 14(3): 659-674.

Williams, A.E. & Rhudy, J.L. (2007) The influence of conditioned fear on human pain thresholds: does preparedness play a role? *J Pain* 8(7): 598-606.

Xu, W.H.; Guo, C.B.; Wu, R.G. & Ma, X.C. (2011) Investigation of the Psychological Status of 162 Female TMD Patients with Different Chronic Pain Severity. *Chin J Dent Res* 14(1): 53-57.

Part 2

Cancer Pain

6

Radiation Mucositis

P. S. Satheesh Kumar
Department of Oral Medicine and Radiology,
Government Dental College, Trivandrum, Kerala
India

1. Introduction

Mucosal injury remains an undesirable, painful, and expensive side effect of cytotoxic cancer therapy and is disheartening for patients and frustrating for caregivers.[1,2] Mucositis and associated outcomes in patients receiving radiotherapy (RT) for head and neck cancer shows that the mean incidence was 80%.[3] Rates of hospitalization due to mucositis are reported to be 16% overall and 32% for RT-AF (altered fraction radio therapy) patients.[3 Patients in the high risk of developing oral mucositis group fall into the head and neck cancer population where the incidence of mucositis is high in this group.[3]

Oral mucositis is a distressing toxic effect of chemotherapy and radiotherapy. It can increase the need for total parenteral nutrition and opioids analgesics, prolong hospital stays, increase the risk of infection, and greatly affect the patient's quality of life [4]. All patients treated with high-dose chemotherapy requiring hematopoietic stem cell or bone marrow transplantation develop oral mucositis of varying severity. In addition, up to 80% of patients receiving radiotherapy for head or neck tumours and almost 90% of pediatric patients treated for cancer also develop oral mucositis[5,6]

2. Mechanism of development

Radiation induced mucositis is initiated by direct injury to basal epithelial cells and cells in the underlying tissue. DNA-strand breaks can result in cell death or injury. Non-DNA injury is initiated through a variety of mechanisms, some of which are mediated by the generation of reactive oxygen species. Radiation and chemotherapy are effective activators of several injury-producing pathways in endothelia, fibroblasts, and epithelia. In these cells, the activation of transcription factors such as nuclear factor-κB (NF-κB) and NRF-2 leads to the upregulation of genes that modulate the damage response. Immune cells (macrophages) produce pro-inflammatory cytokines, such as tumor-necrosis factor-α (TNF-α) and interleukin-6, which causes further tissue injury.[7] These signaling molecules also participate in a positive-feedback loop that amplifies the original effects of radiation and chemotherapy. For example, TNF-α activates NF-κB and sphingomyelinase activity in the mucosa, leading to more cell death. In addition, direct and indirect damages to epithelial stem cells result in a loss of renewal capacity. As a result, the epithelium begins to thin and patients start to experience the early symptoms of mucositis.[8]

An oropharyngeal epithelial surface has a rapid rate of cell turnover and appears to be at high risk of injury from ionizing radiation. A healthy oral mucosa serves to clear microorganism and provides a chemical barrier that limits penetration of many compounds into the epithelium. A damaged mucosal surface increases the risk of a secondary infection. Acute mucositis results from the loss of squamous epithelial cells owing to the sterilization of mucosal stem cells and the inhibition of transit cell proliferation. This leads to a gradual linear decrease in epithelial cell numbers. Normally, cells of the mouth undergo rapid renewal over a 7–14 day cycle. Radiation therapy interferes with cellular mitosis and reduces the ability of the oral mucosa to regenerate. [9]

As radiation therapy continues, a steady state between mucosal cell death and regeneration may occur because of an increased cell production rate from the surviving cells. Usually, however, cell regeneration cannot keep up with cell death, and therefore, partial or complete denudation develops. This presents as patchy or confluent mucositis. As the mucositis becomes more severe, pseudomembranes and ulceration develops. Poor nutritional status further interferes with mucosal regeneration by decreasing cellular migration and renewal. The loss of the epithelial barrier enhances insults from physical, chemical, and microbial agents.

Stages of mode l[10] for the pathogenesis of mucositis are based on the evidence available to date:

1. **Initiation of tissue injury:** Radiation and/or chemotherapy induce cellular damage resulting in death of the basal epithelial cells. The generation of reactive oxygen species (free radicals) by radiation or chemotherapy is also believed to exert a role in the initiation of mucosal injury. These small highly reactive molecules are by-products of oxygen metabolism and can cause significant cellular damage.
2. **Up-regulation of inflammation via generation of messenger signals:** In addition to causing direct cell death, free radicals activate second messengers that transmit signals from receptors on the cellular surface to the inside of cell. This leads to up-regulation of pro-inflammatory cytokines, tissue injury, and cell death.
3. **Signaling and amplification:** Up-regulation of pro-inflammatory cytokines, such as TNF-a, produced mainly by macrophages, causes injury to mucosal cells, and also activates molecular pathways that amplify mucosal injury.
4. **Ulceration and inflammation:** There is a significant inflammatory cell infiltrate associated with the mucosal ulcerations, based in part on metabolic by-products of the colonizing oral microflora. Production of pro-inflammatory cytokines is also further up-regulated as a result of this secondary infection.[10]
5. **Healing:** This phase is characterized by epithelial proliferation, as well as, cellular and tissue differentiation,[11] restoring the integrity of the epithelium.

A number of authors have reported that the oropharyngeal flora may contribute to radiation-induced mucositis. In health, the oral mucosa has a number of distinct habitats which are colonized by micro-organism that are able to establish a homeostatic community.[12] These homeostatic microbial communities are protective for the host by preventing or interfering with the colonization of exogenous pathogens; this potent defense mechanism is called "colonization resistance". When the oral tissues are irradiated, the colonization resistance is practically abolished. Irradiation mucositis is caused by a combination of alteration of the normal oral microflora with concomitant changes in the tissues. However, healing eventually occurs when cells regenerate from the surviving mucosal stem cells.

3. Clinical presentation

Clinically, mucositis presents with multiple complex symptoms. It begins with a symptomatic redness and erythema and progresses through solitary white elevated desquamative patches that are slightly painful to contact pressure. Following this, large, painful contiguous pseudo membranous lesions develop with associated dysphagia and decreased oral intake. The nonkeratinized mucosa is the most affected one. The most common sites include the labial, buccal, and soft palate mucosa, as well as, the floor of the mouth and the ventral surface of the tongue. Oral lesions usually heal within two to three weeks [Figure 1].

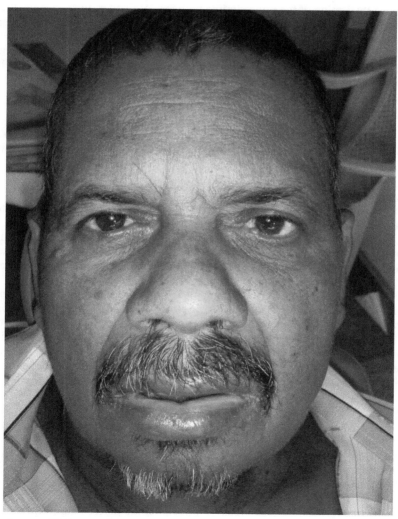

Fig. 1. Oral mucositis in a patient.

Mucositis is an inevitable side effect of radiation. Its severity is dependent on the type of ionizing radiation, the volume of irradiated tissue, the dose per day, and cumulative dose. It has been noted in a considerable number of clinical trials that the severity of acute normal tissue responses, particularly oral mucositis, is significantly increased when the overall treatment time is shortened.[12,13] The clinical course of oral mucositis may sometimes be complicated by local infection, particularly in immunosuppressed patients. Viral infections such as herpes simplex virus (HSV), and fungal infections such as candidiasis can sometimes be superimposed on oral mucositis. Although HSV infections do not cause oral mucositis, they can complicate its diagnosis and management.

Histopathologically, edema of the retepegs is noted, along with vascular changes that demonstrate a thickening of the tunica intima with concomitant reduction in the lumen size and destruction of the elastic and muscle fibers of the vessel walls. The loss of the epithelial cells to the basement membrane exposes the underlying connective tissue stroma with its associated innervations, which, as the mucosal lesions enlarge, contributes to increasing pain. If the patient develops both severe mucositis and thrombocytopenia, oral bleeding may occur, which is very difficult to treat.

4. Clinical management of oral mucositis

Management of oral mucositis can be divided into the following sections: pain control, nutritional support, oral decontamination, palliation of dry mouth, management of oral bleeding, and therapeutic interventions for oral mucositis.

4.1 Pain control

The most common symptom of oral mucositis is pain. Pain significantly affects the nutritional intake, the mouth care, and the quality of life. Thus, management of mucositis pain is a primary component of any mucositis management strategy. Many centers use saline mouth rinses, ice chips, and topical mouth rinses containing an anesthetic, such as 2% viscous lidocaine, which may be mixed with equal volumes of diphenhydramine and a soothing covering agent in equal volumes. Such topical anesthetic agents may provide short-term relief. Sucralfate is the most commonly used and widely studied, even though there is no significant decrease in the pain control.[14,15] In addition to the use of topical agents, most patients with severe mucositis require systemic analgesics, often including opioids, for satisfactory pain relief. Though, the so called 'magic mouthwash' (lidocaine, diphenhydramine, magnesium aluminum hydroxide) has been observed to be beneficial, morphine mouth washes are preferable.[16,17] It was significantly better at reducing intensity and duration of pain and functional impairment, with fewer adverse effects.

4.1.1 Sucralfate

Sucralfate also has been tested in patients receiving radiation therapy. One study compared 21 patients who received standard oral care to the head and neck with 24 patients who received sucralfate suspension four times daily. Results revealed a significant difference in mucosal edema, pain, dysphagia, and weight loss in patients receiving sucralfate [18]. In a pilot study done by Pfeiffer et al. [19], sequential patients who received radiation therapy to the head and neck received sucralfate at the onset of mucositis. Most patients had a decrease in pain following the use of sucralfate. A double-blind, placebo-controlled study with sucralfate in 33 patients who received. irradiation to the head and neck reported no stastitically significant differences in mucositis; however, the sucralfate group reported less oral pain, and other topical and systemic analgesics were started later in the course of radiation [20]. A prospective double-blind study compared the effectiveness of sucralfate suspension versus diphenhydramine syrup plus kaolin-pectin on radiotherapy-induced mucositis. Data were collected daily, including perceived pain, helpfulness of mouth rinses, weekly mucositis grade, weight change, and interruption of therapy. Analysis of the two groups revealed no statistically significant differences between the two groups. In a retrospective review, 15 patients who had not used daily oral rinses were compared with the two groups, and the results suggested that the use of a daily oral rinse with a mouth-coating agent may result in less pain, reduce weight loss, and help prevent interruption of radiation because of severe mucositis[21].

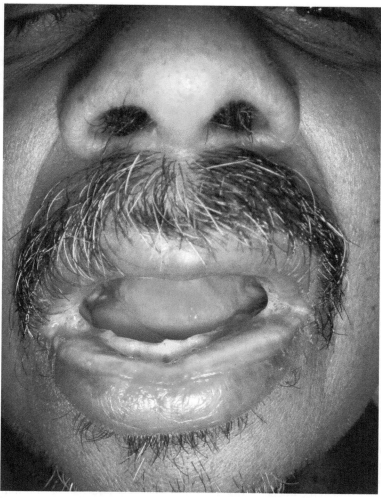

Fig. 2. Oral mucositis in a patient.

4.1.2 Morphine in pain control

In a study to compare the effect of locally applied morphine mouthwash(MO) with Magic mouth wash (MG) on mucositis-related oral pain and on the maintenance of oral intake in patients with tumors of the head and neck area treated with a chemoradiotherapy regimen[51]. Additional objectives were to evaluate the safety of MO by determining the frequency of treatment-emergent drug-related adverse events (local and systemic) or hematologic and biochemical abnormalities, the intensity of chemoradiotherapy administered, tumor response, weight loss, need of a nasogastric tube, and mucositis-related hospitalizations. The duration of severe pain was 3.5 days less in the Morphine group compared with the Magic mouth wash group (P _ 0.032). The intensity of oral pain was also significantly lower in the MO group compared with the MG group .More patients in the MG group needed supplementary (oral or parenteral) analgesia compared with the MO group (P _ 0.019). Nevertheless, the time elapsed before the first supplemental analgesic and the total amount of analgesics taken was similar for both groups. Of 12 patients in the MG group, 3 (25%) and none in the MO group required third-step opiates for alleviation of mouth pain. However, the differences in the maximum WHO step needed for control of pain were not statistically significant. There was a significant difference in duration of severe functional impairment. Nevertheless, the body weight change was similar for both groups. There were no significant differences in documented or highly suspected infections, change in performance status, tumor response rate, and intensity of the chemoradiotherapy delivered between the two treatment groups. No patients required hospitalization due to mucositis during the study. Patients in the MG group reported more local side effects [51].

4.2 Nutritional support

A soft diet or liquid diet was more easily tolerated than a normal diet, when oral mucositis is present; gastrostomy tube is more beneficial, when there is severe mucositis.

4.3 Selective oral decontamination

It has been hypothesized that microbial colonization of oral mucositis lesions exacerbates the severity of oral mucositis and, therefore, decontamination may help to reduce mucositis. Due to the fact that the oral cavity contains a high amount of Gram-negative bacilli and considering its etiological role in mucositis, the concept of 'Selective Decontamination' has been developed. In this regard, lozenges composed of polymyxin E, tobramycin, and amphotericin B have been studied in patients receiving radiation for cancers of head and neck in a randomized trial that compared lozenges with placebo or chlorhexidine rinses, the antimicrobial lozenges provided more effective mucositis prevention in patients receiving head and neck irradiation. Addition of ciprofloxacin or ampicillin with clotrimazole to Sucralfate has shown reduction in mucositis.[22]

4.4 Oral hygiene

Significant reduction in oral mucositis can be attained by proper oral hygiene measures.[23] It was noted that proper oral care also reduced oral toxicity of radiation therapy. Indeed, multiple studies have demonstrated that maintenance of good oral hygiene can reduce the severity of oral mucositis. Furthermore, oral decontamination can reduce infection of the oral cavity by opportunistic pathogens.[24] Therefore, a second function of oral decontamination can be to reduce the risk of systemic sepsis from resident oral and/or opportunistic pathogens. Intensive oral care protocol decreased risk of oral mucositis, but not the percentage of patients with a documented septicemia.[25]

The RTOG and MASCC/ISOO (Mucositis study group of the multinational association for supportive care in cancer and the International society of oral oncology) guidelines recommend use of a standardized oral care protocol, including brushing with a soft toothbrush, flossing, and the use of nonmedicated rinses (for example, saline or sodium bicarbonate rinses). Patients and caregivers should be educated regarding the importance of effective oral hygiene [26, 52, 53].

4.5 Palliation of dry mouth

In cancer therapy, patients often develop transient or permanent xerostomia and hyposalivation. Hyposalivation can further aggravate inflamed tissues, increase risk for local infection, and make mastication difficult. Many patients also complain of a thickening of salivary secretions, because of a decrease in the serous component of saliva. The following measures can be taken for palliation of a dry mouth:

- Sip water as needed to alleviate mouth dryness; several supportive products including artificial saliva are available.
- Rinse with a solution of half a teaspoon of baking soda half in one cup warm water several times a day to clean and lubricate the oral tissues and to buffer the oral environment.
- Chew sugarless gum to stimulate salivary flow.
- Use cholinergic agents as necessary.

4.6 Kaolin pectin

Kaolin pectin, combined with diphenhydramine, which is a H1-histamine antagonist and local anesthetic, was found to reduce oral pain without reducing the degree of mucositis in a double blind randomized and controlled study.[27]

5. Growth factors

One of the problem faced by the therapy is the loss of proliferation of the oral epithelial cells, it has seen that various growth factors that can increase epithelial cell proliferation have been studied for the management of oral mucositis. Recent evidence shows that intravenous recombinant human keratinocyte growth factor-1, Palifermin, significantly reduced incidence of WHO grades 3 and 4 oral mucositis in patients with hematologic malignancies (for example, lymphoma and multiple myeloma) receiving high-dose chemotherapy and total body irradiation before autologous hematopoietic cell transplantation.[28]

Human keratinocyte growth factor-2, Repifermin, was found to be ineffective in reducing the percentage of subjects who experienced severe mucositis.[29] Intravenous human fibroblast growth factor-20, Velafermin, is currently in clinical development for reduction of mucositis secondary to high-dose chemotherapy in autologous hematopoietic cell transplant patients.[30] The safety of this class of growth factors has not been established in patients with nonhematologic malignancies. There is a theoretical concern that these growth factors may promote growth of tumor cells, which may have receptors for the respective growth factor. However, one recent study found no significant difference in survival between subjects with colorectal cancer receiving Palifermin or placebo at a median follow-up duration of 14.5 months.[31] Further studies are ongoing to confirm the safety of epithelial growth factors in the solid tumor setting, including patients receiving radiation therapy for head and neck cancer.

Source	Grade 0	Grade 1	Grade 2	Grade 3	Grade 4
WHO	No change	Soreness/erythema	Erythema,ulcers, can eat solids	Ulcers; requires liquid diet only	Alimentation not possible
RTOG	No change over baseline	May experience mild pain not requiring analgesic	Patchy mucositis may have a serosanguinous discharge. May experience pain requiring analgesics. < 1.5 cm, noncontiguous	Confluent fibrinous mucositis/may include severe pain requiring narcotics, > 1.5 cm, contiguous	Necrosis or deep ulceration, ± bleeding .
NCI CTC	None	Painless ulcers, erythema or mild soreness	Painful erythema,oedema or ulcers, but can eat.	painful erythema, edema or ulcers can not eat.	Requires Parenteral or enteral support
Van der schueren et al	None	Slight erythema	Pronounced erythema	Spotted mucositis	Confluent mucositis patches >0.5cm.
Byfield et al	---	Minimal dysphasia, thinning but no overt break in mucosal integrity.	Significant dysphasia, semi soft foods only, focal mucosal vesicles or denuded patches.	Fluids only tolerated, obviously large confluent patches of mucosal denudation	Parenteral fluids only, severe confluent mucosal denudation with bleeding.
Seto et al	-----	Localized erythema with no pain	Generalized erythema without pain or localized erythema or ulcers with mild pain.	Multiple ulcers or generalized erythema with moderate pain	Generalized erythema or ulcers with moderate to severe pain.
Eilers et al	-----	Pink and moist	Reddened or white film without ulcerations	Ulceration with or without bleeding	-------
NCIC	None	Painless ulcers,erythema,or mild soreness.	Painful erythema,oedema,or ulcers, but can eat	Painful erythema,oedema,or ulcers, but can not eat	Mucosal necrosis and/or requires Parenteral or enteral support,dehydration.
Spijkervet et al	None	White discoloration	Erythema	Pseudomembrane	ulceration
Maceijewski	None	Type: mild erythematous area: <25%	Type : severe erythematous area: 25-50%	Type: spotted mucositis area >50%	Type:confluent mucositis
Hickey et al	No stomatitis	Whitish gingival or slight burning sensation or discomfort.	Moderate erythema and ulcerations or white patches.pain, but can eat, drink and swallow.	severe erythema and ulcerations or white patches. Severe Pain and can not eat, drink or swallow.	-------

Table 1. Comparison of commonly used mucositis scoring system

6. Anti-inflammatory agents

6.1 Benzydamine hydrochloride
It is a nonsteroidal antiinflammatory drug that inhibits proinflammatory cytokines including TNF-a. In a Phase III trial, Benzydamine hydrochloride mouthrinse reduced the severity of mucositis in patients with head and neck cancer undergoing radiation therapy of cumulative doses up to 50-Gy radiation therapy.[32] Based on this and previous studies, the MASCC/ISOO guidelines recommends use of this agent in patients receiving moderate-dose radiation therapy.[33]

6.2 Saforis
It is a proprietary oral suspension of L-glutamine that enhances the uptake of this amino acid into epithelial cells. Glutamine may reduce mucosal injury by reducing the production of proinflammatory cytokines and cytokine-related apoptosis;[34,35] and may promote healing by

increasing fibroblast and collagen synthesis.[36] In a Phase III study, this topical agent reduced the incidence of clinically significant chemotherapy-induced oral mucositis compared to placebo.[37] By comparison, the MASCC/ISOO guidelines recommend that systemically administered glutamine not be used for the prevention of GI mucositis because of lack of efficacy.[38]

6.3 Amifostine

It (phosphothiorate, radiation protection agent) is thought to act as a scavenger for harmful reactive oxygen species that are known to potentiate mucositis.[39] However, because of insufficient evidence of benefit, various guidelines could not be established regarding the use of this agent in oral mucositis in chemotherapy or radiation therapy patients. The use of amifostine has been recommended for the prevention of esophagitis in patients receiving chemoradiation for nonsmall-cell lung cancer.[40]

6.4 RK- 0202 (RxKinetix)

It consists of the antioxidant, N-acetylcysteine, in a proprietary matrix for topical application in the oral cavity. In a placebo-controlled phase II trial in patients with head and neck cancer, this agent significantly reduced the incidence of severe oral mucositis up to doses of 50-Gy radiation therapy.[41]

6.5 Beta carotene

Beta carotene, a vitamin A derivative, is a scavenger of singlet oxygen. Based on the findings of different randomized controlled study, it is of the view that supplemental dietary beta-carotene lead to a mild decrease in the severity of chemotherapy and radiotherapy-induced oral mucositis.[42]

7. Immunomodulatory drugs

7.1 Pentoxifylline

Oral pentoxiphylline reduced the frequency and severity of all major complications after BMT, including reduction of oral mucositis.[43] Contradictory to this, other workers reported a significant aggravation of symptoms when they studied the effect of IV Pentoxiphylline in 92 patients.[44] However, no difference in symptoms was noted in patients who undergone chemo radio therapy.

7.2 Indomethacin

Indomethacin, a nonsteroidal antiinflammatory drug inhibiting prostaglandin synthesis is noted to delay the onset of mucositis.

7.3 Immunoglobulin

Treatment with low-dose intra muscular immunoglobulin is said to decrease the severity and duration of radio therapy-induced oral mucositis. Immunoglobulin has also been tried as a therapeutic agent in radiation-induced mucositis in various clinical trials and the observations were promising.[45]

7.4 Cytokines

Preclinical models have been used to demonstrate that the cytokines interleukin-1, interleukin-2, epidermal growth factor, interleukin-11, and transforming growth factor-beta have direct effect on intestinal or oral mucosa. Interleukin-1 increases thymidine labeling, and protects oral and intestinal mucosa, when given to mice before radiation. Interleukin-11 can decrease mucositis, when given to hamster models.

7.5 G-CSF, GM-CSF

The mucosal protection effects of granulocyte colony stimulating factor G-CSF were observed in patients treated with various chemotherapy regimens by many authors.[46] But controversies to this exist in other clinical trials. In a recent preliminary report of a pilot study found significant reduction in oral mucositis.[47] The study was to evaluate the effect of GM-CSF in reduction of radiotherapy induced oral mucositis. At about second week of radiotherapy, when oral pain was experienced 400 µg of GM-CSF was administered locally once a day, until completion of radiotherapy. The patients were evaluated weekly for mucosal reaction and functional impairment. The result of the study was prompting with reduction and almost healing of oral mucositis in 14 out of 17 patients with completion of radiotherapy within the preplanned schedule. Moreover patients did not show a significant weight loss or functional impairment.

8. Anti-viral drugs

8.1 Acyclovir

Although acyclovir prophylaxis is effective in preventing oropharyngeal shedding of the virus in herpes simplex virus seropositive patients receiving intensive chemotherapy or BMT, it did not influence chemotherapy, radiotherapy and BMT-related oral toxicity.

9. Role of safe radiotherapy

Normal tissue reactions can be reduced in a substantial number of patients with head and neck cancer by the use of computed tomography (CT)-based target delineation, Intensity-Modulated Radiation Therapy (IMRT), and simple, custom-made, intraoral devices that are designed to exclude uninvolved tissues from the treatment portals or to provide shielding of tissues within the treatment area.[43] Stents can be useful in excluding the palate mucosa during treatment of the tongue or floor of the mouth. These shielding stents can decrease the amount of radiation that is delivered to the contra-lateral mucosa. More frequent use of electron-beam and/or sophisticated three-dimensional conformal, multibeam, wedged-pair, or oblique treatment plans will also help to exclude or minimize the radiation dose to uninvolved mucosa. Packing gauze between metallic dental restorations and mucosa of the lateral tongue and buccal area appears to be very beneficial in minimizing the dose from scattered radiation.

9.1 Antifungal therapy

The mucosa of patients undergoing radiation therapy to the oral cavity should be examined at least once a week, and antibiotic or antifungal medications should be prescribed when infections are documented. Clotrimazole troches, dissolved in the mouth five times a day for 14 days, generally works well for oral candidiasis. However, if significant mucositis, altered taste, or xerostomia has developed, the troches might not be tolerated. In this situation, nystatin oral suspension or Fluconazole in tablet or liquid form is often effective. Fluconazole is more effective than nystatin and might need to be given at a higher dose and/or for an extended period of time in patients who are receiving combined chemotherapy and radiation therapy due to infections with resistant species.[48]

9.2 Low-level laser therapy

The mechanism of low-level laser therapy is not understood, but many studies have proved the efficacy of the same in reducing the symptoms related to oral mucositis. Low-level laser therapy may reduce levels of reactive oxygen species and/or proinflammatory cytokines that contribute to the pathogenesis of mucositis.[49] The various guidelines suggest the use of low-level laser therapy for reducing the severity of chemotherapy and radiotherapy-induced oral mucositis.[50]

9.3 AMP-18 (Antral mucosal protein) 18

A study on AMP18 (AMP-18 is a protein constitutively expressed in epithelial cells of the gastric antrum that is cell protective, mitogenic and motogenic in cell culture and in vivo) shows, AMP peptide, by activating CCKBR (cholecystokinin-B/gastrin receptor), targets TJs(Tight Junctions) to maintain mucosal integrity, and sets in motion protective and cell regenerative mechanisms for the prevention and treatment of OM. Treatment with AMP peptide protected the surface epithelium of the mouse oral mucosa. AMP-18 peptide stimulates growth of diverse types of epithelial cells including HaCaT cells [54].

10. Summary

Mucositis is an inevitable side effect of radiation. The severity of the mucositis depends on the type of ionizing radiation, the volume of irradiated tissue, the daily dose, and the cumulative dose. As the mucositis becomes more severe, pseudomembranes and ulcerations develop. Poor nutritional status further interferes with mucosal regeneration by decreasing cellular migration and renewal. Radiation-induced oral mucositis affects the quality of life of the patients and the family concerned. The present day management of oral mucositis is mostly palliative and or supportive care. Management includes good oral hygiene, avoiding irritating or abrasive substances, use of bland rinses, topical anesthetic agents, and systemic analgesics. Though, the newer guidelines are suggesting Palifermin, which is the first active mucositis drug as well as Amifostine, for radiation protection and cryotherapy for symptoms related to high-dose melphalan; the role of safe radiotherapy remains the ultimate goal in reducing the symptoms of radiation-induced oral mucositis. Future research for the newer drugs in the field of radiation-induced oral mucositis is a must, and the current management should focus more on palliative measures, such as pain management, nutritional support, and maintenance, of good oral hygiene.

11. References

[1] Sonis ST. Is mucositis an inevitable consequence of intensive therapy for hematologic cancers? Nat Clin Pract Oncol 2005;2:134-5.
[2] Keefe DM. Mucositis guidelines: What have they achieved, and where to from here? Support Care Cancer 2006;14:489-91.
[3] Trotti A, Bellm LA, Epstein JB, Frame D, Fuchs HJ, Gwede CK, et al. Mucositis incidence, severity and associated outcomes in patients with head and neck cancer receiving radiotherapy with or without chemotherapy: A systematic literature review. Cancer 2008;113:2704-13.
[4] Satheesh Kumar PS, Balan A, Sankar A, Bose T. Radiation induced oral mucositis. Indian J Palliat Care 2009;15:95-102

[5] Satheeshkumar PS, Chamba MS, Balan A, Sreelatha KT, Bhatathiri VN, Bose T. Effectiveness of triclosan in the management of radiation-induced oral mucositis: A randomized clinical trial. J Can Res Ther 2010;6:466-72.

[6] P.S Satheeshkumar, A. Balan.Subjective response of pain on patients treated with aqueous base Hexidine and weekly dentist assisted oral hygiene maintenance for radiation induced oral mucositis- An interventional study." Oral Oncology, Volume 47, Supplement 1, July 2011, Page S82

[7] Logan RM, Gibson RJ, Sonis ST, Keefe DM. Nuclear factor-кappaB (NF-kappaB) and cyclooxygenase-2 (COX-2) expression in the oral mucosa following cancer chemotherapy. Oral Oncol 2007;43:395-401.

[8] Gibson RJ, Bowen JM, Cummins AG, Logan R, Healey T, Keefe DM. Ultrastructural changes occur early within the oral mucosa following cancer chemotherapy [abstract A-373]. Support Care Cancer 2004;12:389.

[9] Sonis ST, Elting LS, Keefe D, Peterson DE, Schubert M, Hauer-Jensen M, *et al.* Perspectives on cancer therapy-induced mucosal injury: Pathogenesis, measurement, epidemiology, and consequences for patients. Cancer 2004;100:1995-2025.

[10] Sonis ST, Elting LS, Keefe D, Peterson DE, Schubert M, Hauer-Jensen M, *et al.* Perspectives on cancer therapy-induced mucosal injury: Pathogenesis, measurement, epidemiology, and consequences for patients. Cancer 2004;100:1995-2025.

[11] Sonis ST, Peterson RL, Edwards LJ, Lucey CA, Wang L, Mason L, *et al.* Defining mechanisms of action of interleukin-11 on the progression of radiation-induced oral mucositis in hamsters. Oral Oncol 2000;36:373-81.

[12] Dorr W, Emmendorfer H, Haide E. Proliferation equivalent of 'accelerated repopulation' in mouse oral mucosa. Int J Radiat Biol 1994;66:157-67.

[13] Epstein JB, Gorsky M, Guglietta A, Le N, Sonis ST. The correlation between epidermal growth factor levels in saliva and the severity of oral mucositis during oropharyngeal radiation therapy. Cancer 2000;89:2258-65.

[14] Dodd MJ, Miaskowski C, Greenspan D, MacPhail L, Shih AS, Shiba G, *et al.* Radiation-induced mucositis: A randomized clinical trial of micronized sucralfate versus salt and soda mouthwashes. Cancer Invest 2003;21:21-33.

[15] Nottage M, McLachlan SA, Brittain MA, Oza A, Hedley D, Feld R, *et al.* Sucralfate mouthwash for prevention and treatment of 5-fluorouracil-induced mucositis: A randomized, placebo-controlled trial. Support Care Cancer 2003;11:41-7.

[16] Barclay L. Morphine mouthwash relieves pain of oral mucositis. Cancer 2002;95:2230-6.

[17] Spijkevet FK, van saene JJ, Panders AK, Vermy A, Mehta DM, Filder V. Effect of selective elimination of the oral flora on mucositis in irradiated head and neck cancer patients. J Surg Oncol 1991;46:167-73.

[18] Matthews RH, Ercal N. Prevention of mucositis in irradiated head and neck cancer patients. J Exp Ther Oncol 1996;1:135-8.

[19] Borowski B, Benhamou E, Pico JL, Laplanche A, Margainaud JP, Hayat M. Prevention of oral mucositis in patients treated with high-dose chemotherapy and bone marrow transplantation: A randomized controlled trial comparing two protocols of dental care. Eur J Cancer B Oral Oncol 1994;308:93-7.

[20] Yoneda S, Imai S, Hanada N, Yamazaki T, Senpuku H, Ota Y, *et al.* Effects of oral care on development of oral mucositis and microorganisms in patients with esophageal cancer. Jpn J Infect Dis 2007;60:23-8.

[21] McGuire DB, Correa ME, Johnson J, Wienandts P. The role of basic oral care and good clinical practice principles in the management of oral mucositis. Support Care Cancer 2006;14:541-7.

[22] Barker G, Loffus L, Cuddy P, Barker B. The effects of of sucralfate suspension and diphenhydramine syrup plus kaolin-pectin on radiotherapy-induced mucositis. Oral Surg Oral Med Oral Pathol 1991;71:288-93.

[23] Spielberger R, Stiff P, Bensinger W, Gentile T, Weisdorf D, Kewalramani T, et al. Palifermin for oral mucositis after intensive therapy for hematologic cancers. N Engl J Med 2004;351:2590-8.

[24] von Bultzingslowen I, Brennan MT, Spijkervet FK, Logan R, Stringer A, Raber-Durlacher JE, et al. Growth factors and cytokines in the prevention and treatment of oral and gastrointestinal mucositis. Support Care Cancer 2006;14:519-27.

[25] Scherlacher A, Beaufort-Spontin E. Radiotherapy of head-neck neo-plasms:prevention of inflammation of the mucosa by sucralafate treatment. HNO 1990;38:24-28.

[26] Pfeiffer P, Hansen O, Madsen el, et al. A prospective pilot study on the effect of sucralafate mouth-swishing in reducing stomatitis during radiotherapy of the oral cavity. Acta Oncol 1990;29:471-3.

[27] Epstein jb, Wong FLW The efficacy of sucralafate suspension in the prevention of oral mucositis due to radiation therapy. Int J Radiat Oncol Biol Phys 1994;28:693-698.

[28] Barker G, Loftus L, Cuddy P, et al. The effects of sucralafate suspension and diphenhydramine syrup plus kaolin-pectin on radiotherapy-induced mucositis. Oral Surg Oral Med Oral Pathol Oral Radiol Endod 1991;71:288-293.

[29] Lalla RV. Velafermin (CuraGen). Curr Opin Investig Drugs 2005;6:1179-85.

[30] Rosen LS, Abdi E, Davis ID, Gutheil J, Schnell FM, Zalcberg J, et al. Palifermin reduces the incidence of oral mucositis in patients with metastatic colorectal cancer treated with fluorouracil-based chemotherapy. J Clin Oncol 2006;24:5194-200.

[31] Epstein JB, Silverman S Jr, Paggiarino DA, Crockett S, Schubert MM, Senzer NN, et al. Benzydamine HCl for prophylaxis of radiation-induced oral mucositis: Results from a multicenter, randomized, double-blind, placebo-controlled clinical trial. Cancer 2001;92:875-85.

[32] Lalla RV, Schubert MM, Bensadoun RJ, Keefe D. Anti-inflammatory agents in the management of alimentary mucositis. Support Care Cancer 2006;14:558-65.

[33] Coeffier M, Marion R, Leplingard A, Lerebours E, Ducrotté P, Déchelotte P. Glutamine decreases interleukin-8 and interleukin-6 but not nitric oxide and prostaglandins e production by human gut in-vitro. Cytokine 2002;18:92-7.

[34] Evans ME, Jones DP, Ziegler TR. Glutamine prevents cytokine-induced apoptosis in human colonic epithelial cells. J Nutr 2003;133:3065-71.

[35] Bellon G, Monboisse JC, Randoux A, Borel JP. Effects of preformed proline and proline amino acid precursors (including glutamine) on collagen synthesis in human fibroblast cultures. Biochim Biophys Acta 1987;930:39-47.

[36] Peterson DE, Jones JB, Petit RG 2nd. A Randomized, placebo-controlled trial of Saforis for prevention and treatment of oral mucositis in breast cancer patients receiving anthracycline-based chemotherapy. Cancer 2007;109:322-31.

[37] Pytlik R, Benes P, Patorkova M, Chocenská E, Gregora E, Procházka B, et al. Standardized parenteral alanyl-glutamine dipeptide supplementation is not beneficial in autologous transplant patients: A randomized, doubleblind, placebo controlled study. Bone Marrow Transplant 2002;30:953-61.

[38] Mantovani G, Maccio A, Madeddu C, Mura L, Massa E, Gramignano G, et al. Reactive oxygen species, antioxidant mechanisms and serum cytokine levels in cancer patients, Impact of an antioxidant treatment. J Environ Pathol Toxicol Oncol 2003;22:17-28.

[39]   Bensadoun RJ, Schubert MM, Lalla RV, Keefe D. Amifostine in the management of radiation induced and chemo-induced mucositis. Support Care Cancer 2006;14:566-72.

[40]   Barasch A, Peterson DE, Tanzer JM, D'Ambrosio JA, Nuki K, Schubert MM, et al. Helium-neon laser effects on conditioning induced oral mucositis in bone marrow transplantation patients. Cancer 1995;76:2550-6.

[41]   Mills EE. The modifying effect of beta-carotene on radiation and radiotherapy and chemotherapy induced oral mucositis. Br J Cancer 1988;57:416-7.

[42]   Bianco JA, Appelbaum FR, Nemunaitis J, Almgren J, Andrews F, Kettner P, et al. Phase I-II trial of pentoxifyline for the prevention of transplant-related toxicities following bone marrow transplantation. Blood 1991;78:1205-11.

[43]   Clift RA, Bianco JA, Appelbaum FR, Buckner CD, Singer JW, Bakke L, et al. A randomized controlled trial of pentoxifylline for the prevention of regimen-related toxicities in patients undergoing allogeneic marrow transplantation. Blood 1993;82:2025-30.

[44]   Mose S, Adametz IA, Saran F, Thilmann C, Hayd R, Knecht R, et al. Can Prophylactic application of immunoglobulin decrease radiotherapy-induced oral mucositis. Am J Clin Oncol 1997;20:407-11.

[45]   Hermann F, Schuiz G, Weser M, Kolbe K, Nicolay U, Noack M, et al. Effect of granulocyte-macrophage colony stimulating factor on neutropenia and related morbidity induced by myelotoxic chemotherapy. Am J Med 1990;88:619-24.

[46]   Gluckman E, Lotsberg J, Devergie A, Zhao XM, Melo R, Gomez-Morales M, et al. Oral acyclovir prophylactic treatment of herpes simplex infection after bone marrow transplantation. J Antimicrob Chemother 1983;12:161-7.

[47]   Kaanders JH, Fleming TJ, Ang KK, Maor MH, Peters LJ. Devices valuable in head and neck radiotherapy. Int J Radiat Oncol Biol Phys 1992;23:639-45.

[48]   Dahiya MC, Redding SW, Dahiya RS, Eng   TY,   Kirkpatrick   WR,   Coco   BJ,   et al. Oropharyngeal candidiasis caused by non-albicans yeast in patients receiving external beam radiotherapy for head-and-neck cancer. Int J Radiat Oncol Biol Phys 2003;57:79-83.

[49]   Bensadoun RJ, Franquin JC, Ciais G, Darcourt V, Schubert MM, Viot M, et al. Low-energy He/Ne laser in the prevention of radiation-induced mucositis: A multicenter phase III randomized study in patient's with head and neck cancer. Support Care Cancer 1999;7:244-52.

[50]   Migliorati CA, Oberle-Edwards L, Schubert M. The role of alternative and natural agents, cryotherapy, and/or laser for management of alimentary mucositis. Support Care Cancer 2006;14:533-40.

[51]   Cerchietti LC, Navigante AH, Bonomi MR, Zaderajko MA, Menéndez PR, Pogany CE, Roth BM. Effect of topical morphine for mucositis-associated pain following concomitant chemoradiotherapy for head and neck carcinoma. Cancer. 2002 Nov 15;95(10):2230-6.

[52]   S.K. Poolakkad Sankaran, A. Balan. Neighbourhood Dental Clinic programme (NDCP) for oral care in patients undergoing head and neck cancer therapy. Support Care Cancer (2011) 19 (Suppl 2):S67–S370.

[53]   S.K. Poolakkad Sankaran, A. Balan. The degree of discomfort due to mucositis is related to the prior patient awareness? Support Care Cancer (2011) 19 (Suppl 2):S67–S370.

[54]   Chen P, Lingen M, Sonis ST, Walsh-Reitz MM, Toback FG. Role of AMP-18 in oral mucositis. Oral Oncol. 2011 Sep;47(9):831-9. Epub 2011 Jul 6

Part 3

Non Pharmacological Treatments

7

Overview of Collateral Meridian Therapy in Pain Management: A Modified Formulated Chinese Acupuncture

Chih-Shung Wong[1], Chun-Chang Yeh[2] and Shan-Chi Ko[3]

[1]*Department of Anaesthesiology, Cathay General Hospital, Taipei,*
[2]*Department of Anaesthesiology, Tri-Service General Hospital, Taipei,*
[3]*Painless Hospital, Ginza, Tokyo,*
[1,2]*Taiwan*
[3]*Japan*

1. Introduction

The Western approach to pain management is focused on the use of pharmacotherapy, physical therapy, nerve blocks, nerve ablations, implantable devices. Even though increasing of understanding of the mechanisms of pain for the treatments; some pains remain intractable (Hariharan et al, 2007; Wagner et al, 2007; Laxmaiah et al, 2009). In contrast, traditional Chinese medicine (TCM) centres primarily on the energy relationship among the environment and the body and organs, without a clear understanding of pathophysiology or the mechanisms of diseases and its effects are varied and inconsistent. The collateral meridian therapy (CMT), offers an alternative treatment for different types of pain by taking a systematic approach to a variant of traditional Chinese acupuncture (TCA). Here, we highlight the recent development of CMT by describing the main theory, discussing the differences between CMT and TCA, defining abbreviations associated with CMT, explaining acupoint localization principles, and providing clinical reports for application in pain management.

2. The theory behind CMT

To achieve an understanding of CMT, it is necessary to revisit the modality on which it is based. In TCA, it is believed that the manipulation of certain points on the skin can affect the movement of energy, or "Qi", throughout the body. It is assumed that "Qi" flows in channels, or meridians, along the body, and that good health is maintained through balancing the circulation of Qi along these channels. In TCA, there are 12 established meridians. On these 12 meridians, a total 361 acupoints are located through which the flow of Qi can be manipulated. The selection of points for treatment, following the "one-needle effect", where therapeutic effect is obtained from manipulation of one strong acupoint, is based on the nature of the disease treated as defined by the five-element theory of TCM, and by a number of personal factors. As a result, the treatment for disease is changed on a case-by-case basis. There has no standard method; the effectiveness of TCA varies from patient to patient.

In CMT, however, two acuponts are manipulated, instead of one. The meridian lines are the same as in TCA, but each meridian has only nice standard acuponits (a total of 108). Two acupoints are used for redirection the flow of Qi from one meridian to another. As such, in CMT, the points selected for treatment are commonly on non-diseased meridians. CMT also follows the use of a standardized set of protocol for treatment, instead of the individual varied treatments given in TCA. The two points manipulated are known as control C-point and functional F-point. These points are specific to each meridian and allow the flow of Qi to be linked from the diseased meridian to a healthy one.

2.1 Two-point theory: C-point and F-point

The C-point is used to connect the diseased meridian and the healthy meridian. In treatment, practitioners manipulate the healthy meridian to relieve the pain or symptoms. Obstructed energy Qi is allowed to flow from the lesion site to the unobstructed healthy meridian, through which the disease will be discharged. Each meridian has its own C-point. For the location of C-points, please see figures 1 and 2. For the abbreviations and anatomical definition of C-points, please see table 1. The C-point is for linking the diseased meridian to the treatment meridian, and the F-point is for the treatment of the disease symptom or painful location. The F-points in the different regions of the body are shown in figure 3. Each region of pain or disease in the body is represented by its own F-point. For instance, if the patient had pain in the neck of shoulder, the practitioner should select "a" as an F-point for treatment (Fig. 3). If a patient has an acute lumbar strain, the F-point over the lumbar L4-5 region would be "4"; the F-point over the lumbar L3-4 region would be "5" (Fig. 3).

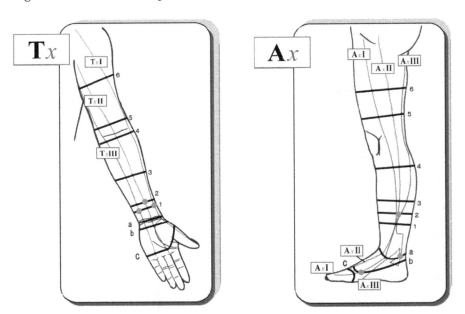

Fig. 1. The numbers 6, 5, 4, 3, 2, 1 and letters a, b, c are the treatment function points of six yin meridians. The blue points indicated control-point of each yin meridian (1, 2, and 1 for TxI, TxII, TxIII; b, 2 and a for AxI, AxII, AxIII).

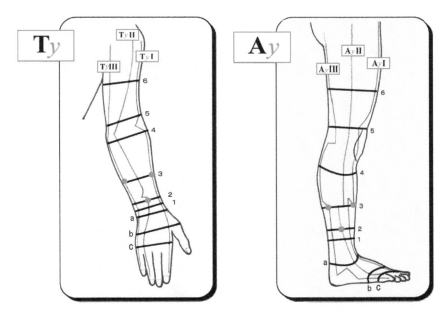

Fig. 2. The numbers 6, 5, 4, 3, 2, 1 and letters a, b, c are the treatment function points of six yin meridians. The blue points indicated control-point of each yang meridian (3, 2, and 3 for both TyI, TyII, TyIII and AyI, AyII, AyIII).

2.2 Abbreviations in CMT

The abbreviations used in CMT are defined as follows: "T" represents the upper extremity (Te is the pronunciation of "arm" in Japanese); "A" represents the lower extremity (Ashi is the pronunciation of "leg" in Japanese); the roman numerals, I, II and III represent the meridians on the radial, median and unlar side of the upper extremities, and the meridians on the anterior, medial (or lateral), and posterior aspect on the lower extremities, respectively. The use of "x" symbolizes the yin aspect, and use of "y" denotes the yang aspect of the extremities. Each extremity had nine acupoints in which point a, b and c are located on the hand or foot, and point 1 to 6 are located on the arm or leg (Figs. 1 and 2). The letters "r" and "l" represent the right and left side of the limb, respectively. For example, "lTyI" describes a meridian on the dorsal aspect (y) of the radial side (I) of the left (l) upper extremity (T) (see Fig. 8a).

2.3 How CMT identifies the diseased meridian and formulates a treatment protocol

For the purpose of simplicity, the symbols "/", "()" and "." are used to describe diseased or treatment meridians. For example, if the diseased region is over the right wrist (corresponding to "a", Fir. 3) of the TyI meridian, it is represented by rTyI/a. If the treatment meridian selected is lTxI/1:a, then constant pressure is applied on the C-point "1' of the lTxI meridian (Fig. 1), while a "remove" manoeuvre at the corresponding "a" point is simultaneously performed on the lTxI meridian. The letter "1" before ":" signifies the C-point of the lTxI meridian, while the letter "a" after ":" expresses the F-point "a". T denote a supplement or enhancement manoeuvre, place "()" around "a" to make the treatment formula lTxI/1:a); otherwise, "a" without "()" represents a removal manoeuvre on point "a". When there is no need to use the C-point, the symbol "0" is used for the treatment meridian. Examples of cases where no C-point is used included yin to yin or yang to yang meridians for namesake (T-A) links, or for the original meridian manipulation. Therefore, the colon symbol ":" is used to differentiate the diseased from the treatment meridian because only the presence of an F-point on the diseased meridian is necessary.

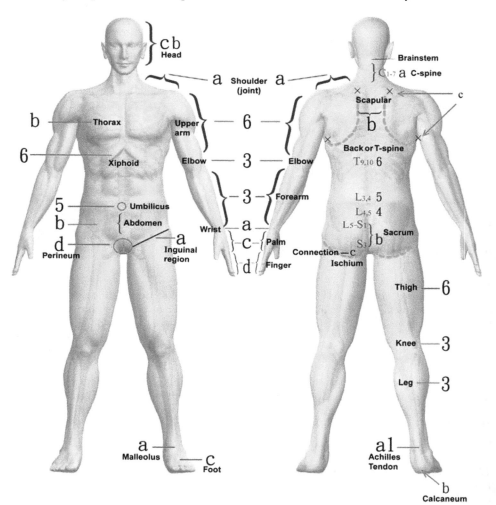

Fig. 3. This figure indicates specific body regions corresponding to F-points. The unique "d" system, different form the ordinary 9-point (6, 5, 4, 3, 2, 1, a, b, c) system on the treatment meridians, corresponds to intracranial, perineum and digits. al: the most painful point between point-a and point-1 on the treatment meridian, ac: the most painful point between point-c and point-b on the treatment meridian.

2.4 How CMT links to channel Qi and diverts the body flow in the meridians

The C-point ensures the link to channel Qi from the diseased meridian to the healthy one. Four different types of links are available to channel Qi: 1) Zang-Fu (TA-xy). 2) Exterior-Interior (x-y), 3) Namesake (T-A), and 4) Original meridian links (Fig. 4). The selection of treatment from the diseased meridian is shown in Figure 4. Zang-Fu (TA-xy) is the most common link for treatment. For example, if the diseased meridian is AxI, the treatment meridian is TyIII (TA-xy link) and vice versa. The determination of the treatment meridian, whether ipsilateral or contralateral, is based on the location of the lesion, as shown in Figure 5. For example, if the diseased meridian is rAyI, the treatment meridian is TxII (according to the TA-xy link in Fig. 4). Figure 5 shows that the treatment side for the TxII meridian is contralateral side to the diseased meridian; thus the left side is selected as the treatment side. Figure 6 illustrates the usage of the C-point to link the diseased meridian (rAyI) to the lTxII meridian by the TA-xy link (visceral Znag-Fu link) for treatment, acting as an area of energy discharge. By simultaneously manipulating the C-point and the F-point that corresponds to the painful site, the pain in rAyI will flow to lTxII, and the pain will be removed or reduced by manipulating the functional F-point pressed against the body flow direction (yin meridian). Similarly for the lAyIII or rAyIII problem in post-regional anesthesia/analgesia backache, the treatment meridian will be chosen as rTxI or lTxI (Yeh et al, 2009). Most acupoints are located along the edge of the bony shaft or on the tendinomuscular grooves. The accurate localization of the acupoint can be achieved through patient reports of soreness or painful sensation when the area is pressed deeply. For detailed anatomical localization of acupoints, please refer to 10b, and book by Ko and Chao (2007).

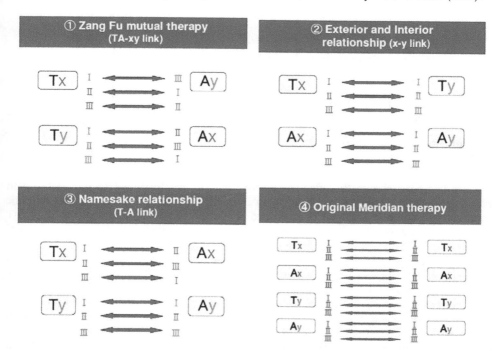

Fig. 4. The four types of links used to choose the treatment meridian.

	Yin (x)		Yang (y)	
T	I	contralateral	I	contralateral
Upper	II		II	
limbs	III	Ipsilateral	III	
A	I		I	ipsilateral
Lower	II	contralateral	II	
limbs	III		III	

Fig. 5. Determination to choose contralateral or ipsilateral side or ipsilateral side of treatment meridian. For yin meridians used as the treatment ones to divert the obstructed flow, all of them must choose the opposite side to the diseased meridian, except for TxIII. On the other hand, for yang meridians used, all must choose the same side as the diseased meridian, except for TyI.

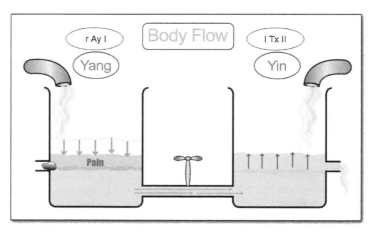

Fig. 6. Illustratin of the proposed mechanism of pain reduction.

2.5 Clinical reports for application in pain management

Case studies have shown the effectiveness of CMT on the treatment of intractable pain (Wong et al, 2006). Patients suffering from intricate chronic pain, such as post-herpetic neuralgia and complex regional pain syndrome, are responded dramatically to the CMT treatment (Wong et al, 2007). Moreover, CMT is also observed effectively on local musculoskeletal pain that resulted from such injuries as sprains or strains and demonstrated positive effect on shoulder pain relief after laparcoscopic surgery (Yeh et al, 2008). CMT is also an effect technique to reduce painful dysmenorrhea (Lin et al, 2010). Moreover, CMT is also highly effective in the treatment of post-neuraxial block backache in patients who were failed to treated by the conventional treatment (Yeh et al, 2009). Over the post few years, Dr. Ko and his team have repeatedly demonstrated positive results of this therapy through workshops, courses and pain clinics throughout Japan., Taiwan, Singapore and the United States (Hoka et al, 2008). A mini-symposium on CMT was also offered in the 13th World Society of Pain Clinicians Congress for the World Institute of Pain Meeting in 2008.

Meridian in CMT	Meridian in TCA	C-Point	Actual anatomical location
TxI	Lung	1	On the junction of the metaphysis and diaphysis over the distal radius. The pressure should be applied on the radial side of the flexor carbi radialis directly on the bone; pressure to the radial artery should be avoided (Fig. 7a).
TxII	Pericardia	2	Approximately three finger breadths proximal to the TxI/a (Fig. 7b).
TxIII	Heart	1	On the radial depression of the flexor carbi ulnaris at the junction of the metaphysis and diaphysis over the distal ulna (Fig. 7a).
AxI	Spleen	b	On the tangent line to the plantar-medial depression at the junction of the metaphysis and diaphysis over the proximal end of first metatarsal bone (Fig. 9a, b).
AxII	Liver	2	Approximately 1 cm posterior to the AxI/2 at the same horizontal level as AxI/2 (Fig. 9a).
AxIII	Kidney	a	On the tangent line to the posterior border of the medial malleolus (Fig. 9a).
TyI	Large Intestine	3	On the tangent line to the ulnar side of the radius at the musculotendinous junction (Fig. 8a).
TyII	Triple Energizer	2	Between the distal ulna and radius about one-sixth of the distance above TyII/a toward the olecranon (approximately three finger breadths proximal to TyII/a) (Fig. 8b).
TyIII	Small Intestine	3	On the tangent line to the radial border of the dorsal ulna at the musculotendinous junction (Fig. 8a).
AyI	Stomach	3	At the same horizontal level as AyIII/3, approximately one finger breadth posterior to the anterior crest of the tibia (Fig. 10a).
AyII	Gall Bladder	2	On the tangent line to the anterior border of the fibula at the same horizontal level as AyIII/3 (Fig. 10a).
AyIII	Bladder	3	First identify the Chinese traditional acupoint BL57 (Chengshan), which is in the depression below the belly of the gastrocnemius when the leg is stretched or the heel is lifted. After pressing BL57, find two lines running from it lateroinferiorly and medioinferiorly; AyIII/3 point is at the lateroinferior end on the tangent line to the posterior surface of the fibula (Fig. 10a, b).

CMT: Collateral Meridian Therapy; TCA: Traditional Chinese Acupuncture

Table 1. Anatomical location of C-points.

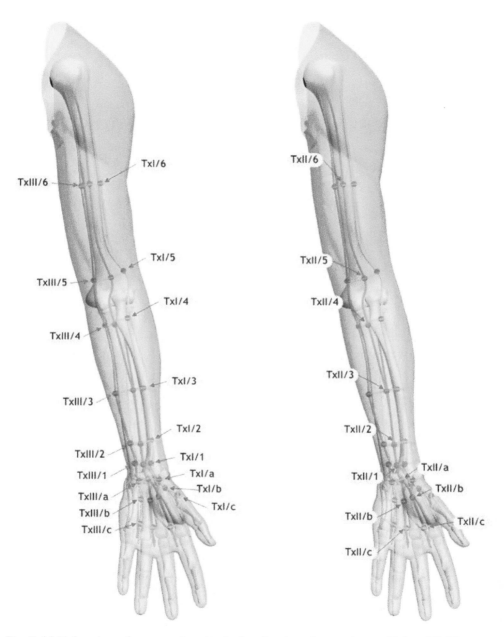

Fig. 7. (a) Volar view of upper extremity for localization of acupoints on TxI and TxIII.
(b) Volar view of upper extremity for localization of acupoints on TxII.

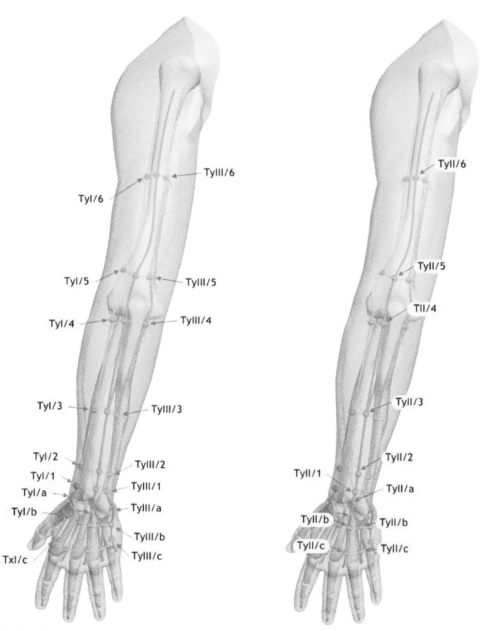

Fig. 8. (a) Dorsal view of upper extremity for localization of acupoints on TyI and TyIII.
(b) Dorsal view of upper extremity for localization of acupoints on TyII.

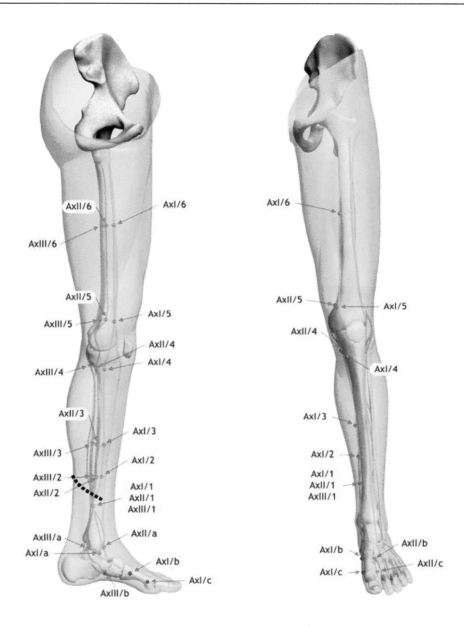

Fig. 9. (a) Medial view of lower extremity for localization of acupoints on AxI and most of AxII and AxIII (except for AxII/b AxII/c and AxIII/c). (b) Anterior view of lower extremity for localization of on AxI and AxII. The dotted line is extended along the curve of the lower border of the medial gastrocnemius belly.

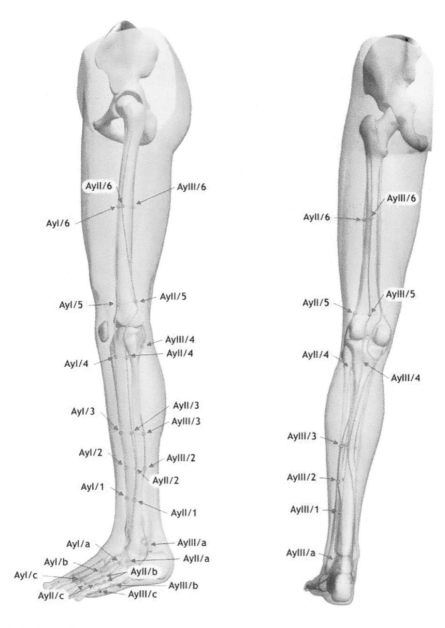

Fig. 10. (a) Lateral view of lower extremity for localization of acupoints on AyI, AyII and AyIII. (b) Posterior view of lower extremity for localization of acupoints on AyII and AyIII.

The National Institute of Health consensus, published in 1998, states that acupuncture shows effectiveness in the treatment of postoperative and chemotherapy induced nausea and vomiting and postoperative dental pain. The statement concludes that acupuncture may be useful in other conditions, including myofascial pain, osteoarthritis, low back pain, menstrual cramps and so on. In addition, we conducted a MEDLINE search and found that acupuncture therapy is also effective for low back pain (LBP) and myofascial pain. From prospective randomized controlled trials published in the peer-reviewed medical literature after 1998, we summarize the acupoints/meridians use for TCA and CMT in the management of LBP in table 2. According to the rules that we have introduced in this article, we can choose the corresponding healthy meridian and formats a set of acupoints for the treatment of LBP, whereas in TCA, one usually uses the diseased meridian, with different acupoints chosen in different reports (Ezzo et al, 2001; Leibing et al, 2002; Meng et al, 2004; Trinh et al, 2007; Wang et al, 2008; Yeh et al; 2009). Based on our literature review, patients with LBP received at lease short-term pain relief after TCA treatment; the CMT also provides significant pain relief via different approach with a standardized formulated protocol. Table 3 shows as summary of published CMT clinical reports for different types of pain (Wong et al, 2006; 2007; Hoka, 2008; Yeh et al, 2008; 2009, Lin et al, 2010). Furthermore to date, no clinical reports described the use of TCA to treat complex regional pain syndrome which patients may not tolerate the direct stimulation/acupuncture to the painful area. In contrast, CMT provides a promising technique for treating complex regional pain syndrome that can be used without touching the painful sites (Wong et al, 2007; Hoka, 2008).

Meridian	TCM [ref]	CMT [ref]
Governing vessel meridian	(+) Wang et al (2008) Leibing et al (2002)	
Urinary bladder meridian (AyIII)	(+) Wang et al (2008) Leibing et al (2002) Meng et al (2004) Ezzo et al (2001) Trinh et al (2007)	
Lung meridian (TxI)		(+) Yeh et al (2008)
Heart meridian (TxIII)		(+) Yeh et al (2008)
Spleen meridian (AxI)	(+) Wang et al (2008) Carlsson & Sjolund (2001)	
Large intestine meridian (TyI)	(+) Wang et al (2008)	

TCM: traditional Chinese medicine; CMT: collateral meridian therapy. (+): treatment meridian. Number: reference number.

Table 2. Acupunture points/meridians used for TCM and CMT in the management of low back pain and lumbar myofascial pain syndrome

First author (year) [Ref]	Condition treated	Post intervention	
		Pain reduction	Physical function recovery
Wong et al (2006)	Acute and chronic intractable pain	+	+
Lin et al (2010)	Primary dysmenorrhea	+	–
Wong et al (2007)	Complex regional pain syndrome	+	+
Hoka et al (2008)	Complex regional pain syndrome	+	+
Yeh et al (2008)	Shoulder-tip pain	+	+
Yeh et al (2009)	Post-regional anesthesia/analgesia backache	+	+

CMT, collateral meridian therapy. +, Yes; –, Not observed

Table 3. Clinical reports of CMT for pain management

3. Conclusion

CMT provides a different approach for managing intractable pain and various illnesses. It may play a role in the field of complementary and alternative medicine. The role of CMT in pain management looks promising for both acute and chronic pain, even including intractable pains, even though published randomized controlled trials are so far lacking. It is our hope that future research can focus on methodologically strong randomized controlled trials to validate the efficacy of CMT with high evidence level. The purpose of this article is to introduce the theory of CMT to interest physicians to achieve a greater awareness and understanding of this technique and theory.

4. Acknowledgment

The authors thank the Ko Medical System Inc. for providing the illustrations and figures for this chapter.

5. References

Carlsson C, Sjolund B. Acupuncture for chronic low back pain: a randomized placebo-controlled study with long-term follow-up. *Clin J Pain* 2001, 17:296-305.

Ezzo J, Hadhazy V, Birch S, Lao L, Kaplan G, Hochberg M, Berman B. Acupuncture for osteoarthritis of the knee: a systematic review. *Arthr Rheum* 2001, 44:819-25.

Hariharan J, Lamb GC, Neuner JM. Long-Term Opioid Contract Use for Chronic Pain Management in Primary Care Practice. A Five Year Experience. J of Gen Intern Med 2007, 22: 485-490.

Hoka S, Kanai A, Ko SC, Suzuki A. Collateral Meridian Therapy Alleviates Intractable Pain and Disablity in CRPS Patients. *ASA meeting* 2008: A904 .

Ko SC, Chao HR. Atlas of Ko medicine pressure points. (ISBN:978-986-83890-0-7, 2007)

Laxmaiah M, Mark VB, Vijay S, Ramsin M. B, Bert F, Salahadin A, Ricardo M B, Ann C, Sukdeb D, Richard D, Frank JE F, Stephanie E, Sudhir D, Salim M. H, Standiford H, Allan T. P, David M S, Howard S S, Lee R W, Joshua A H. Interventional techniques: evidence-based practice guidelines in the management of chronic spinal pain. *Pain Physician* 2009; 12: 699-802.

Leibing E, Leonhardt U, Koster G, Goerlitz A, Rosenfeldt J, Hilgers R, Ramadori G. Acupuncture treatment of chronic low-back pain- a randomized, blinded, placebo-controlled trial with 9-month follow up. *Pain* 2002, 96:189-196.

Lin JA, Wong CS, Lee MS, Ko SC, Chan SM, Chen JJY, Chen TL. Successful treatment of primary dysmenorrhea by collateral meridian acupressure therapy – a time series case report. *J Manipulative Physiol Ther* 2010, 33:70-5.

Meng C, Wang D, Ngeow J, Lao L, Peterson M, Paget S. Acupuncture for chronic low back pain through adjuvant electrical versus manual auricular acupuncture. *Anesth Analg* 2004, 98:1359-64.

Trinh K, Graham N, Gross A, Goldsmith C, Wang E, Careron I, Kay T. Acupuncture for neck pain disorder. *Spine* 2007, 32:236-43.

Wagner E, Ehrenhofer B, Lackerbauer E, Pawelak U, Siegmeth W. Rehabilitation of non-specific low back pain. Results of a multidisciplinary in-patient program. Schmerz 2007, 21: 228-33.

Wang SM, Kain ZN, White PF. Acupuncture Analgesia: II. Clinical Considerations. *Anesth Analg* 2008, 106:611-21.

Wong CS, Kuo CP, Ko SC. Can we do better, in addition to the pharmacological treatment, on pain: collateral meridian therapy. *Acta Anaesthesiol Taiwanica* 2006, 44:59-60.

Wong CS, Kuo CP, Fan YM, Ko SC. Collateral meridian therapy dramatically attenuates pain and improves functional activity of a patient with complex regional pain syndrome. *Anesth Analg* 2007, 104:452.

Yeh CC, Ko SC, Huh BK, Kuo CP, Wu CT, Cherng CH, Wong CS. Shoulder-tip pain following laparoscopic surgery analgesia by collateral meridian acupressure (shiatsu) therapy—report of two cases. *J Manipul Physiol Therap* 2008, 31:484-8.

Yeh CC, Wu CT, Huh BK, Lee SM, Wong CS. Collateral Meridian Acupressure Therapy Effectively Relieves Post-Regional Anesthesia/Analgesia Backache –The Report of Five Cases. *South Med J* 2009, 102:1179-1182.

Non-Pharmacological Therapies in Pain Management

Yurdanur Demir

Abant İzzet Baysal University, Bolu Health Sciences High School,
Turkey

1. Introduction

Pain is an unpleasant feeling and emotional experience that is related to real or potential tissue damage or a damage that is defined similarly. Pain is mostly subjective (Merskey, Bogduk 1986). From many points of view, the pain is a common symptom intended for seeking aid (Dickens et al. 2002). International Association for the Study of Pain (IASP) defines the pain as "an unpleasant emotional situation which is originating from a certain area, which is dependant or non-dependant on tissue damage and which is related to the past experience of the person in question" (Merskey, IASP 1986).

Although there is an increase of knowledge and developments in technological resources regarding the pain, many patients still experience pain (Nash et al. 1999). This situation causes for reduction in living quality and functional situation of the patients, increase in the fatigue levels (Kim et al. 2004) and impairments in daily life activities in working capacity and social interactions (McMillan et al., 2000; Allard et al., 2001). Also this situation will cause loss of workforce and will affect not only the patients but also his/her family members in economical terms thus causing undesired problems in psychological and social well being status (Uçan and Ovayolu 2007). All of these elements have directed both the patients and caregivers to seek for different searches in pain management (Evans and Rosner, 2005). For this reason in addition to the pharmacological treatment options for pain management, today, non-pharmacological treatment options and complementary medical attempts have started to be used (Kwekkeboom et al., 2003; Menefee and Monti, 2005). It is stated that such kind of therapies can be useful in pain management (Uçan and Ovayolu 2007). In a study conducted with the participation of 31.044 adults in United States, Barnes et al. (2004) determined that the usage rate of the complementary methods for the last year has been 36% and back pain and lumbago come first with 16.8% and neck pain comes third with 6.6% in terms of usage reasons of the complementary methods . Sherman et al. (2004) have stated that 24% of the patients with chronic lumbago used massage therapy.

2. Non-pharmacological therapies in pain management

It is considered that these therapies help the standard pharmacological treatment in pain management. While medical drugs are being used for treating the somatic (physiological and emotional) dimension of the pain non-pharmacological therapies aim to treat the affective, cognitive, behavioral and socio-cultural dimensions of the pain (Yavuz 2006).

These therapies can treat the pain as adjuvant or complementary at middle level and severe pain experiences as an adjuvant or complementary treatment. (Delaune & Ladner 2002).

Non-pharmacological methods,

- Increase the individual control feeling.
- Decrease the feeling of weakness.
- Improves the activity level and functional capacity.
- Reduces stress and anxiety.
- Reduces the pain behavior and focused pain level.
- Reduces the needed dosage of analgesic drugs thus decreasing the side effects of the treatment (Yıldırım 2006).

Non-pharmacological methods used in pain management can be classified in different ways. In general; they are stated as physical, cognitive, behavioral and other complementary methods or as invasive or -non-invasive methods. Meditation, progressive relaxation, dreaming, rhythmic respiration, biofeedback, therapeutic touching, transcutaneous electrical nerve stimulation (TENS), hypnosis, musical therapy, acupressure and cold-hot treatments are non-invasive methods (Black & Matassarin Jacobs, 1997). The most famous and common method among the invasive methods is acupuncture (Menifee and Monti, 2005). It is considered that these methods control the gates that are vehicles for pain to be transmitted to the brain and affect pain transmission or the release of natural opioids of the body such as endorphin (Black & Matassarin Jacobs, 1997; Menefee & Monti, 2005; Uçan & Ovayolu 2007).

Non-pharmacological methods used in pain management have been examined below in three groups such as peripheral therapies (physical agents/skin stimulation methods), cognitive-behavioral therapies and other therapies. Some of these methods require special training (Turan et al. 2010).

2.1 Peripheral therapies (physical agents/skin stimulation)

Skin stimulation that provides analgesia is defined as stimulating the patient's skin in a harmless manner to treat the pain (Yıldırım 2006). Skin stimulation attempts (physical therapies) can be classified as hot-cold treatments, exercise, positioning, movement restriction-resting, acupuncture, hydrotherapy, TENS, massage and therapeutic touch. If used in an appropriate manner these methods are effective on secondary pathologies such as inflammation, edema, progressive tissue damage, muscle spasm and function loss which takes part in acute pain. (Yıldırım 2006).

2.1.1 TENS (Transcutaneous Electrical Nerve Stimulation)

TENS has been defined by the American Physical Therapy Association as applying electrical stimulation to the skin to manage the pain (Sluka & Walsh 2003). Usually, it may be used in addition or instead of pharmacological agents to manage acute, chronic and post-operative pain. It is an electro-analgesia method (Mucuk and Başer, 2009). That is to say, thick and rapid transmitting nerve fibers are stimulated artificially with TENS and the pain transmission is tried to be stopped or reduced. TENS, which functions in that way, has an effect to reduce the narcotic drugs usage and pain level (Arslan & Çelebioğlu; Chen et al. 1998). TENS has various mechanisms of action regarding pain. Gate Control Theory is a theory used to define how TENS affects the pain perception which also has a part in improving TENS. Gate control theory regarding pain management is very commonly used by TENS in defining the process to

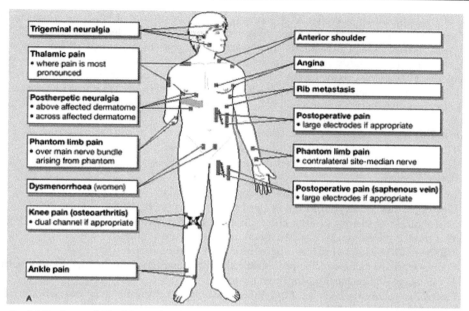

Fig. 1. a) *http://www.ib3health.com/products/TensandEMS/Literature/ApplicationChart.shtml* June/2011

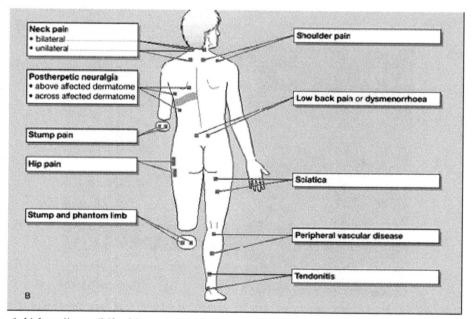

Fig. 1. b) *http://www.ib3health.com/products/TensandEMS/Literature/ApplicationChart.shtml* June/2011

prevent the pain (Sluka & Walsh 2003; Johnson 2002). In a study that has been conducted, it has been determined that the placebo group experienced 2-4 times less pain when TENS is used with pharmacological methods in post-operative pain management (Rakel & Frantz 2003), and in another study it has been determined that TENS usage in post-operative pain management has helped reducing the pain level and dosage of using analgesics (Bjordal et al. 2003). In addition to that, in some other studies it has been determined that first phase of labor in TENS group has been shorter and TENS treatment has been effective in relieving the pain (Kaplan et al. 1998; Simkin and Bolding 2004).

Points to Take into Consideration While Using Tens:

- TENS device should be used under the control of a health personnel.
- TENS devices should be used with caution in the areas where the pain could not be defined exactly.
- Device should be turned off while placing the materials.
- Electrical stimulation should not be used in front parts of the neck.
- You should use the device after controlling machine or motor vehicle producing TENS.
- This device should not be used on metal prostheses or monitors.
- TENS should be kept at places where the children cannot reach.
- People who are using cardiac pacemaker should consult to their doctors about whether TENS usage will be harmful for them or not.
- Electronic materials such as ECG monitors and ECG alarms may not work in full capacity while using TENS.
- It can cause damages on skin. That can be prevented by changing the type of gel and electrodes that are used.
- There are not reliable study results describing TENS usage during pregnancy (Yavuz 2006).

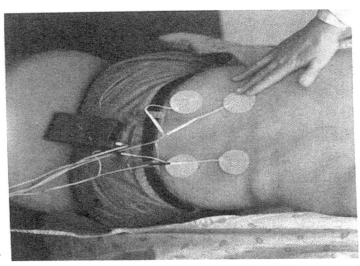

Dewit, S.C., (2009), *Fundamental concepts and skills for nursing*, 3rd Edition, W.B. Saunders Comp. Philadelphia, p.603-614.

Fig. 2. TENS Usage

2.1.2 Hot-cold treatment

Hot treatment moves the reflex arcs that inhibit the pain by means of heat receptors and reduces pain by vasodilatation effect. It is cheap and easy to use and it has a minimum amount of side effects when used regularly. It can be applied deeply or on surfaces. Application to the surface includes hot compresses, warm baths and paraphine usage. Deep applications such as ultrasound may increase the temperature of the tissues which are three to five centimeter deep (Arslan & Çelebioğlu, 2004).

On the other hand, cold treatment consists of applying a cooling material or device on any part of the body. Cold treatment which is a simple and cheap treatment method has an important place in non-drug therapies for pain management(Yavuz, 2006). Cold gel packages and ice packages commonly used in the application should be used by placing a tin towel/gauze between the skin and the package for being able to withstand extreme cold feeling during the first contact of the package, for having a homogenous cooling and providing hygiene. Cold treatment may be done for 15-30 minutes averagely until the anesthesia is felt on the area of application. The cold ice packs should be applied for at least 20 minutes. As a matter of fact, the affect of cold treatment on the human skin reveals itself in 4 stages. The patient will feel the cold within 1 to 3 minutes after the application, then feel a burning and pain sensation within 2 to 7 minutes and the pain and lethargy will decrease within 5 to 12 minutes, a breaking occurs for the pain-spasm vicious-circle and transmission of the nerve fibers in the area will decrease. An increase will occur for the metabolism within 12 to 15 minutes after cold treatment and a reflex vasodilatation occurs on the deep tissue. Thus, the edema and the pain will reduce and the tissue will be nourished with vasodilatation that will develop 15 minutes later (Karagözlüoğlu, 2001). Results of the studies made in the area have shown that the cold treatment has increased the pain threshold (Koç et al. 2006; Raynor et al. 2005; Sarifakioğlu & Sarifakioğlu 2004). So, the cold treatments that are applied locally are used to reduce the edema and treat the pain by taking the inflammation process under control (Saeki 2002; Sarifakioğlu & Sarifakioğlu 2004; Van der Westhuijzen et al. 2005).

It has been stated that cold treatment over the area where surgical sutures are found after lumbar disc surgery reduces both the pain during first 24 hours and the need for morphine (Brandner et al. 1996). Also, it has been shown that fluoromethane spray applications are a cheap method that are rapidly effective in managing the injection pain due to vaccination (Mawhorter et al. 2004) and cold package and ice applications have reduced the pain due to heparin injections (Kuzu ve Uçar 2001; Ross and Soltes 1995). In the study that they conducted, Demir and Khorshid (2010) have stated that cold treatment that is applied to the skin around the chest tube reduced the severity of the pain that is felt due to exclusion of chest tube and it has extended the time between exclusion of chest tube and taking an analgesic. It is stated that cold treatment is contraindicated for the situations such as urticaria/hypersensitivity, hypertension, Reynaud's phenomenon and sickle cell anemia which are related to cold (Mucuk & Başer, 2009).

2.1.3 Acupuncture and acupressure

Acupuncture which is one of the important components of traditional Chinese medicine has become a largely complementary in the West together with the conventional medicine. Acupuncture is accepted as a scientific treatment method that provides the body to restore its balance by means of stimulating some special points on the body with needles (Taşçı & Sevil 2007). Mechanism of action for the acupuncture could not be completely understood until now. Effect of the acupunctures is tried to be explained by Gate Control Theory. According to this theory, effect of a sensory stimulant (for example lumbago) can be suppressed with another stimulant (picking a needle) within a neural system. Another theory that explains the effect of acupuncture is Raising Pain Threshold Theory. That is a theory in which inhibitor effect of acupuncture is defined. In this theory, it is predicted to stimulate the analgesia mechanisms of the body by causing various pains on the area where an individual is feeling the pain to be treated. In addition to these, it has also been evidence that the acupuncture stimulates the production of endorphin, serotonin and acetyl choline within the central nerve system (Van Tulder et al. 2005). It has been shown in the studies that have been conducted that the acupuncture had positive effects on post-traumatic somatic pain, patella-femoral pain, rheumatoid arthritis and idiopathic head pain. (Snyder & Wieland 2003). It is sated in the literature that the acupuncture is especially useful in treating the lumbago but it is underlined that the patients should be informed in terms of increasing or carrying on the activities (Öztekin, 2005). Although there are some strong evidences showing the benefit of acupuncture in acute pain, the evidence regarding the cancer pain is limited (Black & Matassarin Jacobs, 1997; Filshie & Thompson 2004; Menefee & Monti, 2005). In spite of that, Alimi et al. (2003) stated that the acupuncture applied to cancer patient has decreased the pain level.

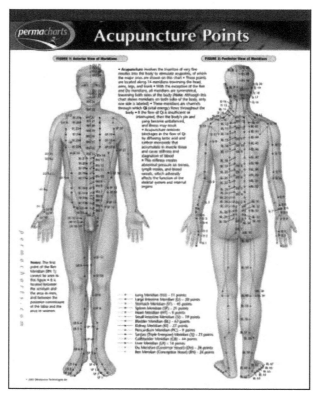

Fig. 3. http://suphecimelek.wordpress.com/2010/10/31/akupunktur June/2011

Acupressure is one of the traditional Chinese medicine approaches used for pain relief, diseases and injuries. Acupressure is a therapy that is conducted by applying physical pressure on various points on body surface by means of energy circulation and balance in cases of pain symptoms. This therapy is similar to the acupuncture and it is conducted by applying pressure on selected points of the body by fingers, hands, palms, wrists and knees in order to provide internal flow of energy. Acupressure technique is a noninvasive, safe and effective application (Hakverdioğlu, & Türk, 2006). It is suggested that acupressure reduces back, head, osteoarthritis, musculoskeletal and neck pains, pre-operative and post-operative pains, nausea-vomiting and sleeping problems (Tsay, Rong and Lin 2003; Tsay & Chen 2003; Hakverdioğlu, & Türk 2006).

2.1.4 Exercise
Exercise includes active-passive movements, bed movements and ambulation. Exercise increases the movement and provides continuity thus increasing the blood flow, preventing spasm and contractures of the muscles and relieving the pain (Musclow et al., 2002).

2.1.5 Positioning
It is applied to help or support the patient. This application can be supported by pillows, special beds and weight lifting. Position changes, which prevent the subsequent development of pain and reducing the acute pain, also increase the blood flow and prevent muscle contraction and spasms (Akdağ & Ovayolu, 2008). Positioning has been determined as the most common post-operative non-pharmacological method (Carroll 1999).

2.1.6 Restriction of movement /resting
These are applied for the patients who need certain bed rest and which are in traction. However, it should not be used alone for pain management. It can be used for fractures and back surgeries. Restriction of movement can also decrease edema development (Arslan & Çelebioğlu, 2004).

2.1.7 Massage
Massage is a manipulation applied on the soft tissue with various techniques (such as friction, percussion, vibration and tapotement) for recovery and supporting health. It is thought that the massage relieve the mind and muscles and increase the pain threshold (Karagöz 2006). Peripheral receptors on the body are stimulated with massage and stimulants reach the brain by means of spinal cord. In addition to pleasant feeling, a general relief is provided here (Turan et al. 2010). It is underlined that especially therapeutic massage is effective on chronic lumbago and that effect is stated to be a short term effect (Hsieh et al. 2004). Melancon and Miller (2005) draw attention to the fact that pain management in patient groups with lumbago that are treated with massage and pharmacological therapies are similar and they recommend the sue of massage as an alternative treatment option for the patients with lumbago within the framework of a integrated care. Nixon et al (1997) has stated that massage played a role in reducing the pain. In addition to that it is determined in some randomized controlled studies that massage made during labor decreases pain and anxiety; it also improves the general well being and progression of birth process and less reaction is given to the pain (Caton et.al 2002; Simkin & O'Hora 2002).

2.1.8 Hydrotherapy (Balneotherapy)
Using water for treatment by means of thermal springs, potable water resources and other methods is defined as "hydrotherapy" while using the water for therapy by means of temperature effect is defined as "hydrothermal treatment". Effect of hydrotherapy is related to its mechanical or thermal effect. Hot application stimulates the immune system, provides hormones that are suppressing the stress to be released, stimulates the circulation and digestion systems, increases the blood flow and provides muscle relaxation thus reducing the sensitivity developed against the pain (Karagöz, 2006). It is stated in the literature that hydrotherapy is effective while treating back and chronic lumbago (Balogh et al. 2005; Hartel & Volger 2004).

2.2 Cognitive-behavioral therapies
Cognitive-behavioral therapies are a part of multimodal approach in pain management. These attempts affect not only the pain level but also helps the patients to establish a management feeling of theirselves while dealing with pain and develop management behaviors and improved self-esteem. Cognitive-behavioral therapies can generally be applied by all members of the pain team. Most of the special techniques can be learned and applied by doctors, nurses, social service specialists and psychologists (Yıldırım 2006). These therapies should be thought and applied as early as possible before the patient experiences pain (Delaune & Ladner 2002).

2.2.1 Relaxation - respiration techniques and dreaming
Relaxation techniques cause an increase in slow brain waves in EEG by decreasing oxygen consumption, blood pressure, respiration amount and the number of pulse. Therefore, it is stated that the sensitivity developed against the pain should be prevented by means of these techniques (Karagöz, 2006).
Techniques used in providing the spiritual and physical relaxation are summarized below:
- *Respiration providing the relaxation:* It is provided to focus on the respiration and avoid disturbing thoughts by taking a deep breath slowly through the nose and giving it back in a long time through the mouth. These techniques can be applied for 5-10 minutes per day (Nordin 2002).
- *Advanced muscle relaxation treatment:* It is aimed to relax the unwanted contractions by determining them through making the patient contract and relax certain muscle groups on his body (Nordin 2002).
- *Dreaming:* After relaxation is provided, the patient is made to focus on a stimulant that makes the patient happy (light, color, sound, pattern etc.) in order to get the patient far away from his pain for a short period of time (Karagöz 2006). In a study made by Lewandowski et al (2005) it has been stated that an effective pain management can be obtained by directing the patients to dreaming for more than 4 days.

2.2.2 Distraction
Getting the attention away from the pain reduces its severity. The aim in using that technique is to increases the tolerance for pain and decrease the sensitivity for pain. This method includes listening to music, watching television, reading books and dreaming (Arslan & Çelebioğlu, 2004). There are some sources which supports that distraction is a method used in decreasing the pain (Seers & Carroll 1998; Petry 2002).

2.2.3 Praying

Most of the individuals with chronic pains use the praying method. It is indicated that praying has positive results for decreasing the body pain in old people and relieving their physical functional disorders and it is suggested to use the praying method in order to reduce the depression and anxiety that is caused by chronic pain (Meisenhelder & Chandler, 2000; Karagöz, 2006).

2.2.4 Meditation

In the traditional meaning, meditation is generally focusing on the moment. Meditation; can also be defined as focusing on the present. This act is realized with an individual focusing on his own respiration, a word or picture. Duration of the meditation can last from a few minutes to 30 minutes or take more (Snyder & Wieland, 2003; Gray, 2004). Considering the fact that meditation helps relaxation, it is thought to be effective in relieving the pain (Gray, 2004). Carson et al (2005) have stated that an 8-week meditation is useful for relieving the pain for patients with chronic lumbago.

2.2.5 Yoga

Yoga is providing relaxation by using respiration exercises and meditation with slow movements. It is considered that it can be useful against musculoskeletal pain in terms of using physical stretching moves and increasing strength (Dillard & Knapp, 2005). Individuals that use yoga have stated that they believe in the benefit of this method and it is a cost-effective method. It is stated in a study that applying yoga for 16 weeks has cured the chronic lumbago (Williams et al. 2005). Also, in a study conducted by Williams et al (2005) it has been stated that functional insufficiency experienced with chronic lumbago and use of pain killers have been reduced by means of yoga.

2.2.6 Hypnosis

Hypnosis; it is the state of conscious change similar to sleep. Hypnosis requires the body to relax and the patient to focus on an object, a stimulant or memory. Hypnosis is *"the deep physical relaxation state during which subconscious can be reached and important abilities are suspended"*. In this state, ability of people to be dominated increases (Taşçı & Sevil, 2007). Besides mechanism of action of hypnosis over the pain is not known exactly and it is mentioned that the pain is reduced with some physiological changes that occur as a result of hypnosis. Hypnosis has been used in a positive manner in terms of cancer pain, pains in head-neck region and phantom pain which is the sensations felt by amputees (Black & Matassarin Jacobs, 1997). Jensens and Patterson (2006) has stated that hypnotherapy/hypnosis is used for analgesia in various types of chronic pains and it has been stated that hypnosis has been effective for neck pain. Also Liossi et al (2006) has made a study with pediatric cancer patients in which it has been determined that hypnosis application has decreased pain and anxiety level in patients (Liossi et al. 2006).

2.2.7 Bio-feedback

Biological feedback is based informing the patient in order to help relaxation or control a physiological function. For example, in cases of tension type headache, it is provided for the electrical activity received by means of head muscles and facial muscles to be perceived as colors or sounds by the patient. Thus, observing the color changes or decreases in the sound, the patient understands whether the relaxation occurred or not (Uçan & Ovayolu 2007). Bio-feedback is used for treatment in the cases of pain, migraine pain, spinal cord injuries and movement disorders. It is aimed to control of physiological reactions such as muscle tension, body temperature, heart rate, brain wave activity and other vital parameters. Efficiency of the treatment depends on the desire that a patient shows for learning of how controlling of these functions and participation of patient in the process. Biofeedback appliers train the patient in terms of mental and physical exercises, visualization and deep breaths (Eidelson, 2005). In many types of chronic pain the bio-feedback has been shown to be effective (Moseikin 2003; Teyhen et al. 2005).

2.2.8 Behavioral therapy

Aim of this therapy is to increase the functional level of the patient decrease the maladaptive behaviors and firstly reduce and then completely stop painkiller usage. The family is trained by the treatment team; description of pain (grimacing, moaning, and remaining motionless) is avoided and well-adaptive behaviors such as physical activities are reinforced (Brietbart et al. 2004).

2.3 Other non-pharmacological therapies
2.3.1 Reflexology

Reflexology is a technique that is based on the principle that suggests there are reflex points on our feet corresponding to all parts of our bodies , all organs and systems and these points are the mirrors of the body anatomy. Pressure applied to these reflex points by special hand and finger techniques provides the stress to be relieved and cause physiological changes and a reduction in pain perception (Yıldırım, Fadıloğlu and Uyar, 2006). There are totally five pressurizing techniques to make massage on reflex areas: Thumb move, finger move, rubbing move, patting move and compressing move. These moves are applied to ears, hands and feet similarly. The important thing here is to know how this technique will be applied to whom. Physical structure of an individual, age and current health status are taken into consideration. Treatment consists of applying pressure with the side of a thumb or other fingers and turning it clockwise. This pressure is generally deep but it does not have to be painful. A good reflexologist prefers repetition of short and painless seances to a single but painful seances for the whole disease. Intensity of the pressure can be low at the beginning and increased as the treatment progresses. Each seance takes from 10 minutes to 30 minutes and it is decided according to the situation of the person how many seance will be necessary (Stephenson et al. 2000; Bolsoy 2008).

It is stated in the literature that reflexology is used especially for reducing migraine pain, back pain, muscle pain, end stage cancer pain and side effects of chemotherapy and to increase living quality (Long et al. 2001; McNeill et al. 2006; Mollart 2003; Quattrin et al.2006; Wringht et al.2002) In spite of that, it is stated that it is unfavorable to use reflexology in acute infections and fever situation, deep venous thrombosis, surgical situations and in cases of open scars, malign melanoma and during first trimester of the pregnancy or with the patients that has miscarriage or premature birth risks (Long et al. 2001; Lett 2002).

2.3.2 Herbal treatments

Herbal medicine is using the chemical materials obtained from inside, root, leave, seed and flower parts of the herbs for treatment (Karagöz 2006). Today, most individuals use herbal products in addition to their medical treatments with drugs without consulting to any professional (Turan et al. 2010 ; Deng et al. 2005). It is stated in the literature that herbal medicine has been commonly used to treat lumbago and back pains (Gray, 2004; Gagnier et al. 2006; Hartel & Volger 2004).

2.3.3 Aromatherapy

Aromatherapy is using the essential oils that are obtained from flowers, herbs and trees to improve health and well being. These oils are applied by being respired through oily gauze that is placed under the nostrils of the patient or as massage oils being applied on skin. It has been evidenced that the aroma oils reached the lymph system by means of blood circulation and provided recovery by means of intercellular fluids (Turan et al. 2010). It is thought that aromatherapy may be able to help reducing stress, treating cold, sniffles, skin and menstruation problems and relieving pain (Karagöz, 2006; Jennings, 2004; Yıldırım et al. 2006; Deng et al. 2005). It is known that lavender oil is used in treating migraine pain, osteoarthritis, rheumatoid arthritis and lumbago. It is also known that eucalyptus, black pepper, ginger, daisy, licorice, rosemary and myrrh oils are used in relieving pain. But it is stated that lavender oil can cause hypersomnia and using licorice for long time can cause hypertension (Delaune & Ladner 2002). Although the usage of aromatherapy within health system increases day by day it is seen that the researches in this meaning is quite insufficient. Data regarding the efficiency of essential oils depend only on individual experiences. For this reason, it is necessary to conduct studies with large samples and high level of evidence to determine the efficiency of essential oils in pain management (Snyder & Wieland 2003; Tseng 2005)

2.3.4 Chiropractics

Chiropractics is the neck-pulling movement used in treatment of the disorders in connective tissues and musculoskeletal system which consists of muscles, joints, bones, tendon, cartilage and ligaments. The main principle of this approach is the fact that to relieve the pain and to improve health with the applications made on spine and joints which have had a positive effect on neural system and natural defense mechanisms (Gray, 2004). Chiropractics have focused on the connection between body structure and the functions of the neural system and manipulation of bones and joints to regain the health. It is known that the application that is taken, decreases the amount of burden on the neck and relives the pain. However, the individuals who have serious disorders such as severe cervical disc hernia, complaints due to rheumatoid arthritis , tumors and infection have to avoid from these applications (Turan et al. 2010; Karagöz 2006; Deng et al. 2005).

2.3.5 Musical therapy

Many studies that have been conducted have sown that the music had positive effects on pain and anxiety and increased the living quality of the patient or healthy individuals. Music reduces heart rate, blood pressure, body temperature and respiration rate and it distraction the attention of the patient to another point thus reducing the pain perception and reducing especially the nausea due to chemotherapy so that increasing living quality of patients in terminal period of cancer (Chase, 2003; Hilliard, 2003; Deng et al. 2005; Stefano et al. 2004, Uçan & Ovayolu 2007). In a study that states listening to music stimulates the alpha waves of brain which have been determined as a stimulator for the release of endorphin and creates a relaxation state and therefore music has played a role not only in relieving the pain but also decreasing blood pressure, heartbeat rate and other physiological responses (Henry, 1995). A point to be taken into consideration here is to let the music type to be prefered by the patient (Delaune & Ladner, 2002). New studies show that slow music creates a relaxing effect. According to the literature musical therapy should not be used continuously to be an effective method. Applying musical therapy form 25 to 90 minutes per day will provide sufficient treatment period.

Attempt	Advantage	Disadvantage
Relaxation Bio-feedback Distraction	• It may reduce the pain and anxiety without having drug-related side effects. • It can be used more likely as an adjuvant therapy together with other methods. It may increase the management feeling of the patient. • Most of them are not expensive, they do not require special equipment and they are easily applicable.	• The patients should be aware of using the management strategies by theirselves. • An appropriate time zone is needed to teach the attempts.
Psychotherapy, Hypnosis	• It may reduce the pain and anxiety of the patients who have pains that are relatively difficult to manage. • It may increase the number of methods that the patient uses to manage.	• It requires an experienced therapist.
Skin Stimulation/Cutaneous Stimulation (superficial hot-cold application and massage)	• It may reduce muscle spasms, inflammation and pain. • It can be used more likely as an adjuvant therapy together with other methods. • It may increase the controlling ability of pain feeling of the patient. • It is so easy to use. • It may be applied by the patients or families. • It is a cheap method.	• Hot application can increase the bleeding or edema after acute injuries. • Cold application is contraindicate for the situations such as uritcaria/hypersensitivity, hypertension, Reynaud's phenomenon and sickle cell anemia which are related to cold.
Transcutaneous Electrical Nerve Stimulation (TENS)	• It reduces the pain without having any drug-related side effects. • It can be used more likely as an adjuvant therapy together with other methods. • It gives the feeling of pain management to the patient.	• It requires an experienced therapist. • There is a risk for bleeding and infection. • There are no reliable results for use in cases of pregnant women.
Aromatherapy	• It has an analgesic effect. • It has a sedative and relaxing effect.	• It may cause hypersomnia. • Some herbs should not be used with other anti-depressants and alcohol.
Acupuncture	• It may provide pain reduction without any side effects. • It can be used more likely as an adjuvant therapy together with other methods.	• It requires an experienced therapist.

Table 1. Advantages and Disadvantages of Some Non-pharmacological Methods

In a study they conducted, Nilsson et al (2003) have stated that listening to music for one hour in earl post-operative period may reduce post-operative pain and morphine consumption of the patients. In a study conducted by Sahler and Hunter (2003) with the patients who had bone marrow transplantation, the patients were made to listen music which has a relaxing effect, at least twice a week for 45 minutes and it has been determined that the group which was not included to music therapy has a higher pain score when compared to the one that has received musical therapy. It has been stated that the musical also has positive effects during labor period. In a study that is conducted by Browning (2000) related to the mother's pain and anxiety levels to evaluate the effect of musical therapy applied to primipar mothers before delivery, the mothers have stated that the musical therapy relives their pain and it made them feel themselves more comfortable and calm.

Advantages and disadvantages of some non-pharmacological methods used in pain management have been specified below (Table 1).

3. Conclusion

As a result, the pain can be managed in a more effective manner with the combination of pharmacological and non-pharmacological therapies. Developments in pain management may provide different opportunities to the patients and their families thus providing the patients to carry on a more comfortable and productive life. Both health personnel and caregivers need to have important responsibilities while following these developments. For an effective care to be provided to patients, developments regarding pain management and updated pharmacological and non-pharmacological approaches regarding pain management and pain should be followed. Also these techniques may help reducing pain and it must be encouraged as a part of the comprehensive pain management efforts. For this reason, abilities and preferences of the patient regarding the use of non-pharmacological methods should be taken into consideration; it should be underlined for the patients that these are used together with medical and pharmacological treatments and the use of non-pharmacological methods should be included to the care plan when patient is appropriate and willing. From this point of view, it is recommended to use various non-pharmacological methods for pain management but we need more study results that support the efficiency of these methods. For this reason, it will provide the evidence-based results to be put forward if randomized controlled experimental studies, which examine the efficiency of these methods in taking the pain under control, are conducted.

4. References

Akdağ, R. G. & Ovayolu, N. (2008). Hemşirelerin Ağrı Yönetimi ile İlgili Bilgi, Tutum ve Klinik Karar Verme Durumlarının Değerlendirilmesi. *Gaziantep Üniversitesi Sağlık Bilimleri Enstitüsü,* Master's Thesis.

Alimi, D.; Rubino, C.; Pichard-Leandri, E.; Fernand, B.S.; Dubreuil-Lemaire, M.L. & et al. (2003). Analgesic effect of auricular acupuncture for cancer pain: randomized, blinded, controlled trial. *Journal of Clinical Oncology*, 15;21(22): 4120-4126; Nov 2003.

Allard, P.; Maunsell, E.; Labbe, J. & Dorval, M. (2001). Educational interventions to improve cancer pain control: a systematic review . *Journal of Palliative Medicine*, Vol.4 , No:2 , pp.191-203.

Arslan, S. & Çelebioğlu, A. (2004). Postoperatif Ağrı Yönetimi ve Alternatif Uygulamalar. *International Journal of Human Sciences*, 1(1): 1-7.

Balogh, Z.; Ordogh, J.; Gasz, A.; Nemet, L. & Bender, T. (2005). Effectiveness of balneotherapy in chronic low back pain -- a randomized single-blind controlled follow-up study. *Forsch Komplementarmed Klass Naturheilkd*, 12(4): 196-201; Aug 2005.

Barnes, P.; Griner, E.; Mcfann, K. & Nahin, R.L.(2004). Complementary and alternative medicine use among adults: United States, 2002. *Adv Data.*, Vol.27, pp.1-19.

Bjordal, M.J.; Johnson, I.M. & Ljunggreen, A.E. (2003). Transcutaneous Electrical Nerve Stimulation (TENS) Can Reduce Postoperative Analgesic Consumption: A Meta-Analysis With Assesment Of Optimal Treatment Parameters For Postoperative Pain. *The European Journal Of Pain*, 7(2): 181-188.

Black, J.M. & Matassarin Jacobs, E. (1997). Pain , In: *Medical-Surgical Nursing: Clinical Management for Continuity of Care. 5.th edition*, J.M. Black, E.M. Jacobs & J. Luckmann(Edts.) pp: 342-365, W.B. Saunders Co., ISBN: 978-0721663999.

Bolsoy, N. (2008). Perimenstrüel Distresin Hafifletilmesinde Refleksolojinin Etkinliğinin İncelenmesi. Ege Üniversitesi Sağlık Bilimleri Enstitüsü, PhD Thesis.

Brandner, B.; Munro, B.; Bromby, L.M. & Hetreed, M. (1996). Evaluation of the Contribution to Postoperative Analgesia by Local Cooling of the Wound. *Anaesthesia*, 51(11): 1021-1025; Nov 1995.

Brietbart, W.; Payne, D. & Passik, S.D. (2004). Psychological and psychiatric interventions in pain control. In: *Oxford Textbook of Palliative Medicine. 3rd ed.* Doyle D, Hanks NC, Calman K (eds), pp: 424-438 NY: Oxford University Pres, New York; ISBN:9780198566984.

Browning, C.A. (2000) Using musiv during childbirth. *Birth*,27(4),272-276.

Carroll, C.et al.(1999). Pain Assessment and Management in Critically ill Postoperative and Trauma Patients: A Multisite Study . *American Journal of Critical Care.* Vol.8 (2),March 1999..

Carson, J.W.; Keefe, F.J.; Lynch, T.R.; Carson, K.M.; Goli, V.; Fras, A.M. & et. al. (2005). Loving-kindness meditation for chronic low back pain: results from a pilot trial.*J. Holist. Nurs.*, 23(3): 287-304; Sep 2005.

Caton, D.; Corry, M.P.; Frigoletto, F.D.; Hopkins, D.P.; Lieberman, E.; Mayberry, L.; Rooks, J.P.; Rosenfield, A.; Sakala, C.; Simkin, P. & Young, D. (2002). The nature and management of labor pain: executive summary. *American Journal of Obstetrics And Gynecology*, 186(5 Suppl Nature):S1-15;May 2002.

Chase, K.M. (2003). Multicultural music therapy: A review of literature. *Music Therapy Perspectives*, 21(2):84-88;ISSN : 0734-6875.

Chen, L.; Tang, J.; White, P. F.; Slonınsky, A.; Wender, R. H.; Naruse, R. & Kariger, R. (1998). The Effect of Location of Transcutaneous Electrical Nerve Stimulation on Postoperative Opioid Analgesic Requirement: Acupoint Versus Nonacupoint Stimulation. *Anesth Analg*, 87(5): 1129–34; Nov 1998.

Delaune, S.C.& Ladner, P.K. (Eds.) (2002). *Fundamental of Nursing : Standard And Practice (2nd Edition)*, pp.916-941,Newyork, Thomson Delmar Learning. ISBN: 978-076824522.

Demir, Y. & Khorshıd, L. (2010). The Effect of Cold Application in Combination with Standard Analgesic Administration on Pain and Anxiety During Chest Tube Removal: A Single-Blinded, Randomized, Double-Controlled Study. *Pain Management Nursing*, (11)3: 186-196; Sep 2010.

Deng, G. & Cassileth, B.R. (2005). Integrative oncology: complementary therapies for pain, anxiety, and mood disturbance. *CA: A Cancer Journal for Clinicians*, 55(2):109-116;May/April 2005.

Dewit, S.C. (2009). *Fundamental concepts and skills for nursing, 3rd Edition*, p.603-614, W.B. Saunders Comp. Philadelphia,; ISBN : 978-1-4160-5228-9.

Dickens C, Jayson M, Creed F (2002) Psychological Correlates Of Pain Behavior in Patients With Chronic Low Back Pain. *Psychosomatics*, 43:42–48;February 2002.

Dillard, J.N. & Knapp, S. (2005). Complementary and alternative pain therapy in the emergency department. *Emerg Med Clin North Am*, 23(2): 529-549; May 2005.

Eidelson, S.G. (2005). *Advanced Technologies to Treat Neck and Back Pain, A Patient's Guide*; Eidelson's book; http://www.spineuniverse.com/displayarticle.php/article224.html; March 2005.

Evans, R. & Rosner, A. (2005). Alternative in cancer pain treatment: the application of chiropractic care . *Seminars in Oncology Nursing* , Vol.21 , No:3 , pp.184-189.

Filshie, J. & Thompson, J.W. (2004). Acupuncture; In: *Oxford Textbook of Palliative Medicine. 3rd ed,* D. Doyle ; NC. Hanks & K. Calman (eds), pp: 410-424.. NY: Oxford University Press, New York. ISBN-13: 978-0198510987

Gagnier, J.J.; Van Tulder, M.; Berman, B. & Bombardier, C. (2006). Herbal medicine for low back pain. *Cochrane Database Syst Rev,*19(2); CD004504 April 2006

Gray, D.P. (2004). Complementary and alternative therapies. In : *Medical Surgical Nursing,* S.M., Lewis, ; L. Heitkemper, & S.R. Dirksen, (Eds). pp:94-109, St. Louis : Mosby Inc; ISBN-13: 978-0323016100.

Hakverdioğlu G. & Türk, G. (2006). Acupressure. *Journal of Hacettepe University School of Nursing,*43-47.

Hartel, U.; Volger, E. (2004). Use and acceptance of classical natural and alternative medicine in Germany--findings of a representative population-based survey. *Forsch Komplementarmed Klass Naturheilkd*, 11(6): 327-334; Dec 2004.

Henry, L.L. (1995). Music therapy: a nursing intervention for the control of pain and anxiety in the ICU: a review of the research literature. Dimensions of Critical Care Nursing, 14(6):295-304.

Hilliard, R.E. (2003). The effect of music therapy on the quality and length of life people diagnosed with terminal cancer. *Journal of Music Therapy*, 40(2):113-117.

Hsieh, L.L.; Kuo, C.H.; Yen, M.F. & Chen, T.H.A. (2004). A Randomized controlled clinical trial for low back pain treated by acupressure and physical therapy. *Prev Med*, 39(1): 168-176; Jul 2004.

http://suphecimelek.wordpress.com/2010/10/31/akupunktur-ise-yarar-mi; June/2011

http://www.ib3health.com/products/TensandEMS/Literature/ApplicationChart.shtml, June 2011.

Jennings, W.M. (2004). Aromatherapy practice in nursing: literature review. *Journal of Advanced Nursing*, 48 (1): 93–103.

Jensen, M. & Patterson, D. (2006). Hypnotic treatment of chronic pain. *J. Behav. Med.,*29(1): 95-124;Feb 2006.

Johnson MI. (2002). Transcutaneous Electrical Nevre Stimulation. In: *Electrotherapy: Evidence-Based Practice(11th edition),* S. Kitchen.(Ed.), pp.:259-286; Edinburgh: Churchill Livingstone, ISBN : 0443072167.

Kaplan, B.; Rabinerson, D.; Lurie, S.; Bar, J.; Krieser, U.R. & Neri, A. (1998). Transcutaneous electrical nevre stimulation (TENS) for adjuvant pain-relief during labor and delivery. *International Journal of Gynecology & Obstetrics*, 60(3): 251-255; Mar 1998.

Karagöz, G. (2006). Sırt, boyun, bel ağrıları olan ve ameliyat programına alınan nöroşürurji hastalarının ağrı gidermede kullandıkları tamamlayıcı ve alternatif tedaviler. *İstanbul Üniversitesi Sağlık Bilimleri Enstitütüsü. İstanbul* Master's Thesis.

Karagözoğlu, Ş.A. (2001). Intravenöz Sıvı Tedavısı Komplikasyonu Olarak Gelişen Tromboflebitte Hemşirelik Bakımı Ve Sıcak - Soğuk Uygulamanın Yeri. *C.Ü. Hemşirelik Yüksekokulu Dergisi*, 5(1):18-25.

Kim, J.E.; Dodd, M. & West, C. (2004). The PRO-SELF Pain control program improves patients knowledge of cancer pain management. *Oncology Nursing Forum*, Vol. 31 , No:6 , pp.1137-1143.

Koç, M.; Tez, M.; Yoldaş, Ö.; Dizen, H. & Göçmen, E. (2006). Cooling for the Reduction of The Postoperative Pain. Prospective-Randomized Study. *Hernia*, 10(2):184-186; Apr 2006.

Kuzu, N. & Uçar, H. (2001). The Effect of Cold on The Occurence of Bruising, Haematoma and Pain at the Injection Site in Subcutaneous Low-Molecular Weight Heparin. *International Journal of Nursing Studies*, 38(1):51-59; Feb 2001.

Kwekkeboom, K.; Kneip, J. & Pearson, L. (2003). A pilot study to predict success with guided imagery for cancer paitent . *Pain Management Nursing*, Vol. 4 , No.3 , pp.112-123.

Lett, A. (2002). The Future of Reflexology. *Complementary Therapy in Nursing & Midwifery*, 8(2): 84-90; May 2002.

Lewandowski, W.; Good, M. & Draucker, C.B. (2005). Changes in the Meaning of pain with the use of Guided Imagery. *Pain Manag Nurs*, 6(2): 58-67; Jun 2005.

Liossi, C.; White, P. & Hatira, P. (2006). Randomized clinical trial of local anesthetic versus a combination of local anesthetic with self-hypnosis in the management of pediatric procedure-related pain. *Health Psychology*, 25(3):307-315; May 2006.

Long, L.; Huntley, A.& Ernst, E. (2001) Which Complementary and Alternative Therapies Benefit Which Conditions? A Survey of Opinions Of 223 Professional Organizations. *Complementary Therapy in Medicine*, 9: 178-185.

Mawhorter, S.; Daugherty, L.; Ford, A.; Hughes, R.; Metzger, D. & Easley, K. (2004). Topical Vapocoolant Quickly and Effectively Reduces Vaccine- Associated Pain: Results of Randomized Single-Blinded, Placebo-Controlled Study. *J. Travel Med*, 11(5), 267-272; Sep-Oct 2004.

McMillan, S.C.; Tittle, M.; Hagan, S. & Laughlin, J. (2000). Management of pain and pain-related symptoms in hospitalized veterans with cancer . *Cancer Nursing*, Vol. 23 , No:5 , pp.327-336.

McNeill, J.A.; Alderdice, F.A. & Mcmurray, F. (2006). A Retrospective Cohort Study Exploring the Relationship Between Antenatal Reflexology and İntranatal Outcomes. *Complementary Therapies in Clinical Practice*;12(2): 119-125; May 2006.

Meisenhelder, J.B. & Chandler, E.N. (2000). Prayer and health outcomes in church members. *Altern. Ther. Health Med.*, 6(4): 56-60; Jul 2000.

Melancon, B. & Miller, L.H. (2005). Massage therapy versus traditional therapy for low back pain relief: implications for holistic nursing practice. *Holist Nurs Pract*, 19(3): 116-21;May-Jun 2005.

Menefee, L.A. & Monti, D.(2005).Nonpharmacologic and complementary approaches to cancer pain management . *The Journal of the American Osteopathic Association*, Vol.105, No.11 , pp.15-20.

Merskey, H. & Bogduk, N. (editors.).(1986). Pain, In:*Classification of chronic pain : description of chronic pain syndromes and definition of pain terms , Prepared by the İnternational Association for the study of Pain,(IASP), Subcommittee on Taxonomy.* Pain Suppl 3:S1-226., IASP Press, ISBN-13: 978-0-931092-05-3

Mollart, L. (2003). Single-Blind Trial Addressing the Differential Effects of Two Reflexology Techniques Versus Rest, On Ankle and Foot Oedema in Late Pregnancy. *Complementary Therapy in Nursing & Midwifery*, 9(4): 203-208; November 2003.

Moseikin, I.A . (2003). Use of biofeedback in combined treatment of low spine pain. *Zh Nevrol Psikhiatr Im S S Korsakova*, 103, 32-6.

Mucuk, S. & Başer, M. (2009). Doğum ağrısını hafifletmede kullanılan tensel uyarılma yöntemleri. Journal of Anatolia Nursing and Health Sciences, 12(3),61-66.

Musclow, SL.;Sawhney, M. & Watt-Watson, J. (2002). The emerging role of advanced nursing practice in acute pain management throughout Canada. *Clinical Nurse Specialist* 16(2):63-67.

Nash, R.; Yates, P.; Edwards, H.; Fentiman, B.; Dewar, A; Mcdowell, J. & Clark, R. (1999). Pain and administration of analgesia: what nurses say. *Journal of Clinical Nursing,* 1999; 8(2):180.

Nilsson, U.; Rawal, N.; Enqvist, B.& Unosson, M.(2003) Analgesia following music and therapeutic suggestions in the PACU in ambulatory surgery; a randomized controlled trial. *Acta Anaesthesiol Scand;*47(3):278-83.

Nixon, M. et al.(1997). Expanding the nursing repertoire: The effect of massage on post-operative pain *.Australian Journal of Advanced Nursing,* 14(3):21-26,March-May 1997.

Nordin, M. (2002). Self-care techniques for acute episodes of low-back pain. *Best Practice & Research Clinical Rheumatology,* 16(1): 89-101;Jan 2002.

Öztekin, İ. (2005). Bel ağrısı: Primer tedavide bütünleyici yaklaşım. *Akupunktur Dergisi,* 15(55-56): 7-11.

Petry, JJ.(2002). Surgery and complementary therapies: A review. *Alternative Therapies in Health and Medicine,*6(5):64-74.

Quattrin, R.; Zanini, A.; Buchini, S.; Turello, D.; Annunziata, M.A.; Vidotti, C.; Colombatti, A. & Brusaferro, S. (2006). Use of Reflexology Foot Massage to Reduce Anxiety in Hospitalized Cancer Patients in Chemotherapy Treatment: Methodology and Outcomes. *Journal of Nursing Management*, 14(2): 96-105; March 2006.

Rakel, B. & Frantz, R.(2003). Effectiveness Of Transcutaneous Electrical Nerve Stimulation On Postoperative Pain With Movement. *The Journal of Pain*, 4(8); 455-464.

Raynor, M.C.; Pietrobon, R.; Guller, U. & Higgins, L.D. (2005). Cryotherapy After ACL Reconstruction: a Meta Analysis. *J. Knee Surgery*, 18(2),123-9; Apr 2005.

Ross, S. & Soltes, D. (1995). Heparin and Haematoma: Does Ice Make a Difference?. *Journal of Advanced Nursing*, 21(3), 434-439; Mar 1995.

Saeki, Y. (2002). Effect of Local Application of Cold or Heat for Relief of Pricking Pain. *Nursing and Health Sciences.* 4(3):97-105; Sep 2002.

Sarifakioğlu, N. & Sarifakioğlu, E. (2004). Evaluating the Efffect of Ice Application on The Pain Felt During Botilinum Toxin Type-a Injections: a Prospective, Randomized, Single-blind, Controlled Trial. *Ann Plast Surg,* 53(6),543-546; Dec 2004.

Seers, K.& Carroll, D.(1998) Relaxation techniques for acute pain management : a systematic review. Australian *Journal of Advanced Nursing,* 27(3)466-475,March 1998.

Sherman, K.J.; Cherkin, D.C.; Connelly, M.T.; Erro, J.; Savetsky, J.B. & Davis, R.B.(2004). Complementary and alternative medical therapies for chronic low back pain:What treatments are patient willing to try? *BMC Complement Altern Med,* Jul 19;4-9.

Simkin, P. & Bolding, A. (2004). Update on nonpharmacologic approaches to relieve labor pain and prevent suffering. *Journal of Midwifery & Women's Health,* 49 (6), 489- 504; Nov-Dec 2004.

Simkin, P.P.& O'Hara, M. (2002). Nonpharmacologic relief of pain during labor: systematic reviews of five methods, *American Journal of Obstetrics and Gynecology*, 186 (5 Suppl Nature):S131-159; May 2002.

Sluka, K.A. & Walsh, D. (2003). Transcutaneous Electrical Nevre Stimulation: Basic Science Mechanism and Clinical Effectiveness. *The Journal of Pain*, 4(3): 109-121. Apr 2003.

Snyder, M. & Wieland, J. (2003). Complementary and alternative therapies: What is their place in the management of chronic pain? *Nurs Clin North Am*. 38(3): 495-508; Sep 2003.

Stefano, G.B.; Zhu, W.; Cadet, P.; Salamon, E. & Mantione, K.J. (2004). Music alters constitutively expressed opiate and cytokine processes in Listeners. *Medical Science Monitor*, 10(6):18-27.

Stephenson, N.L.N.; Weinrich, S.P. & Tavakoli, A.S. (2000). The Effects of Foot Reflexology on Anxiety and Pain in Patients with Breast and Lung Cancer. *Oncol Nurs Forum*, 27(1):67-72.

Taşçı, E. & Sevil, Ü. (2007). Doğum ağrısına yönelik farmakolojik olmayan yaklaşımlar. *Genel Tıp Dergisi*, 17(3): 181-186.

Teyhen, D.S.; Miltenberger, C.E.; Deiters, H.M.; Del Toro, Y.M.; Pulliam, J.N. & Childs, J.D. (2005). The use of ultrasound imaging of the abdominal drawing-in maneuver in subjects with low back pain. *J Orthop Sports Phys Ther*, 35(6): 346-355;Jun 2005.

Tsay, S.L. & Chen, M.L.(2003). Acupressure and quality of sleep in patients with end- stage renal disease-a randomized controlled trial. *International Journal of Nursing Studies*; 40(1): 1-7; Jan 2003.

Tsay, S.L. ; Rong, J.R. & Lin, P.F.(2003). Acupoints massage in improving the quality of sleep and quality of life in patients with end-stage renal disease. *Journal of Advanced Nursing*; 42 (2): 134-142; April 2003.

Tseng, Y.H. (2005). Aromatherapy in nursing practice. *Hu Li Za Zhi*, 52(4):11-5;PMID 16088776.

Turan, N.; Öztürk, A. & Kaya, N.(2010).Hemsirelikte Yeni Bir Sorumluluk Alanı: Tamamlayıcı Terapi. *Maltepe Üniversitesi Hemsirelik Bilim ve Sanatı Dergisi*, 3(1):.93-98.

Uçan, Ö. & Ovayolu, N. (2007). Kanser ağrısının kontrolünde kullanılan nonfarmakolojik yöntemler. *Fırat Sağlık Hizmetleri Dergisi‚* Vol.2 , No:4 , pp.123-131.

Van der Westhuijzen, A. J.; Becker, P.J.; Morkel, J. & Roelse, J.A. (2005). A Randomized Observer Blind Comparison of Bilateral Facial Ice Pack Therapy with No Ice Therapy Following Third Molar Surgery. *Int J Oral Maxillofac Surg*, 34(3): 281-286; May 2005.

Van Tulder, M.W.; Furlan A.D. & Gagnier J.J. (2005). Complementary and alternative therapies for low back pain. *Best Pract Res Clin Rheumatol*, 19(4): 639-654; Aug 2005.

Williams, K.A.; Petronis, J.; Smith, D.; Goodrich, D.; Wu J.; Ravi, N.; Doyle, E.J.; Juckett, G.; Kolar, M.M.; Gross, R. & Steinberg, L. (2005).Effect of Iyengar yoga therapy for chronic low back pain. *Pain*;115(1-2):107–17; May 2005

Wringht, S.; Courtney, U.; Donnelly, C.; Kenny, T.; Lavin, C. (2002). Clients'perceptions of the benefits of reflexology on their quality of life. *Complementary Therapy in Nursing & Midwifery*, 8(2): 69-76; May 2002.

Yavuz, M.(2006). Ağrıda Kullanılan Nonfarmakolojik Yöntemler, In: *Ağrı Doğası ve Kontrolü*, 1st edition , F.E. Aslan (Editor), , Vol.42, pp.135-147., Avrupa Tıp Kitapçılık Ltd. Şti. Bilim Yayınları, ISBN: 975-6257-17-2.

Yıldırım, Y.K. (2006).Kanser Ağrısının Nonfarmakolojik Yöntemlerle Kontrolü, In: *Kanser ve Palyatif Bakım*, In M. Uyar, R. Uslu, YK. Yıldırım, (Eds), pp.97-126; Meta Press Matbaacılık, İzmir.

Yıldırım, Y.K.; Fadıloğlu, Ç.& Uyar, M. (2006). Palyatif Kanser Bakımında Tamamlayıcı Tedaviler. *Ağrı*, 18(1), 26–32.

Part 4

Nursing and Pain

9

When Theoretical Knowledge Is Not Enough: Introduction of an Explanatory Model on Nurse's Pain Management

Katrin Blondal[1] and Sigridur Halldorsdottir[2]
[1]Landspitali -National University Hospital of Iceland, University of Iceland,
School of Health Sciences, Faculty of Nursing, Reykjavik,
[2]School of Health Sciences, University of Akureyri, Akureyri,
Iceland

1. Introduction

Relieving the suffering of patients is a paramount responsibility for all health professionals. The fact that hospitalised patients still suffer from pain despite increasing technology and a wealth of research during recent decades, calls for an audit and new approaches in pain management. Nurses are professionally responsible for pain assessment and the administration of analgesia and are often considered the key persons in the management of pain. However, for many reasons nurses are unable to achieve the desired results of pain relief. Our study on nurses' experiences of caring for patients in pain indicates that previous studies in this field have often been limited to isolated aspects of pain management (Blondal & Halldorsdottir, 2009). Furthermore, they have been rather negative towards nurses. Our position is that many researchers have not appreciated the complexity of the nurse's multifaceted assignment of caring for patients in pain. We suggest that knowledge, in this respect, may often have been too narrowly defined. We challenge statements that propose that nurses do not believe that pain relief is a priority for nurses (Brockopp et al., 1998) or their responsibility (Twycross, 2002). Successful pain relief may provide satisfaction for the nurses involved (Blondal & Halldorsdottir, 2009), which is a rarely identified outcome by means of professional achievements. Various research results indicate that nurses' knowledge is less than adequate (Howell et al., 2000; Kuuppelomäki; 2002a; Van Niekerk & Martin, 2002). Therefore, the main methods that have previously been employed in order to improve nurses' performance and to achieve better pain control are formal education about pain assessment and the use of pain medication. Interestingly, programmes that aim at increasing this knowledge, however, often fail to help in diminishing patients' pain. Some programmes may demonstrate changes in practice (e.g. Carr, 2002) where other findings are contradictory regarding their effectiveness, indicating that the effect of nurses' re-education is not maintained over time (Howell et al., 2000) and that more theoretical knowledge does not necessarily correlate with patients reporting less pain (Watt-Watson et al., 2001). Furthermore, Wilson's (2007) survey on nurses' knowledge of pain also indicates that nurses may be incapable of managing pain, despite their knowledge of the existence of the patients' pain. It is, therefore, important to search for other explanations for inadequate pain management of nurses. Therefore, perhaps other patterns of knowledge are needed in addition to the often traditional emphasis on formal education about pain assessment and analgesics.

1.1 Aim of the theory

Theory is the acknowledged foundation to practise methodology, professional identity and the growth of formalized knowledge. Practice must not only be evidence based but also theory based. Hence, pain management must be theory based because theories serve as a broad framework for practice and may also articulate the goals of a profession and its core values. Our aim was to develop a theory, an explanatory model, which can explain nurses' complex task of pain management.

2. Methodology

In our evaluation of the various methods for this theory development we found *theory synthesis* as described by Walker and Avant (2004) a good method for constructing our explanatory model. They posit that more theory synthesis is needed to advance practice disciplines so we found a perfect fit. In the theory synthesis the theorists combine isolated pieces of information that may even be theoretically unconnected. Theory synthesis entails constructing a theory from study findings and scholarly writings, which may be numerous. It enables the theorist to organise and integrate a large number of findings into a single theory which can be presented as a model. The theory put forth in this chapter is based on 11 study findings, e.g. on our own phenomenological study on nurses' experience of taking care of patients in pain and ten other research findings from various researchers about: nursing advocacy; moral obligation; organisational barriers; patient based hindrances; and the nurse-doctor relationship (see Table 1). All these different studies helped us to clarify the manifold task of a nurse's pain management. This method can be compared with painting a picture where in step one the picture is drawn and step two (the literature in this case) is used to compare the "picture" drawn with other similar "pictures" for confirmation and clarification. In step three the picture is presented (Figure 1).

3. Findings

The theory provides a holistic view of the complicated task of relieving pain. The main tenets of this theory are: *the role of the nurses as the patient's advocates, multiple patterns of knowledge* and *the doctor-nurse relationship*. The theory is introduced in the form of an exploratory model which illustrates the main tenets, how they interact and how other aspects simultaneously mould nurses' actions and reactions while taking care of patients in pain (Figure 1).

3.1 The explanatory model

To understand and explain the nurses' central role of caring for patients in pain and their potential for providing adequate pain management, their position may be portrayed as that of *patients' advocates* (Mallik, 1997) within a goal-directed mission aimed at patients' pain relief. In figure 1, this journey is presented in an explanatory model where its main tenets have been arranged into a figure with a definite beginning and an end from top to bottom. As may be seen from the four central tenets of the model, acting as *patient's advocate, moral obligation, formal and tacit knowledge, knowing persons* and *the system,* initially dominate, followed by the concepts of *internal and external hindrances,* as well as *potential outcomes.*

Authors, published	Research	Participants, N	Data collection
Blondal & Halldorsdottir, 2009	The challenge of caring for patients in pain: from the nurse's perspective	Nurses caring for patients with pain in hospital wards, N= 10	20 in-depth interviews
De Schepper et. al, 1997	Feelings of powerlessness in relation to pain: ascribed causes and reported strategies	Community nurses caring for cancer patients with pain, N= 24	13 individual and 3 group interviews
Jenks, 1993	The pattern of personal knowing in nurse clinical decision making	Nurses working in various hospital settings, N= 23	Four focus groups/ participant observation
Kuuppelomäki, 2002	Pain management problems in patients' terminal phase as assessed by nurses in Finland	Nurses on inpatient wards of 32 municipal health centres, N= 328	Questionnaire and an open end question
Mallik, 1997	Advocacy in nursing – perceptions of practising nurses	Experienced nurses from various settings, N= 104	Focus group interviews
Malloy et al, 2009	Culture and organizational climate: nurses' insights into their relationship with physicians	Nurses from various settings in 4 countries, N= 42	Focus groups
Nagy, 1999	Strategies used by burns nurses to cope with the infliction of pain on patients	Nurses within paediatric and adult burn units, N= 32	84 unstructured interviews
Nash et al., 1999	Pain and the administration of analgesia: what nurses say	Registered nurses and BSc nursing students in acute and community settings, N= 19	Three focus group interviews
Oberle & Hughes, 2001	Doctors' and nurses' perceptions of ethical problems in end-of-life decisions	7 doctors and 14 nurses working in acute care adult medical-surgical areas, N= 21	Unstructured interviews
O'Connor & Kelly, 2005	Bridging the gap: a study of general nurses' perceptions of patient advocacy in Ireland	Practicing nurses in hospitals, N= 20	3 focus group interviews
Van Niekerk & Martin, 2002	The impact of the nurse-physician professional relationship on nurses' experience of ethical dilemmas in effective pain management	Nurses within public and private settings, N= 1,015	Questionnaire

Table 1. Key research used to develop the theory

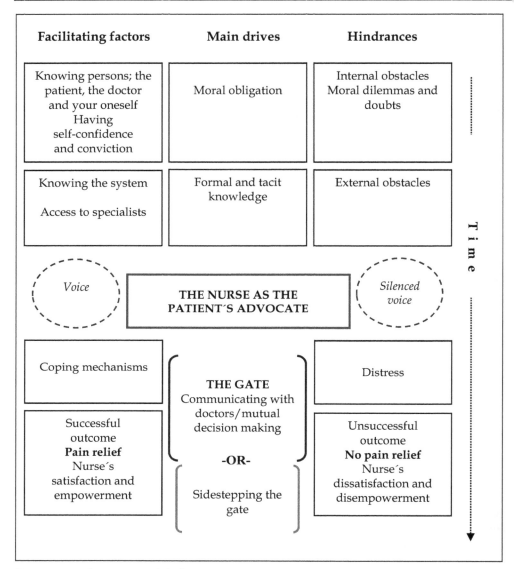

Fig. 1. An explanatory model of nurses' pain management

3.2 Nurses' two main drives: Moral obligation and formal and tacit knowledge

The first two concepts we introduce in our explanatory model are *moral obligation* (Mallik, 1997; Oberle and Hughes, 2001) and *formal and tacit knowledge* (Blondal & Halldorsdottir, 2009; Mallik, 1997; Nash et al., 1999). We propose that on the nurses' journey to fulfil their mission of relieving patients' pain these two important drives prevail, as illustrated in figure 2 in the shadowed boxes.

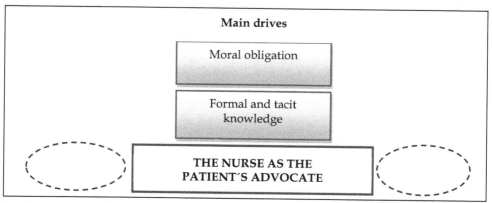

Fig. 2. Nurses' moral obligation and formal and tacit knowledge

The nurses' moral orientation is displayed in accounts like this one: "If the patients report pain, then they're in pain ... and of course you must do something about it" (Blondal & Halldorsdottir, 2009, p. 4). Possessing *formal or theoretical knowledge* about pain assessment, pain management and medication is of importance but *tacit knowledge* is no less important, as experience and learning from other colleagues creates a sense of self confidence and increased empowerment in following their convictions to be the *patient's advocate* (Blondal & Halldorsdottir, 2009; Mallik, 1997; Nash et al., 1999). "I suppose I believe advocacy is utilizing our own clinical knowledge as well as our own knowledge of the patient and putting the two of them together and then doing what you feel is best for the patient." (O'Connor & Kelly, 2005, p. 460). This approach assists nurses to keep on advocating and relating with patients and doctors (Blondal & Halldorsdottir, 2009).

3.3 The nurse as the patient's advocate

As may be seen from our model, its central tenet portrays the position of the nurse as the *patient's advocate* (Figure 3). Here, the mission's journey begins with the nurse's assessment of the patient's pain, which leads to further decisions and reactions and where the nurse will direct his or her responses; what she or he can solve alone and what problems must be referred to physicians (Blondal & Halldorsdottir, 2009).

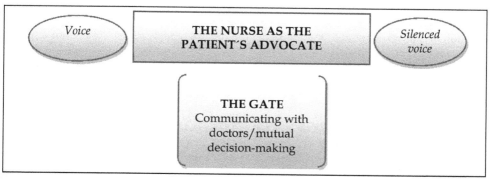

Fig. 3. Central position of the nurse as the patient's advocate

3.3.1 Communicating with doctors at the gate/mutual decision-making

Since medication is often the major pain treatment, and physicians are required to be responsible for all drug prescriptions, a crucial element in this process is the nurses' contribution to mutual *decision-making with the doctor*, where nurses assume the responsibility of advocates (Blondal & Halldorsdottir, 2009). At this point, which may be referred to as *"the gate"*, *having a voice* is pivotal for nurses (Blondal & Halldorsdottir, 2009; Van Niekerk and Martin, 2002) because they represent the patient, and by using their influence they try to fulfil their mission (Blondal & Halldorsdottir, 2009; Jenks, 1993; O'Connor & Kelly, 2005). As two different nurses put it: "Well, unfortunately the decision-making is not ours. We are restricted to what's ordered... I mean, if the doctor's ordered it, you can't very well make a decision" (Nash et al., 1999, p. 186), and further: "I don't stand by and watch the patients and do nothing if I think they are wild with pain, I keep on pushing until something is done." (Blondal & Halldorsdottir, 2009, pp. 5-6). If the nurse and the doctor do not reach reciprocal decision or agreement the nurses may have to keep on insisting or else give up -- feeling *silenced* (Malloy, 2009; Blondal & Halldorsdottir, 2009). "We don't have any final authority – perhaps that's what's most difficult...and we have to put up with that, naturally, but it's very important, of course, that we feel we are listened to, that our voice is heard." (Blondal & Halldorsdottir, 2009, p. 2901). Furthermore, to maintain trust between all involved, the nurses sometimes take on the role of a mediator or intermediary (Blondal & Halldorsdottir, 2009; O'Connor & Kelly, 2005), but the importance of co-operation and holding a mutual vision crystallises in this description: "I just think it's lot of give and take between doctors and nursing staff and patients; you've got to work together to actively relieve pain." (Nash et al., 1999, p. 185).

3.4 Facilitating factors for a successful outcome

The main drives, moral obligation and formal and tacit knowledge may not be enough for successful pain management. There are several facilitating factors which are necessary to make use of, together with the main drives, in order to achieve a positive outcome of pain management (See Figure 4).

3.4.1 Knowing the patient

One of the *facilitating factors* that are important motivating factors for advocacy (Mallik, 1997), requires that the nurse *knows the patient as a person,* that is, as an individual, which allows the nurse to interpret information and select individualised interventions (Jenks, 1993). "I think, knowing the patient's background and seeing more than just, say, a medical condition or a surgical wound, that makes you more able to advocate." (O'Connor & Kelly, 2005, p. 459).

3.4.2 Knowing the doctor

In the explanatory model we propose that *to know the gatekeeper,* i.e. the doctor, greatly influences the nurse's success (Jenks, 1993). "Sometimes I think the nurses are underheard if you go and you're telling the doctor, this patient is in pain. This patient is in pain, ah yeah, we'll change this. The patient is still in pain. Sometimes they don't actually listen to what you're saying. It depends on how you say it, or who you're actually saying it to." (Malloy et al., 2009, p. 726). Then on the other hand, "It's a good feeling when you know that someone respects your opinion and respects your assessment of the patient also." (Jenks, 1993, p. 403).

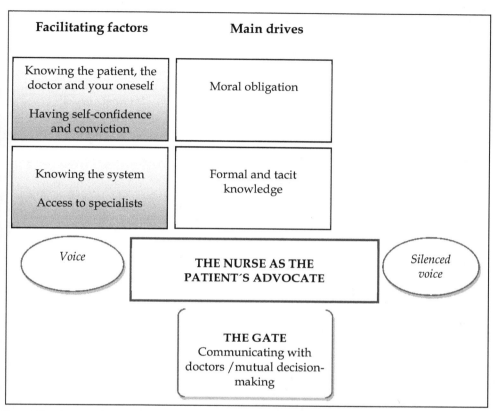

Fig. 4. Facilitating factors; Knowing persons and knowing the system

3.4.3 Knowing your own self, having self-confidence and conviction

It is no less important for nurses to know their own potential and believe in themselves, since experience creates a *sense of self-confidence* and increased empowerment in following their own *convictions*. Therefore, individual factors influence nurses' decisions on pain management; "I'm quite happy to make those decisions, because I'm happy to be answerable for them...so I do things that I am comfortable with and I feel that I am doing the best for the patient." (Nash et al., 1999, p. 185)

3.4.4 Knowing the system and access to specialists

Organizational knowledge, to *know how the system works*, together with knowledge of the wishes of patients, allows nurses to advocate in an effective way; therefore "[A]n advocate to me would be somebody who uses whatever knowledge they have in a situation to do the best for the patient." (O'Connor & Kelly, 2005, p. 460). Then *having access to a specialist in pain management* and pain teams within the organisation is of utmost importance as they serve as nurses' guides and help to turn distress into satisfaction (Blondal & Halldorsdottir, 2009).

3.5 Hindrances to successful pain management

This journey is complicated, however, by several obstacles that emerge either as *internal* or *external obstacles* (see figure 5).

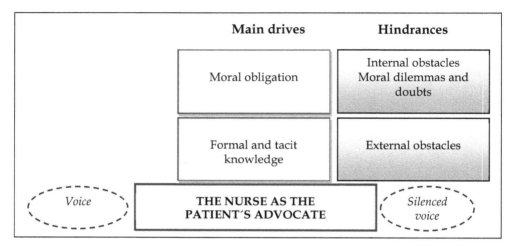

Fig. 5. Internal and external obstacles

3.5.1 Internal obstacles

Internal obstacles that can complicate this process are the nurses' inner struggle of *moral dilemma and doubt*, of doing right and trusting one's own judgement, that appear to be the result of tension between doubt and duty. Here a prevailing feature includes the fear of giving too much medication and caring for addicts (Blondal & Halldorsdottir, 2009; Nash et al., 1999). "I felt it [to give pain medication to an addict] was a strain, really, on human nature – are you doing something wrong? Or are you doing right? Or are you just cruel to refuse to give it to him? – really, what should you do?"(Blondal & Halldorsdottir, 2009, p. 5).

3.5.2 External obstacles

External obstacles are connected to organisational structures (Kuuppelomäki, 2002a) such as absence of or an inadequate prescription, lack of access to accountable physicians, and the lack of directions and clear rules. Moreover, decisions regarding palliative care are imperative for successful pain relief (Blondal & Halldorsdottir, 2009; Kuuppelomäki, 2002a); "Accepting death and the transition from acute care to terminal care are a problem." (Kuuppelomäki, 2002a, p. 706). External hindrances may also be patient related, such as their unwillingness to report pain and to accept analgesics (Blondal & Halldorsdottir, 2009; Kuuppelomäki, 2002a), which further complicates the assessment of pain and pain relief. "He was a difficult man and so withdrawn. You just couldn't get through [to] him and you don't know why not. Cases like that make me feel so uncertain, I start to doubt myself." (De Schepper et al., 1997, p. 424).

3.6 Coping mechanisms

Further action can involve the use of various *coping mechanisms* in order to share the burden, seek better solutions for the patient and/or control their feelings (Blondal & Halldorsdottir, 2009; Nagy, 1999). (See figure 6.)

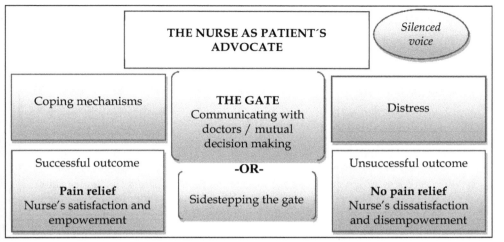

Fig. 6. Coping mechanisms

The most important factor is support provided by colleagues (De Schepper et al., 1997; Nagy, 1999) and specialists in pain management that serve as their guides (Blondal & Halldorsdottir, 2009). "The people that we work with. You can go up and say 'So-and-so, I can't cope with this any longer! Can you either give me a hand or do it for me?' And people where we are working at the moment will do that. So if we're getting too fed up someone else will either help you out or do it for you so you can go and have a rest. They understand what it's like!" (Nagy, 1999, p. 1433). Furthermore, "I get a lot of support from the team here. They give me [the] feedback I need and I can have a good moan." (De Schepper et al., 1997, p. 426). Assistance can, therefore, like other coping strategies, transform *distress* into *satisfaction* (Blondal & Halldorsdottir, 2009) which may keep them satisfied despite unfavourable outcomes. Some nurses do *sidestep the gate* by using independent nursing interventions, take control and thread the risky road of bypassing the gate by altering the medication on their own initiative or bend existing rules and directions (Blondal & Halldorsdottir, 2009). But this also may be the result of the distress mentioned above.

3.7 Potential outcomes
As suggested by this model, the nurse's journey has two potential outcomes, based on the degree to which nurses are able to fulfil their commitments (see figure 7).
Successful pain relief leads to nurses' *satisfaction* and *empowerment* and *patients' satisfaction* and possibly mutual trust (Blondal & Halldorsdottir, 2009). Conversely, pain management is burdensome when the patients' sufferings are not relieved (Nagy, 1999) or the nurses are *silenced*, with consequent *dissatisfaction and distress* (De Schepper et al., 1997; Oberle and Hughes, 2001), *disempowerment* and possibly mutual distrust. "I think, really, it's one of the more difficult things one experiences... I was so upset inside... so angry inside, not being able to help and not really knowing where to turn, because the doctors said just that [dose of medication], and it didn't work at all, so I was somehow defenceless about what to do." (Blondal & Halldorsdottir, 2009, p. 6). However, importantly, we want to point out that perceived discomfort or *dissatisfaction* with the outcome can serve as a drive for further action (Blondal & Halldorsdottir, 2009; Mallik, 1997).

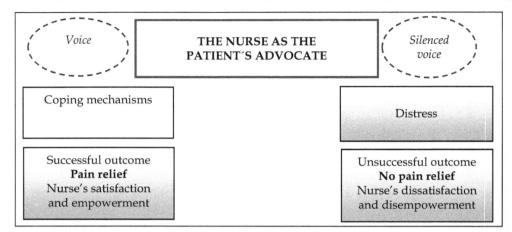

Fig. 7. Potential outcomes

From this overview we conclude that theoretical knowledge is only one aspect of nurses' pain management. They require knowledge from various other sources, ethical, personal, and aesthetic, as well as many skills, e.g. communication and negotiation skills, in order to fulfil their obligations and role. In our view, lack of recognition of these other kinds of knowledge may stem from the fact that many studies focus only on isolated aspects of pain management. All too commonly the studies provide only a somewhat fragmented analysis of isolated factors of pain management. In contrast, the explanatory model presented here provides a more holistic view of the nurses' complex situation when caring for patients in pain and may reveal that neglecting these other facets may have contributed to the permanent inadequacy in pain management of patients that is so widely described.

4. Discussion

This explanatory model clarifies how nurses require various coexisting patterns of knowledge, within a favourable organisational environment, to be able to perform in accord with their role as key persons in pain management and how their performance may predict a positive or negative outcome for the patient and the nurse. This model further explains the relationships of nurses with patients and physicians where nurses seek to act as patients' advocates and how having a voice is pivotal for nurses. Furthermore, we depict how internal and external barriers can hinder the performance of nurses and how an unsuccessful outcome that evokes profound distress may concurrently stimulate further actions and turn a negative outcome into a more favourable one. This explanatory model of a nurse's journey therefore denotes nurses' encounters with, and reactions to, the multiple demanding assignments they continually meet on their mission towards pain relief.

4.1 Nurses´ two main drives: Moral obligation and formal and tacit knowledge
4.1.1 Knowledge of ethical origins
According to our explanatory model *the role of ethical knowledge in pain management must be highlighted,* as it may be the fundamental component needed for nurses to act as advocates

and to initiate the process of pain management. Our notion of nurses' obligation to relieve pain is supported by several studies (Oberle and Hughes, 2001; O'Connor & Kelly, 2005; Rejeh et al., 2009). However, it may have been underestimated up till now because even if nurses possess the relevant theoretical knowledge, they may not necessarily make use of it without the requisite motivation.

We want to emphasize that non-professional and professional *moral values* that motivate and direct individuals' choices can be inculcated through education or socialisation (Omery, 1989), and nurses recognise that a sense of responsibility in pain management needs to be learned (Rejeh et al., 2009). Taylor et al. (1993) also conclude that nurses' education about pain management must include professional ethical obligations and the suitability of their professional values. Importantly, moral values may also be generated by an organisation's philosophy statement or policy (Omery, 1989) and moral values should, therefore, be part of nursing education as well as organisational statements.

4.1.2 Formal and tacit knowledge

In accordance with our propositions, professional responsibility and moral obligation are considered key initiates for advocacy. Twycross (2002) posits that in order to advocate, a theoretical knowledge base is needed. Vaartio et al. (2006) and O'Connor & Kelly (2005) add to this by stating that theoretical as well as practical knowledge of pain management is a necessary antecedent of advocacy. Where sound empirical knowledge about pain assessment and various methods for management of pain are vital, it must be kept in mind that nurses learn no less through experience, where they learn to utilise their own potential and personal knowledge through their own practice and role modelling. This drive for taking action by using theoretical or formal knowledge along with experience and self-confidence is congruent with Mallik's (1997) statement that 'intervening conditions' facilitate advocacy. These factors have also been found important for nurses' decision-making (Nash et al., 1999). Where knowledge of theoretical origins may be the type of knowledge that is most easily recognised and is emphasised during formal education at school and in continuous education, we stress that the role of tacit knowledge gained through experience and role modelling has more rarely been pointed out, perhaps because it is rather of personal and aesthetic origins. Importantly, as we see it, this knowledge supplements formal knowledge, for instance in the early stages of the process where nurses assess the patient's pain.

4.2 The nurse as patient's advocate in pain management

Patients in pain have been recognised as a vulnerable group of patients that are in need of nurses to advocate on their behalf (Ware et al., 2011), and nurses see it as their role to safeguard their interests (Blondal & Halldorsdottir, 2009; Ware et al., 2011). As portrayed in our explanatory model nurses assume a central role in assessing and managing patients' pain. However, since doctors are responsible for prescribing analgesia, nurses' concerns about pain relief are often affected by their relationship with the doctors (Kuuppelomäki, 2002a; Taylor et al., 1993; Van Niekerk and Martin, 2002).

4.2.1 Communicating with doctors at "*the gate*" and mutual decision-making

On the nurses' journey *the gate*, where they enter these relations with *the gatekeeper* — the doctor, is an important turning point (Blondal & Halldorsdottir, 2009). Having a *voice* at the gate is pivotal, because there the nurses represent the patient, and by using their influence try to fulfil their mission. Subsequently, the doctor decides what medication the patient can or cannot receive; i.e. whether the nurses pass through the gate (Blondal & Halldorsdottir, 2009). Within the *gate* the nurses can also assume the role of 'conciliator' or 'intermediary'. Nurses' accounts of their advocating position have, therefore, also been described as 'bridging the gap' between the patients and the medical profession. This involves the translation of information between patients and doctors and in both directions (O'Connor & Kelly, 2005). As we envision it, yet another aspect of personal knowledge is revealed here where, inevitably, nurses must communicate with doctors to achieve the best outcome for patients.

Many nurses do not find it difficult to communicate with doctors or to confront them and are ready to push boundaries to acquire what the patient needs (Blondal & Halldorsdottir, 2009; Vaartio et al., 2008; Ware et al., 2011). For others, communicational problems are a matter of fact and they feel uncomfortable about trespassing on the doctors´ domain (De Schepper et al. 1997; Willson, 2000). Nurses in cancer-related home care, for instance, complain about physicians' lack of knowledge and collaboration, and problems with contacting them (Ferrell et al., 1993). Nurses then also describe physicians' fear of overmedicating patients with dementia or delirium in medical wards (Coker et al., 2010). Communicational problems cause feelings of powerlessness and distress (Blondal & Halldorsdottir, 2009; Malloy et al., 2009) and ethical dilemmas and they are sometimes punished for their advocating activities (Clabo, 2008; Mallik, 1997; Malloy et al., 2009). Mallik (1997) maintains that to achieve their goals, advocates often play the doctor-nurse game of recommending actions without appearing to do so (Stein et al., 1990) or assume the attitude of a 'stubborn rebel' with an over-determined and even hostile behaviour (Stein et al., 1990). In our study, however, the nurses emphasise assertiveness, rather than pushiness, for success (Blondal & Halldorsdottir, 2009). When nurses are straightforward in their requests, this could be explained by their perceptions of being respected and *having a voice*, and therefore in keeping with Van Niekerk and Martin (2002) that nurses who feel adequately consulted by physicians are more likely to initiate the consultation process. The use of assertiveness further matches the argument of Keenan et al. (1998) that conveying ideas in a forceful and confrontational manner increases the likelihood for successful collaboration. We claim that when nurses choose to bypass the *gate* by bending rules (Blondal & Halldorsdottir, 2009; Ware et al., 2011) despite the risk of jeopardising their career, this might indicate a lack of self-confidence, negotiating competence or communicational competence skills. For nurses, ethical problems may often be related to their hierarchical position, where their voices are not heard or they are being silenced in spite of their professional knowledge (Blondal & Halldorsdottir, 2009; Malloy et al., 2009; Oberle and Hughes, 2001). From this, it might be understood that the views of nurses and doctors are incompatible, for instance because of the different orientation of *care* versus *cure* (Malloy et al., 2009). However, doctors can also experience an inability to exercise moral agency and experience powerlessness, because of hierarchical structures, and they are faced with the same kinds of ethical dilemmas as nurses. Furthermore, the obligation to respond is the same for all and this difference could rather be explained by different roles and responsibilities and unawareness of each others' responses (Oberle and Hughes, 2001). This also may reflect the reality that nurses and doctors act independently, without mutually agreed principles or practices rather than as a team in managing pain (Kuuppelomäki, 2002a). Although this statement is made in regard to end-of-life situations, we conclude that this could also apply to other pain management decisions and call for more discussions about the ethical aspects of pain management across professions.

4.3 Facilitating factors for a successful outcome

As represented in our explanatory model, facilitating factors for successful advocacy and a favourable outcome require knowing persons and the system. Jenks' (1993) exploration of nurses' clinical decision-making, proposing that clinical decisions depend on the quality and dynamics of nurses' interpersonal relationships is in harmony with our interpretation of the process from pain assessment to reaction. However, we also want to add the dimension of knowing your own self and the organisation that also are essential facilitating factors. These important features that enhance nurses' possibilities for using their knowledge and moral motivation are opposed to the factors that hinder them in making use of their potential, and may, to some degree, be used to overcome their negative effects.

4.3.1 Knowing the patient

As repeatedly has been pointed out, insufficient pain assessment by nurses interferes with successful pain relief (Carr, 2002). According to McCaffery (Pasero et al., 1999, as cited in McCaffery, 1968) "[P]ain is whatever the experiencing person says it is, existing whenever he says it does" (p. 17). However, because individuals express pain very differently, this definition creates some problems for nurses. For instance, although the risk of addiction is minor (McCaffery et al., 1990), caring for a patient who is, or is suspected of being, an abuser can be very stressful (Blondal & Halldorsdottir, 2009; Nash et al., 1999). Moreover, McCaffery and Ferrell (1997) assert that nurses must appreciate that "the only scientific tool for measuring pain intensity is the patient's report using a pain rating scale" (p. 183). These scales may, however, be difficult to use with patients that are disoriented (Coker et al., 2010) or unconscious (Kuuppelomäki, 2002a) and many nurses are hesitant to use them (Schafheutle et al., 2001). Then many elderly patients suffer in silence with their pain and discomforts and do not seek help and more effort is required if those with pain are to be identified, supported and cared for as Gudmannsdottir & Halldorsdottir (2009) suggest. Whereas the use of various pain scales for pain assessment build on theoretical knowledge, conversely, *knowing the patient* as a person can greatly assist nurses to assess the patient's pain (Blondal and Halldorsdottir, 2009); this approach is more related to personal and aesthetic knowledge. Knowing the patient as a person strongly facilitates the assessment of patients' needs and clinical decision-making (Liaschenko, 1997), and allows nurses to interpret information and select individualised interventions (Takman and Severinsson, 1999). Furthermore, the nurse-patient relationship is a motivating factor for advocacy (Mallik, 1997; O'Connor & Kelly, 2005) and analysing the patient and the situation is a fundamental element of advocacy (Vaartio et al., 2008). Therefore, we suggest that more emphasis is given to this special aspect of pain management. Still, yet another pattern of knowledge may also be needed here; *unknowing the patient*. When nurses admit to themselves that they do not know the patient and his or her point of view, it allows them to hold their former biases and prejudices in abeyance (Munhall, 1993). We suggest that assuming this type of knowledge is of utmost importance as it may prevent nurses from making assumptions about patients´ pain intensity that is based on diagnosis and course of treatment (Clabo, 2008; Manias, 2003; Schafheutle et al., 2001) that is associated with underestimation of pain (Sjöström et al., 2000), and a barrier to effective pain relief (Schafheutle et al., 2001). Adopting this stance of unknowing could also avoid the stereotyping of patients, such as those who may be addicts, homeless or prisoners (Rejeh et al., 2009) or with a lifestyle that may affect nurses' pain management behaviours (Wilson, 2007). Therefore, we advise that strategies nurses use to connect to patients which may be based on personal knowledge (Carper, 1978) and unknowing (Munhall, 1993) are highlighted along with the current emphasis on using pain rating scales (e.g. Paice and Cohen, 1997).

According to our model, competent communication with patients may be a powerful way to overcome internal hindrances in addition to theoretical knowledge about pain assessment, addiction, respiratory depression and other possible side effects of pain medication that also may stem from the ethical orientation of preventing harm to the patients. When nurses' emphasise individualised pain management, knowing the patient as a person, recognising his/her special needs and responding to these needs on the basis of envisioned results, portrays the importance of aesthetic knowledge and comprehension of the particularity of the situation (Carper, 1978). Empathy is also an important component mode of the aesthetic pattern in nursing (Carper, 1978), and apparent in nurses' accounts of pain management (Blondal & Halldorsdottir, 2009; Rejeh et al., 2009) and should be not only acknowledged but utilised more often.

4.3.2 Knowing the doctor

Since nurses call for equality, mutual decision-making and respect for their judgement (Blondal & Halldorsdottir, 2009), knowing the doctor is a factor worth further exploration. In accordance with our explanatory model Jenks (1993) maintains that *knowing the doctor* creates mutual trust in each others' perceptions. Therefore, a good nurse-physician relationship, in accordance with our metaphor of nurses passing through the *gate*, knowing *the gatekeeper* may add to optimal pain relief and consequently affects nurses' and patients' wellbeing. It is, therefore, imperative that both doctors and nurses be aware of the need for good rapport and be knowledgeable about good communication techniques and that both groups of professionals make every effort to encourage collaboration and to find ways to get to know each other as persons. Again, we propose that personal knowledge and communicational skills that nurses must use in relations with patients and doctors is vital because, as before, possessing theoretical knowledge and the motivation to use it (moral orientation) may become of little use if not employed because of lack of communication or negotiating abilities or lack of self-confidence or if nurses cannot react because their voice is silenced. Therefore, nurses must be taught to act as the patients' advocates, represent themselves and act like the patients' representative.

4.3.3 Knowing oneself, having self-confidence and conviction

We further want to draw attention to how nurses' awareness of their feelings such as distress and empathy, recognition of their own capabilities, self-confidence and persistence may be important facilitating factors. As mentioned before, motivational factors such as experience and self-confidence are congruent with Mallik's (1997) 'intervening conditions' that facilitate advocacy and are important for nurses' decision-making (Nash et al., 1999). As further discussed later, emotional responses such as anger and frustration are also potent motivators for advocacy (Mallik, 1997). Such knowledge is of both personal and aesthetical origins and nurses must learn to identify and accept such feelings and be empowered to use them to be capable of following their convictions, both for their own sakes and for the good of the patient. According to our model, nurses that hold such knowledge and believe in themselves are more capable of entering into and coping positively with difficult relations with others — patients, families and doctors, and are more likely to gain what is needed for a positive outcome both for the patients and themselves.

4.3.4 Knowing the system

Yet another facet that is worth more consideration is nurses´ knowledge of the organisation. Knowing the system and the environment is part of nurses' advocacy, for instance when nurses must mediate between the patient and the system through interpretation of medical terminology or advocating for a group of patients (O´Connor et al., 2005). It also seems necessary to recognise what options or resources are available within the organisation, for instance whom to turn to for assistance. Here, the support of professionals — specialists in pain management within organisations, must be present at all times to assist them in dealing with difficult cases (Blondal and Halldorsdottir, 2009; Nash et al., 1999). Moreover, nurses must recognise the availability of specialists and when they should be contacted and involved.

4.4 Hindrances for successful pain management

As the model portrays, some inhibiting factors hinder nurses´ potentials for taking action and therefore interfere with their drives, moral obligation, and formal and tacit knowledge. It may also be seen that these factors are somewhat in opposition to the facilitating factors. The main obstacles are grouped as external — originating in the nurses´ environment, or internal — concerned with inner doubts or dilemmas. This gives an example of how these model elements are interconnected and should not be taken out of the immediate context.

4.4.1 Internal hindrances

As previously mentioned, nurses´ moral motivation is complicated by some dilemmas as the nurses encounter variable decisional and ethical conflicts (Taylor et al. 1993) that directly affect the pain management process and its outcome. The dilemma of inflicting pain to serve other goals of treatment (De Schepper, 1997; Willson, 2000), fear of giving too much pain medication because of respiratory depression (Ferrell et al., 1991; Howell et al., 2000; Wilson, 2007), sedation (Howell et al., 2000), fear of the addictive properties of narcotics (Brockopp et al., 1998), and doubt whether the pain is real (Nash, 1999; Rejeh et al., 2009) has repeatedly been described. So are the difficulties of distinguishing between physical pain and psychological distress (Kuuppellomäki, 2002a), patients' non-compliance in accepting analgesia (Kuuppellomäki, 2002a), patients' reticence (De Schepper et al 1997; Rejeh et al., 2009) and nurses' concerns about giving a dying person the last dose (Brockopp et al., 1998), as for some, hastening death through pain relief is morally unacceptable (O'Rourke, 1992). Ethical problems may also arise from a lack of permission to be honest with patients (Rejeh et al., 2009) or because of the attitudes of family members towards pain medication (Kuuppelomäki, 2002a). Nurses also frequently describe how difficult it is for them to care for patients that are known abusers or suspected of being addicts, and believing their words (Blondal & Halldorsdottir, 2009; Nash et al., 1999; Rejeh et al., 2009). Dilemmas may also be caused by preconceived notions about certain groups of patients that negatively interfere with nurses' decision-making (Brockopp et al., 2003). Interestingly, Van Niekerk and Martin (2002) point out that nurses with greater knowledge of pain assessment are less likely to experience ethical conflicts regarding overmedication, addiction or doubt about the existence of pain. Hence, more knowledge could prevent such ethical conflicts. Accounts like this further sustain our claims about how the separate parts introduced in our model are interconnected and cannot be separated from the complete picture.

4.4.2 External obstacles
Organisational barriers have formerly been extensively described, where lack of time, workload (Ware et al., 2011; Rejeh et al., 2009) financial restraints and staffing cutbacks (Oberle and Hughes, 2001; Rejeh et al., 2009), restraints of routine (Willson, 2000), insufficient prescribing of analgesics (Schafheutle et al., 2001; Kuuppelomäki, 2002a) based on habits instead of individualised needs (Boer et al, 1997), and unavailability of physicians (Kuuppelomäki, 2002a; Rejeh et al., 2009) interfere with pain relief. Other related hindrances that are part of the system have also been identified such as unavailable non-pharmacological pain relief measures and disorganised systems of care (Coker et al., 2010). Rejeh et al. (2009) also point out that defective equipment and interruptions can lead to ethical problems in pain management. The importance of a decision on palliative care for good pain relief is endorsed by Kuuppelomäki (2002b) who reports physicians' hesitancy about starting terminal care, and delayed decisions of using a strong analgesia (Kuuppelomäki, 2002a). The organisation must, therefore, provide an *optimal organisational environment* since organisational barriers such as unclear rules, lack of prescriptions or time and resources such as specialised pain services, may hinder nurses from acting according to their best knowledge, potential and goals. The presence of prescriptions, rules and directives are important to be able to give the patient what she or he needs. Inflexible protocols and strict policies or routines, on the other hand, impede good pain management (Rajeh et al., 2009; Willson, 2000) resulting in the nurses giving up and leaving them feeling silenced and disempowered (Blondal & Halldorsdottir, 2009; Malloy et al., 2009). Alternatively, nurses may feel compelled to choose to bypass the *gate*, by bending rules (Blondal & Halldorsdottir, 2009; Ware et al., 2011), to obtain favourable results for the patient, as is portrayed in our model. Our emphasis on organisational structures is supported by the results of Willson's (2000) participant observation study on factors affecting analgesia administration; Willson suggests that because of the interplay between multiple organisational and interpersonal features, more education of the nurses will not necessarily improve the administration of analgesics.

4.5 Coping mechanisms
How nurses *cope* with their challenges predicts to some extent how they perceive the outcome of pain relief and they seem to use various methods to cope and protect themselves. Applying methods such as concentrating on patients' positive attributes is a component of strategies that prevent burnout (Simoni and Paterson, 1997), and sharing feelings with colleagues (De Schepper et al., 1997; Nagy, 1999) and having the opportunity to stand back from situations (De Schepper et al., 1997; Rejeh et al., 2009) are consistent with strategies that reduce powerlessness (De Schepper et al., 1997). Seeking and receiving support from pain teams and specialists in pain management is vital, and such assistance can transform distress into satisfaction. Ironically, those who accept the responsibility as seeing to pain relief run the risk of experiencing ethical problems which may lead to a sense of loss of control and subsequently burnout, resulting in decreased quality of care (Schmitz et al., 2000). If nurses give up their advocating efforts and instead assume *coping methods* such as avoidance, which indicates unsuccessful coping (Simoni and Paterson, 1997), it may desensitise them to patients' needs (Nagy's, 1999), which means in turn that they may not be

willing or able to attend to patients' suffering. Such strategies should, therefore, be detected, and those nurses helped to adopt more constructive coping strategies.

4.6 Potential outcomes of pain management and advocacy

Effective pain relief may provide *satisfaction*, both by means of professional achievements and benefits for the patient and the nurse (Blondal & Halldorsdottir, 2009; De Schepper et al. 1997; Vaartio et al., 2008). However, such positive outcomes are seldom mentioned. We believe that this aspect should receive more attention and nurses should be enabled to reap satisfaction from overcoming challenges and learning from them. As successful pain relief may enhance autonomy and a sense of *empowerment*, this is relevant to both quality of pain management and job satisfaction. Conversely, much more attention is given to the negative aspects: dissatisfaction, distress and frustration (e.g. Nagy, 1998; Söderhamn and Idvall, 2003) following insufficient or unsuccessful pain management that leads in turn to nurses' suffering and *disempowerment* (Blondal & Halldorsdottir, 2009; Oberle and Hughes, 2001).

4.6.1 Dissatisfaction and distress as motivators for a successful outcome

Since *dissatisfaction* and nurses´ *distress* may be the inevitable results of nurses' inability to ease the patients' pain, for instance because of silencing or lack of resources, it is important to note that nurses' distress can impel further actions. This is in agreement with Mallik's (1997) argument that emotional responses of anger and frustration can be potent motivators for advocacy. It, therefore, seems important that nurses accept and recognise such feelings, not least because those who acknowledge and try to deal with feelings of powerlessness are more capable of coping (De Schepper et al., 1997). All these responses require, once again, both personal and aesthetic knowledge where nurses as individuals must learn to know themselves and their reactions and be able to develop and maintain a view of what they want to achieve with their actions. Here we come back to earlier discussion about nurses' requirements of knowing their own "selves", their own feelings and capabilities.

5. Further development of this theory

Theory provides a more complete picture of practice than factual knowledge alone, and theories formulate, identify, and articulate the science and practice of every discipline (Butcher, 2006). Nursing scholars need to identify and articulate the processes and components of the art and science of pain management. This theory is an attempt to do so in an endeavour to continue the discipline's development by assisting in the understanding and practice of creating further theoretical discourse, processes and products for pain management, similar to what Kagan (2006) has described. All theories are reconstructed in the light of new data. The theory presented here is, therefore, seen as always being in the process of emerging, as is our world view. According to Walker and Avant (2004), the next steps in the phases of our theory development are: theory testing involving concept revision, statement revision, and theory revision, followed by further theory testing. We encourage our colleagues to critique the theory and use it to generate research questions and take part in testing the theory as well as in concept, statement and theory revision.

6. Implications for practice and future research

From our explanatory model many suggestions can be made about how to contribute to changes in the education of nurses, their work environment and future research.

6.1 Nurses' knowledge and formal education

Firstly, we propose that alterations should be made within nurses' basic education at school and continuous education at the institutional level. Nurses' formal education at school must include extensive knowledge about pain assessment and pain management and it is also necessary that courses are offered regularly within all health care settings on pain assessment, analgesia, adverse reactions, and respiratory depression. However, in addition to the traditional emphasis on the use of pain scales for the assessment of patients' pain, it is also important to emphasise *personal and aesthetic knowledge* that contains strategies that contribute to knowing and involving the patient, and nurses' availability. Then education about the pain management of dying patients, addiction and prejudices must also be increased, both at schools and within organisations. The *ethical aspects of pain management* should be included in all courses along with empirical knowledge and should contain discussions about moral responsibility, bioethical principles, nurses' professional code of conduct and the Patients' Rights Act together with religious discussions about pain management. Furthermore, despite differences in educational programmes and the cultures of nurses and doctors, these professions must reach a mutual understanding to achieve suitable and consistent care for their patients (Malloy et al., 2009). One method to bring together their views could, therefore, be to organise courses that these professionals attend together. That said, as nurses' socialisation occurs to a great extent during their nursing education (Stein et al., 1990), nursing students should be taught to make claims for mutual decision-making, to recognise their own potential, and be *empowered* to make claims for resources and improvements. As many nurses may lack the vocabulary for ethical decision-making, thus contributing to the silenced voices of nurses (Malloy et al., 2009), *advocating competence* should be taught at school. Moreover, they should be prepared for the need for *negotiation*, assertiveness, and effective *communication*. It is necessary that nurses are encouraged to reflect on their experience both as nurse students and as practicing nurses and also to establish positive working relationship with doctors. Moreover, since nurses seem to learn strategies such as self-confidence through role modelling we emphasize that during their nursing education and as novice nurses they should have access to role models for guidance that relate to their use of personal and aesthetic knowledge. During courses about pain management nurses' coping methods should be addressed, and they should be taught to recognise destructive methods and adopt more constructive ones. The method of *structured reflection* (Johns, 1995), for instance, could be used to assist nurses in learning about their own abilities and responses. However, not only should negative aspects of their practice or difficult cases be inspected, but also the positive ones.

6.2 Organisational environment

Firstly, it is imperative that pain relief is highlighted within all health care settings and organisational nursing policies or visions for nursing, which must reflect this important aspect of care. It should be stressed that pain management is a priority and recognised that time and adequate resources are important aspects of pain management. Protocols that exemplify the responsibility of each member of the health care team should exist, but all rules that are created should also be flexible; for instance nurses must be enabled to choose an analgesic from a range of individualised prescriptions. It also seems vital that clear directives exist for the pain relief of addicts and access to support from specialists in the management of this group of patients available at all times. Support from specialists in pain management and psychological support at all times are also fundamental. Moreover, the opportunity to discuss difficult cases with philosophers or leaders from different faiths and denominations should be provided in every health care setting. Subsequently, conversations about nurses' ethical responsibilities and dilemmas should be offered and should be open for both nurses and doctors. As pain assessment is partly dependent on positive nurse-patient relationships and knowing the patient as a person, nursing models and interventions that encourage such relations should be introduced and supported. Another aspect of organisational culture that may enhance successful pain management is good collaboration and maintenance of trust between nurses and in the nurse-physician relationships. All efforts that strengthen dialogue and a culture that enables nurses to seek support and advice from colleagues and encourages open discussions about feelings and coping may therefore have positive outcomes in this respect. Lastly, an atmosphere of persistence and seeking the best available solution should be supported.

6.3 Future research

The explanatory model can be a great source of ideas for future research. Firstly, a quantitative study could be conducted, to assess nurses' level of empirical, aesthetic and ethical knowledge along with personal knowledge regarding pain relief; including communication, collaboration and coping. Secondly, it would be interesting to explore the ethical component of the nursing and medical curricula and further to investigate to what extent nurses and doctors are guided by moral values in their pain relief at work. Thirdly, studies on how nurses' moral orientation is balanced with the effectiveness of the pain relief they provide could also be conducted. Fourthly, it seems necessary to conduct more studies where the communication of nurses and doctors connected with pain management is explored, for instance by using an ethnographic approach. Fifthly, it seems important to run more field studies within each organization to identify the main obstructions for effective pain management. It seems vital to begin with identifying what hindrances are most prominent before embarking on a campaign for better pain management within organisations. A part of these studies could be to inspect the effects of workload, lack of time and constraining directives on nurses' potentials for providing optimal pain relief.

7. Conclusion

Our explanatory model is at odds with statements proposing that pain relief is not the nurses' priority (Brockopp et al., 1998) or their responsibility (Twycross, 2002). We assert, however, that various reasons inhibit the nurses' potential for taking action. We conclude that nurses are the patients´ advocates in pain management and successful pain management is rewarded with a sense of satisfaction, empowerment and fulfilment of their duty. They are in a key position to assess and manage pain and their mediatory position within the hospital is unique. It is vital that nurses are adequately prepared for their role educationally by possessing multidimensional knowledge about pain management. We assert that good theoretical knowledge may be inadequate if the nurse does not have the right motivation, i.e. the *moral inclination* to use it in practice. Furthermore, *personal knowledge* that nurses must use in relations with patients and doctors is also necessary because theoretical knowledge alone may be of little use if it cannot be employed because of lack of communication or negotiation competence or because their voice is silenced. They also need personal knowledge for self-knowledge, and to reflect on their own strengths and weaknesses in order to make better use of their own abilities. Therefore, nurses must be taught to act as the patient's advocate and the patients' representative. This also requires nurses to use their *aesthetic knowledge* to appreciate the needs of every individual patient. Furthermore, nurses must acknowledge how little they know about some patients who could beforehand be labelled as "difficult". These patterns of knowledge in pain management are interrelated and should therefore be assessed as a whole if pain management is to be enhanced within an organisation or pain management skills in nurses' primary or continuing education. The organisation in turn must provide an *optimal environment*; a clear statement about pain management and clear but flexible rules on pain management, and provide ample time and resources such as specialised pain services, that otherwise may hinder nurses from acting according to their best knowledge, potentials, and nursing goals. Teamwork and good collaboration between health care professionals must also be supported. The structure and prevailing culture of organisations must therefore be scrutinised before organising improvements in pain management.

All the factors previously mentioned coexist and are interdependent and cannot be taken out of the immediate context, as may be seen from our model. Therefore, developments in pain management that focus only on one aspect of pain management may be ineffective, as many factors affect this process. We, therefore, propose that knowledge in this respect has often been too narrowly defined and we call for a more holistic approach in pain management by nurses and other health care personnel where multiple types of knowledge and skills as well as the organisational context are included and taken into consideration during educational efforts and reform of pain management within organisations.

8. References

Blondal, K. & Halldorsdottir, S. (2009). The challenge of caring for patients in pain: From the nurse's perspective. *Journal of Clinical Nursing*, Vol.18, No.20, pp. 2897–2906, ISSN 0962-1067

Boer, C., Treebus, A.N., Zuurmond, W.W.A. & de Lange, J.J. (1997). Compliance in administration of prescribed analgesics. *Anaesthesia*, Vol.52, No.11, pp. 1177- 1181, ISSN 1365-2044

Brockopp, D.Y., Ryan, P. & Warden, S. (2003). Nurses' willingness to manage the pain of specific groups of patients. *British Journal of Nursing*, Vol.12, No.7, pp. 409-415, ISSN 0966-0461

Brockopp, G., Warden, S., Wilson, J., Carpenter, J.S. & Vandeveer, B. (1998). Barriers to change: A pain management project. *International Journal of Nursing Studies*, Vol.35, No.4, pp. 226-232, ISSN 0020-7489

Butcher, H.K. (2006). Review of Walker and Avant's newest theory development text. *Nursing Science Quarterly*, Vol.19, No.2, pp.174-177, ISSN 0894-3184

Carper, B.A. (1978). Fundamental patterns of knowing in nursing. *Advances in Nursing Science*, Vol. 1, No. 1, pp. 13–23, ISSN 0161-9268

Carr, E.C.J. (2002). Refusing analgesics: Using continuous improvement to improve pain management on a surgical ward. *Journal of Clinical Nursing*, Vol.11, No.6, pp. 743-752, ISSN 0962-1067

Clabo, L.M.L. (2008). An ethnography of pain assessment and the role of social context on two postoperative units. *Journal of Advanced Nursing*, Vol.61, No.5, pp. 531–539, ISSN 0309-2402

Coker, E., Papaioannou, A, Kaasalainen, S., Dolovich, L., Turpie, I. & Taniguchi, A. (2010). Nurses' perceived barriers to optimal pain management in older adults on acute medical units. *Applied Nursing Research*, Vol.23, No.3, pp. 139-146, ISSN 0897-1897

De Schepper, A.M.E., Francke, A.L. & Abu-Saad, H.H. (1997). Feelings of powerlessness in relation to pain: ascribed causes and reported strategies: A qualitative study among Dutch community nurses caring for cancer patients with pain. *Cancer Nursing*, Vol.20, No.6, pp. 422-429, ISSN 0162-220X

Ferrell, B.R., Eberts, M.T., McCaffery, M. & Grant, M. (1991). Clinical decisionmaking and pain. *Cancer Nursing*, Vol.14, No.6, pp. 289-297, ISSN 0162-220X

Ferrell, B.R., Taylor, E.J., Grant, M., Fowler, M. & Corbisiero, R.M. (1993). Pain management at home: Struggle, comfort, and mission. *Cancer Nursing*, Vol.16, No.3, pp. 169-178, ISSN 0162-220X

Gudmannsdottir, G.D. & Halldorsdottir, S. (2009). Primacy of existential pain and suffering in residents in chronic pain in nursing homes: A phenomenological study. *Scandinavian Journal of Caring Sciences*, Vol.20, No.3, pp. 317-327, ISSN 0283-9318

Howell, D., Butler, L., Vincent, L., Watt-Watson, J. & Stearns, N. (2000). Influencing nurses' knowledge, attitudes, and practice in cancer pain management. *Cancer Nursing*, Vol.23, No.1, pp. 55-63, ISSN 0162-220X

Jenks, J.M. (1993). The pattern of personal knowing in nurse clinical decision making. *Journal of Nursing Education*, Vol.32, No.9, pp. 399–405, ISSN 1938-2421

Johns, C. (1995). Framing learning through reflection within Carper's fundamental ways of knowing in nursing. *Journal of Advanced Nursing*, Vol.22, No.2, pp. 226-234, ISSN 0309-2402

Kagan, P. (2006). Review of Walker and Avant's newest theory development text. *Nursing Science Quarterly*, Vol.19, No.2, pp. 177–179, ISSN 0894-3184

Keenan, G.M., Cooke, R. & Hillis, S.L. (1998). Norms and nurse management of conflicts: Keys to understanding nurse-physician collaboration. *Research in Nursing and Health*, Vol.21, No.1, pp. 59-72, ISSN 1098-240X

Kramer, M. & Schmalenberg, C. (1993). Learning from success: autonomy and empowerment. *Nursing Management*, Vol.24, No.5, pp. 58-64, ISSN 0744-6314

Kuuppelomäki, M. (2002a). Pain management problems in patients' terminal phase as assessed by nurses in Finland. *Journal of Advanced Nursing*, Vol.40, No.6, pp. 701-709, ISSN 0309-2402

Kuuppelomäki, M. (2002b). The decision-making process when starting terminal care as assessed by nursing staff. *Nursing Ethics*, Vol.9, No.1, pp. 20-35, ISSN 0969-7330

Liaschenko, J. (1997). Knowing the patient? In Thorne S.E. & Hayes, V.E. (Eds.), *Nursing Praxis: Knowledge and Action*, pp. 23–38, Sage, ISBN 0761900101, London

Mallik, M. (1997). Advocacy in nursing – perceptions of practising nurses. *Journal of Clinical Nursing*, Vol.6, No.4, pp. 303-313, ISSN 0962-1067

Malloy, D.C., Hadjistavropoulos, T., McCarthy, E.F., Evans, R.J., Zakus, D.H., Park, I., Lee, Y. & Williams, J. (2009). Culture and organizational climate: Nurses' insights into their relationship with physicians. *Nursing Ethics*, Vol.16, No.6, pp. 719-33, ISSN 0969-7330

Manias, E. (2003). Pain and anxiety management in the postoperative gastro-surgical setting. *Journal of Advanced Nursing*, Vol.41, No.6, pp. 585-594, ISSN 0309-2402

McCaffery, M. & Ferrell, B.R. (1997). Nurses' knowledge of pain assessment and management: How much progress have we made? *Journal of Pain and Symptom Management*, Vol.14, No.3, pp. 175-188, ISSN 0885-3924

McCaffery, M. & Pasero, C. (1999). Assessment: Underlying complexities, misconceptions, and practical tools. In McCaffery, M. & Pasero, C. (Eds.), *Pain: clinical manual* (2nd ed.), pp. 35-102, Mosby, ISBN 081515609X, St. Louis

McCaffery, M., Ferrell, B., O'Neil-Page, E., Lester, M. & Ferrell, B. (1990). Nurses' knowledge of opioid analgesic drugs and psychological dependence. *Cancer Nursing*, Vol.13, No.1, pp. 21-27, ISSN 0162-220X

Munhall, P.L. (1993) 'Unknowing': toward another pattern of knowing in nursing. *Nursing Outlook*, Vol.41, No.3, pp. 125-128, ISSN 0029-6554

Nagy, S. (1999). Strategies used by burns nurses to cope with the infliction of pain on patients. *Journal of Advanced Nursing*, Vol.29, No.6, pp. 1427-1433, ISSN 0309-2402

Nash, R., Yates, P., Edwards, H., Fentiman, B., Dewar, A., McDowell, J. & Clark, R. (1999). Pain and the administration of analgesia: What nurses say. *Journal of Clinical Nursing*, Vol.8, No.2, pp. 180-189, ISSN 0962-1067

O'Rourke, K. (1992). Pain relief: The perspective of catholic tradition. *Journal of Pain and Symptom Management*, Vol.7, No.8, pp. 485-491, ISSN 0885-3924

Oberle, K. & Hughes, D. (2001) Doctors' and nurses' perceptions of ethical problems in end-of-life decisions. *Journal of Advanced Nursing*, Vol.33, No.6, pp. 707-715, ISSN 0309-2402

O'Connor, T. & Kelly, B. (2005). Bridging the gap: A study of general nurses' perceptions of patient advocacy in Ireland. *Nursing Ethics*, Vol.12, No.5, pp. 453-67, ISSN 0969-7330

Omery, A. (1989). Values, moral reasoning, and ethics. *Nursing Clinics of North America*, Vol.24, No.2, pp. 499-508, ISSN 0029-6465

Paice, J.A. & Cohen, F. L. (1997) Validity of a verbally administered numeric rating scale to measure cancer pain intensity. *Cancer Nursing*, Vol.20, No.2, pp. 88-93, ISSN 0162-220X

Pasero, C., Paice, J.A. & McCaffery, M. (1999). Basic mechanisms underlying the causes and effects of pain. In McCaffery, M. & Pasero, C. (Eds.), *Pain: Clinical manual* (2nd ed.), pp. 15-34, Mosby, ISBN 081515609X, St. Louis

Rejeh, N., Ahmadi, F., Mohamadi, E., Anoosheh, M. & Kazemnejad, A. (2009). Ethical challenges in pain management post-surgery. *Nursing Ethics*, Vol.16, No.2, pp. 161-72, ISSN 0969-7330

Schafheutle, E.I., Cantrill, J.A. & Noyce, P.R. (2001). Why is pain management suboptimal on surgical wards? *Journal of Advanced Nursing*, Vol.33, No.6, pp. 728-737, ISSN 0309-2402

Schmitz, N., Neumann, W. & Oppermann, R. (2000). Stress, burnout and loss of control in German nurses. *International Journal of Nursing Studies*, Vol.37, No.2, pp. 95-99, ISSN 0020-7489

Simoni, P.S. & Paterson, J.J. (1997). Hardiness, coping, and burnout in the nursing workplace. *Journal of Professional Nursing*, Vol.13, No.3, pp. 178-185, ISSN 8755-7223

Sjöström, B., Dahlgren, L.O. & Haljamäe, H. (2000). Strategies used in post-operative pain assessment and their clinical accuracy. *Journal of Clinical Nursing*, Vol.9, No.1, pp. 111-118, ISSN 0962-1067

Söderhamn, O. & Idvall, E. (2003). Nurses' influence on quality of care in postoperative pain management: A phenomenological study. *International Journal of Nursing Practice*, No.9, Vol.1, pp. 26-32, ISSN 1322-7114

Stein, L.I., Watts, D.T. & Howell, T. (1990). The doctor-nurse game revisited. *New England Journal of Medicine*, Vol.322, No.8, pp. 546-549, ISSN 0028-4793

Takman, C. & Severinsson, E.I. (1999). A description of health care professionals' experiences of encounters with patients in clinical settings. *Journal of Advanced Nursing*, Vol.30, No.6, pp. 1368-1374, ISSN 0309-2402

Taylor, E.J., Ferrell, B.R., Grant, M. & Cheyney, L. (1993). Managing cancer pain at home: The decisions and ethical conflicts of patients, family caregivers, and homecare nurses. *Oncology Nursing Forum*, Vol.20, No.6, pp. 919-927, ISSN 0190-535X

Twycross, A. (2002). Educating nurses about pain management: The way forward. *Journal of Clinical Nursing*, Vol.11, No.6, pp. 705-14, ISSN 0962-1067

Vaartio, H., Leino-Kilpi, H., Salanterä, S. & Suominen, T. (2006). Nursing advocacy: How is it defined by patients and nurses, what does it involve and how is it experienced? *Scandnavian Journal of Caring Sciences*, Vol.20, No.3, pp. 282-92, ISSN 0283-9318

Van Niekerk, L.M. & Martin, F. (2002). The impact of the nurse-physician professional relationship on nurses' experience of ethical dilemmas in effective pain management. *Journal of Professional Nursing*, Vol.18, No.5, pp. 276-288, ISSN 8755-7223

Walker, L.O. & Avant, K.C. (2004). *Strategies for theory construction in nursing* (4th ed.). Prentice Hall, ISBN 0838586880, Englewood Cliffs, NJ

Ware, L.J., Bruckenthal, P., Davis, G.C. & O'Conner-Von, S.K. (2011). Factors that influence patient advocacy by pain management nurses: Results of the American society for pain management nursing survey. *Pain Management Nursing*, (Epub 2010 Jul 24), Vol.12, No.1, 25-32., ISSN 1524-9042

Watt-Watson, J., Stevens, B., Garfinkel, P., Streiner, D. & Gallop, R, (2001). Relationship between nurses' pain knowledge and pain management outcomes for their postoperative cardiac patients. *Journal of Advanced Nursing*, Vol.36, No.4, pp. 535-545, ISSN 0309-2402

Willson, H. (2000). Factors affecting the administration of analgesia to patients following repair of a fractured hip. *Journal of Advanced Nursing*, Vol.31, No.5, pp. 1145-1154, ISSN 0309-2402

Wilson, B. (2007). Nurses' knowledge of pain. *Journal of Clinical Nursing*, Vol.16, No.6, pp. 1012–1020, ISSN 0962-1067

Wilson, B. (2009). Can patient lifestyle influence the management of pain? *Journal of Clinical Nursing*, Vol.18, No.3, pp. 399–408, ISSN 0962-1067

Part 5

Complex Regional Pain Syndrome and Reflex Sympathetic Dystrophy

10

Complex Regional Pain Syndrome

Gabor B. Racz[1] and Carl E. Noe[2]
[1]Department of Anesthesiology, Pain Center,
Texas Tech University Health Sciences Center,
[2]Department of Anesthesiology and Pain Management,
Eugene McDermott Center for Pain Mangement,
Univerisity of Texas Southwestern Medical Center,
USA

1. Introduction

Complex regional pain syndromes (CRPS) are pain syndromes characterized by pain out of proportion to an inciting injury, swelling, discoloration, stiffness, hyperhidrosis (sudomotor), temperature (vasomotor) and trophic changes. Also commonly seen are fine tremor and less often spasms involving upper and lower extremities. Dr. Silas Wier Mitchell described CRPS II, or causalgia, during the American Civil War. CRPS I was described about the end of the 19th century by Sudek (Sudek's atrophy). Evans described reflex sympathetic dystrophy (RSD). Numerous other terms used to describe similar syndromes include algodystrophy and shoulder- hand syndrome. Bonica described 3 stages of RSD. Roberts described sympathetically maintained pain.

2. Diagnostic criteria

Specific inclusion criteria are needed for research studies but from a clinical perspective, many patients seem to have a constellation of signs and symptoms of CRPS without meeting strict criteria. The diagnosis is made by the process of exclusion. While avoiding over diagnosing and over treatment, the patients need to be treated.

3. Prognosis

The prognosis for CRPS is highly variable and to a large extent is influenced by the treatment. Functional restoration and involving the patient in ongoing range of motion and resistive exercises is helpful. Timely pain relief and interventional pain procedures, as well as psychological support, are important. Patients need to be followed closely and treatments adjusted accordingly. Timely and appropriate referral to experienced pain physicians that are able to offer multimodal therapies may prevent costly delays and complications.

4. Theories of mechanisms

Multiple possible mechanisms exist for CRPS including psychological, inflammatory, vascular, neurogenic and combinations of several mechanisms. Debate regarding definitions of neuropathic pain has led to the notion that CRPS may not be neuropathic pain. Psychogenic pain could be construed as being "pain arising as a direct consequence of a lesion or disease affecting the somatosensory system" but few would think of it as neuropathic pain which should be treated with anticonvulsants.

CRPS II is generally agreed to be caused by an injury to a peripheral nerve. CRPS 1 is caused by a lesion in or injury to a small nerve or multiple small nerves. It is difficult to accept that it is not neuropathic pain since it resembles CRPS II so closely. Denial of care based on psychological explanations is neither reasonable nor justifiable yet in rare instances pain can be of psychological origin. Commonly the onset of CRPS is 1- 3 months after the injury.

5. History

The diagnosis is made by process of exclusion following history of pain that is out of proportion to an injury or period of immobilization. Swelling, temperature asymmetry, stiffness, atrophy, hair, skin nail, bone changes. Tremor or spasms and asymmetry in sweat function are all potential signs. It is important to remember that many injuries are associated with pain, discoloration and swelling without being CRPS. Infection and other causes of inflammation are sometimes mistakenly thought to be CRPS. A number of patients have CRPS symptoms following stroke and classifying this as central pain or CRPS is problematic.

6. Physical exam

Observation of upper extremity guarding or antalgic gait for lower extremity is important. Range of motion of affected joints is particularly important as many patients develop permanent stiffness without analgesia for specific range of motion therapy. Discoloration or asymmetrical coloration, swelling, atrophy and allodynia are other physical findings. The allodynia may be tactile or cold induced.

7. Diagnostic tests

Bone scans, sweat tests and sympathetic blocks have been used but the diagnosis is a clinical one and can be made without confirmatory tests. Thermography has been used, but more commonly, the documentation of temperature differences is adequate. Early on in the evolution of the condition there may increased temperature and later reduction with the increased sympathetic activity. Three phase bone scan often show corresponding changes.

Comparing contra lateral x-ray images can show osteopenia in the involved area. EMG usually does not change from the CRPS but may show nerve injury.

8. Differential diagnosis

While it important to be vigilant in diagnosing CRPS, as is important to avoid misdiagnosis and over- diagnosis. Many patients have "pain out of proportion", swelling and discoloration after injuries and will improve within a month with usual therapeutic interventions.

Infection is always a concern after surgery or other penetrating trauma. Other causes of acute inflammation, swelling and discoloration need to be considered such as malignancy, deep venous thrombosis as well as peripheral nerve entrapment, peripheral neuropathy and other neuropathic pains.

9. Stages

3 stages of RSD have been described however it is unclear that staging has much value regarding decision making.

10. Timing

Much has been made about early sympathetic blocks and failure to diagnose early. There is no data to support "emergent" sympathetic blocks and some patients have a favorable natural history.

11. Spreading

Pain from CRPS can spread, in rare instances, proximally and contra- laterally. (Shah, Racz) Lower extremity pain can spread to upper extremities and vice versa.

12. Bone loss

Osteopenia and fractures can occur in severe cases and aquatic therapy is useful to rehabilitate these patients.

13. Natural history

The natural history of CRPS 1 is variable but in an interesting report, approximately 25% of patients that had Colles' fractures developed signs of CRPS. (Atkins) Approximately 40% of these patients improved in 6 months. This suggests that mild cases may not require extensive treatment. Not treating the patients early can be problematic if the condition worsens. Appropriate examination and follow up is important where the disease can take a benign course. Patients obtain information on the Internet that is usually about catastrophic cases that needs to be dealt with by educating patients in an appropriate and caring manner where therapy is timely yet one can avoid catastrophizing based on inaccurate information.

14. Dogma

Much of "standard care" is not evidence based, but good outcome based. Additionally, it is based on physician experience and the outcome is superior in the hands of better-trained physicians. As new information becomes available, dogma can be weeded out and treatments based on randomized controlled trails can be incorporated into treatment guidelines.

15. Cases

One lady had not worn high-heeled shoes for a long time and then wore a pair for several hours at an event. She developed classic signs and symptoms of RSD. She experienced profound analgesia with sympathetic blockade and the condition resolved completely.

Another case was a woman who had a paper cut on her distal index finger on the job. She had classic signs and symptoms of CRPS, which resolved with a series of blocks. Both of these cases were challenged by insurance companies since the inciting injury was so minor but both patients were legitimate. The point is that physicians caring for these patients must be willing to serve as advocates for the patient even in an environment of cost containment. We have to be mindful of our "report cards" but not at the expense of a patient's outcome.

16. Overmedication pain syndrome (OPS)

Approximately 20 years ago, a movement began to improve the quality of pain care for cancer patients worldwide. The WHO analgesic ladder was promoted for cancer pain and then it was applied for other types of pain. Many patients are now taking large doses of opioid for chronic pain.

Overmedication pain syndrome is characterized by a chronic treatment program consisting of high doses of multiple analgesic medications without associated functional productivity and psychological coping ability.

Opioids are the most important class of drugs in pain management; however, it is clear that they are two edged swords and overmedication with opioids and other drugs classes have become a problem. Abuse may not be the largest problem. Lack of efficacy, unintended overdose, diversion, development of drug dependence, habituation and resistance to recovery and other unintended consequences may be more common.

Opioid induced hyperalgesia is a real clinical phenomenon and may be a subtle barrier to analgesia in many patients. Pain that is only incrementally responsive to opioid is also common.

Pseudo-addiction is defined in behavioral terms which are similar to addiction but related to pain and not addiction. The problem is that there are not good means to differentiate behaviors between the setting of pain and the setting of addiction.

Some have reported a lack of data to support doses of opioid over 200 mg/day of morphine equivalents. Also, there are no long term randomized controlled trials of opioid versus placebo. Additionally, fracture rates have been reported to be increased in patients on doses above 100 mg/day. (Sullivan) Overdose rates have been reported to increase above 50 mg/day. (Dunn) Drug interactions with other medications, reported and unreported to the treating physician, have been causes of fatalities.

Urine drug testing, opioid contracts and extensive documentation guidelines fail to help answer the clinical question: is the dose just too high?

Patients who are taking opioids chronically should be considered for an evaluation for a lack of meaningful efficacy, fall and fracture risk and overdose risk. An interdisciplinary evaluation may be a way to accomplish these objectives. Patients who are clearly doing well may be less likely to accept dose reductions. Patients who are working or similarly productive and are without signs of poor coping and physical disability may need to continue taking the effective dosages. On the other hand, patients, who have been on stable doses for a long time may need age related dose reductions.

Washington State has new guidelines limiting the dose of opioid to 120 mg/day of morphine equivalents. Patients, who require doses above this level, are guided to seek a pain management consultation. The purpose and intervention of a medical pain management consultation is unclear. The practitioner doing the evaluation needs to have additional training and qualification as well as be informed and knowledgeable in treatment options in addition to opioid management.

JCAHO, Press Gainey and other organizations have changed the environment with respect to patient rights regarding pain. In the past, if a patient wasn't happy with their opioid dose, their recourse was limited. Now, patient satisfaction is used as a factor to determine healthcare provider's compensation. The implication is that patients can pressure providers to prescribe more opioid, which is dangerous for patients and providers.

Regulators have become more active due to the increased rate of diversion and its consequences. However, the accidental overdose rate increase is even more concerning.

Most drugs have dose limits. For example, antibiotics and drugs for hypertension are increased to upper limits but there are limits. Perhaps it is time to limit doses of opioids regardless of pain severity for patients with non palliative care pain syndromes and find another way to treat the patient.

Other drugs classes that are problematic include benzodiazepines, muscle relaxers, sleeping pills and even anticonvulsants and antidepressants. Benzodiazepines are not prominent in the pain literature as analgesics. Baclofen and tizanidine are probably the first line muscle relaxers of choice. Hypnotic drugs are used too often for chronic sleep disturbances without sleep hygiene treatment or other medications which are better for long term use. Anticonvulsant use for chronic pain has exploded as opioids have. Antidepressants, even those not associated with analgesia, are prescribed for pain.

The costs of these drugs are significant and usually of incremental benefit. Most patients with chronic pain go without an interdisciplinary evaluation and many who receive an evaluation do not complete treatment with cognitive behavioral therapy, education and conditioning physical therapy. Treatment goals are frequently not established and some patients just go through the motions and are considered as a treatment failure. There is very little evidence for the multidisciplinary and physical therapy based treatments specifically for CRPS. Reimbursement has suffered for these kinds of therapies.

The cognitive effects and psychological effects of chronic opioid treatment are not well known.

Testosterone levels in males are known to decrease with chronic opioid administration.

It is proposed that patients with chronic pain have a short term trial of low dose opioid to access functional improvement before a treatment plan is finalized. Blinding patients to their drug and dose may be very helpful but has its critics on ethical and regulatory grounds.

Patients who are on doses above 50 mg/day of morphine equivalents need to have access to interdisciplinary pain and addictionology evaluations and treatment if needed. Treatment goals should include dose reduction to below 200mg/day of morphine equivalents for those taking more than that. Intermediate term treatment goals for patients taking less than 200 mg/day should strive for less than 100 mg/day and patients taking less than 100 mg/day, 50 mg/day.

There is no data to support this approach but there was no data 20 years ago to support using the WHO analgesic ladder for headaches, fibromyalgia, back pain or any other condition. Data for limited doses of opioid for arthritis and neuropathic pain exists and prescribing for opioid responsive pain should not be overly scrutinized by regulators. Never the less, diversion, addiction, opioid induced hyperalgesia and other adverse events associated with opioids need to be avoided more effectively before the first prescription is written.

Many patients in drug treatment programs were initially treated with opioid for perfectly legitimate pain. The patient and the doctor may not be the biggest problems. The biggest problem may be the drug and the dosage.

17. Treatment guideline history

In 1994, the International Association for the Study of Pain (IASP) revised the terminology from RSD and causalgia to CRPS type I and II. 15 years ago we proposed an analgesic ladder for CRPS /RSD which included 3 steps. (Racz) Since then, well-respected groups have advanced other guidelines. (Van Eijs) (Stanton-Hicks)

Our initial proposal was:

Step 1. TENS, opioids, topicals, Tricyclic antidepressants, supportive psychotherapy, vocational rehabilitation, patient education, physical therapy and occupational therapy

Step 2. Regional or sympathetic block, evaluation and treatment of the emotional component of pain, IV regional block, peripheral block-infusion, carbamazepine, baclofen, clonidine, corticosteroid, NSAID, mexiletine, other drug trials

Step 3. Sympathectomy/sympatholysis, peripheral nerve decompression, lysis, continuous local anesthetic infusion epidural and or regional for five to seven days, Spinal Cord Stimulation (SCS), Peripheral Nerve Stimulation (PNS), intrathecal/epidural analgesia.

At that time, little data existed to guide treatment and the initial analgesic ladder was based on opinion. Since that time, additional data has been produced leading to modifications to the analgesic ladder. This is categorically not intended to estabish a standard of care since data to do such is inadequate. Rather, our intention is to share our beliefs in hopes of helping patients with this disorder.

18. New principles and information

Our current analgesic ladder promotes several concepts:

1. Interdisciplinary pain treatment is recommended rather than multidisciplinary care which tends to be fragmented. Interdisciplinary treatment specifically provides coordinated medical care, education, cognitive behavioral therapy for pain, physical therapy and outcome documentation by the interdisciplinary team. Patients who receive care at different clinics for each component of care by a group of providers who do not meet on a weekly basis nor document comprehensive outcomes are not receiving interdisciplinary pain management.

2. Interdisciplinary care is not isolated from medical pain management. Analgesic treatments are necessary to provide pain relief and allow functional restoration.
3. The course of an individual patient is highly variable and adjustments to the treatment plan should be made in a highly flexible manner.
4. Limiting opioid doses to below 200mg/day morphine equivalents
5. Numerous randomized controlled trials have been performed since our initial analgesic ladder was proposed and these findings are incorporated.
6. However if there is treatment failure and functional restoration failure the patient needs to be referred to centers or individuals with recognized experience to be specialists in the field.

Sympathetic blocks have been recommended early on in the management of the disorder but little data exists to support this practice. Only recently has any data from a randomized controlled trial been published to demonstrate efficacy of sympathetic blockade. (Meier) Spinal cord stimulation has been shown to produce significant analgesia even after 5 years of treatment. (Klemer) Cortical stimulation has been shown to have some benefit. (Velasco) Deep brain stimulation has been shown to be ineffective. Vitamin C has been studied by multiple investigators for the prevention of CRPS and has some effect. (Besse) Intravenous magnesium has been reported to be effective in an initial study. (Collins) Clodronate has been shown to be partially effective. (Varenna) Mirror therapy has been reported to have benefit in stroke patients with CRPS. (Cacchio) Multicenter comparison of spinal cord stimualtion and peripheral nerve stimulation showed that PNS is more effective than SCS but the best outcome was where both modalities were utilized. (Calvillo)

Intravenous regional anesthesia with the addtion of vasodilators such as phentolamine, reserpine and bretylium allow manipulation of hands without post procedure edema and speed up functional restoration without the pain associated with physical therapy. (Heavner, Calvillo, Racz)

An evidenced based review endorses bisphosphonates (alendronate, pamidronate, clodronate), corticosteroid, gabapentin, physiotherapy and psychotherapy/relaxation techniques as treatments. (Baron) Additionally intrathecal baclofen for associated dystonia and spinal cord stimulation for refractory caes are recommended. Topical DMSO and sympathetic blocks are not strongly recommended. Intravenous regional blocks with guanethidine are not recommended as specific treatment (Van Eijs)

19. Treatments to avoid

Amputation is less common nowadays because it was rarely effective and usually resulted in a phantom pain plus different pain of greater severity

IV regional with guanethidine has been shown to be ineffective in several studies as sole agent.

Deep brain stimulation has been shown to be ineffective.

High dose opioid should be avoided if possible due to possible opioid induced hyperalgesia, addiction, diversion risk and over-dosage.

20. Proposed treatment

Step 1.
Screening for substance abuse, affective disorders and disability
Education

Physical therapy
Occupational therapy
Vocational rehabilitation
Topical lidocaine for allodynia
Tricyclic antidepressants
Gabapentin
Tramadol
Opioid doses limited to less than 200mg morphine equivalents per day and below 50mg/day if possible
Corticosteroid
Step 2.
Interdisciplinary pain evaluation including psychological testing (MMPI-RF) and treatment (cognitive behavioral therapy, group psycho educational therapy and psychotropic medication management, addictionology, physical and occupational therapy, in a coordinated goal directed, outcome documenting rehabilitation program)
Sympathetic block
IV Regional block
Peripheral block
Other drug trials
Step 3.
Spinal cord stimulation
Sympathectomy/sympatholysis
Peripheral nerve stimulation
Peripheral nerve decompression/lysis
Intrathecal/epidural analgesia

21. Interdisciplinary care

Interdisciplinary pain management is a term that is poorly understood. It is best reserved to describe a team of healthcare professionals led by a physician and including a psychologist and physical therapist at a minimum. A care team of multiple physicians from different specialties is not an interdisciplinary team for pain management nor is a psychologically based treatment program in isolation from medical pain management. Cognitive behavioral therapy, education and functional rehabilitation must be provided in an interdisciplinary pain care model in addition to medical pain management therapies. Case management, psychiatry, outcome database management, nursing, vocational rehabilitation, occupational therapy, medical direction and program direction and administrative support are key disciplines to include in a mature pain program. Nutrition, chaplaincy and other medical specialties are needed for tertiary programs.

22. Conclusion

Complex regional pain syndrome is a challenging pain problem that frequently requires a comprehensive interdisciplinary assessment and treatment plan. Until a mechanism is discovered and a specific treatment for the syndrome is developed, an interdisciplinary approach, including pharmacologic and interventional pain management in a step wise fashion, will likely remain as the best route to follow.

23. References

Atkins, R.M., Duckworth, T., Kanis, J.A.: Algodystrophy following Colles' Fracture.Journal of Hand Surgery (British Volume, 1989) 14B: 161-164

Baron, R., Naleschinski, D., Hullemann, P., Mahn, F.: Complex Regional Pain Syndrome: A neuropathic disorder? Pain 2010- An updated Review: Refresher Course Syllabus. IASP Press p. 109-117. 2010

Besse, J., Gadeyene, S., Galand-Desme, S., et.al: Effect of vitamin C on prevention of complex regional pain syndrome in foot and ankle surgery. Foot and Ankle Surgery 15:179-182, 2009

Cacchio, A., De Blasis, E., De Blasis, V., at.al.:Mirror Therapy in Complex Regional Pain Syndrome Type 1 of the Upper Limb in Stroke Patients. Neurorehabilitation and Neural Repair 23: 792-799, 2009.

Calvillo O, Racz GBN, Diede J, Smith K: Neuroaugmentation in the treatment of complex regional pain syndrome of the upper extremity. Acta Orthopaedica Belgica, 64-1, 57-63, 1998.

Collins, S., Zuurmond, W.W.A., de Lange, J.J., et.al.: Intravenous Magnesium for Complex Regional Pain Syndrome Type 1 (CRPS 1) Patients: A Pilot Study. Pain Medicine 10:930-940, 2009.

Dunn KM, Saunders KW, Rutter CM, et al.: Opioid prescriptions for chronic pain and overdose: a cohort study. Annals of Internal Medicine 2010; 152:85-92

Heavner JE, Calvillo O, Racz GB: Thermal grill illusion and complex regional pain syndrome Type I Reflex Sympathetic Dystrophy. Regional Anesthesia 22(3): 257-259, 1997.

Klemer M.A., de Vet, H.C., Barendse, G.A.M., et.al.: Effect of spinal cord stimulation for chronic complex regional pain syndrome Type I: five–year follow-up of patients in a randomized controlled trial. Jounal of Neurosurgery 108:292-298, 2008.

Meier, P.M., Zurakowski, D., Berde, C. B., Sethna, M.B.: Lumbar sympathetic blockade in Children with Complex Regional Pain Syndromes. Anesthesiology 2009, 111: 372-80.

Racz, Gabor B., Heavner, James E., Noe, Carl E.: Definitions, classification and Taxonomy: an overview Sympathetic pain syndromes: reflex sympathetic dystrophy and causalgia. Physical Medicine and Rehabilitation: State of the Art Reviews Vol 10 No 2 June 1996 Hanley and Belfus, Philadelphia

Shah RV, Racz GB. Recurrence and spread of complex regional pain syndrome due to distant site surgery: a case report. Am J Orthop (Belle Mead NJ). 2006 Nov; 35(11): 523-6.

Stanton-Hicks, M., Baron, R., Boas, R., et.al: Complex regional pain syndromes: guidelines for therapy. Clinical Journal of Pain 14:155-166, 1998.

Sullivan, M.D.: Who gets high dose opioid therapy for chronic non-cancer pain? Pain 151:567-568, 2010.

Van Eijs, F., Stanton –Hicks, M., Van Zundert, J., et. al.: Complex Regional Pain Syndrome. Pain practice 11:70-87, 2010.

Varenna, M., Zucchi, F., Ghiringhelli, D., et.al.: Intravenous clodronate in the treatment of reflex symathetic dystrophy syndrome. Journal of Rheumatology 27:1477-83, 2000

Velasco, F., Carrillo-Ruiz, J.D., Castro, G., et.al.: Motor cortex stimulation applied to patients with complex regional pain syndrome. Pain 147:91-98, 2009.

Permissions

The contributors of this book come from diverse backgrounds, making this book a truly international effort. This book will bring forth new frontiers with its revolutionizing research information and detailed analysis of the nascent developments around the world.

We would like to thank Gabor B. Racz, MD, FIPP, ABIPP, for lending his expertise to make the book truly unique. He has played a crucial role in the development of this book. Without his invaluable contribution this book wouldn't have been possible. He has made vital efforts to compile up to date information on the varied aspects of this subject to make this book a valuable addition to the collection of many professionals and students.

This book was conceptualized with the vision of imparting up-to-date information and advanced data in this field. To ensure the same, a matchless editorial board was set up. Every individual on the board went through rigorous rounds of assessment to prove their worth. After which they invested a large part of their time researching and compiling the most relevant data for our readers. Conferences and sessions were held from time to time between the editorial board and the contributing authors to present the data in the most comprehensible form. The editorial team has worked tirelessly to provide valuable and valid information to help people across the globe.

Every chapter published in this book has been scrutinized by our experts. Their significance has been extensively debated. The topics covered herein carry significant findings which will fuel the growth of the discipline. They may even be implemented as practical applications or may be referred to as a beginning point for another development. Chapters in this book were first published by InTech; hereby published with permission under the Creative Commons Attribution License or equivalent.

The editorial board has been involved in producing this book since its inception. They have spent rigorous hours researching and exploring the diverse topics which have resulted in the successful publishing of this book. They have passed on their knowledge of decades through this book. To expedite this challenging task, the publisher supported the team at every step. A small team of assistant editors was also appointed to further simplify the editing procedure and attain best results for the readers.

Our editorial team has been hand-picked from every corner of the world. Their multi-ethnicity adds dynamic inputs to the discussions which result in innovative outcomes. These outcomes are then further discussed with the researchers and contributors who give their valuable feedback and opinion regarding the same. The feedback is then collaborated with the researches and they are edited in a comprehensive manner to aid the understanding of the subject.

Apart from the editorial board, the designing team has also invested a significant amount of their time in understanding the subject and creating the most relevant covers. They scrutinized every image to scout for the most suitable representation of the subject and create an appropriate cover for the book.

The publishing team has been involved in this book since its early stages. They were actively engaged in every process, be it collecting the data, connecting with the contributors or procuring relevant information. The team has been an ardent support to the editorial, designing and production team. Their endless efforts to recruit the best for this project, has resulted in the accomplishment of this book. They are a veteran in the field of academics and their pool of knowledge is as vast as their experience in printing. Their expertise and guidance has proved useful at every step. Their uncompromising quality standards have made this book an exceptional effort. Their encouragement from time to time has been an inspiration for everyone.

The publisher and the editorial board hope that this book will prove to be a valuable piece of knowledge for researchers, students, practitioners and scholars across the globe.

List of Contributors

Kathryn Nicholson Perry
University of Western Sydney, Australia

Gabor B. Racz, Miles R. Day, James E. Heavner, Jeffrey P. Smith and Hana Ilner
Texas Tech University Health Sciences Center, Lubbock, Texas, USA

Jared Scott
Advanced Pain Medicine Associates, Wichita, Kansas, USA

Carl E. Noe
University of Texas Southwestern Medical Center, Dallas, Texas, USA

Laslo Nagy
Texas Tech University Health Sciences Center, Covenant Medical Center, Department of Pediatric Neurosurgery, USA

Renata Ferrari, Michela Capraro and Marco Visentin
Hospital Psychology Service, Pain Relief and Palliative Care Unit, Vicenza Hospital, Italy

Gillian R. Lauder
Department of Anesthesia, British Columbia Children's Hospital (BCCH), Canada

Nicholas West
Pediatric Anesthesia Research Team, University of British Columbia (UBC), Canada

FuZhou Wang
Department of Anesthesiology and Critical Care Medicine, The Affiliated Nanjing Maternity and Child Health Care Hospital, Nanjing Medical University, Nanjing, China

P. S. Satheesh Kumar
Department of Oral Medicine and Radiology, Government Dental College, Trivandrum, Kerala, India

Chih-Shung Wong
Department of Anaesthesiology, Cathay General Hospital, Taipei, Taiwan

Chun-Chang Yeh
Department of Anaesthesiology, Tri-Service General Hospital, Taipei, Taiwan

Shan-Chi Ko
Painless Hospital, Ginza, Tokyo, Japan

Yurdanur Demir
Abant İzzet Baysal University, Bolu Health Sciences High School, Turkey

Katrin Blondal
Landspitali -National University Hospital of Iceland, University of Iceland, School of Health Sciences, Faculty of Nursing, Reykjavik, Iceland

Sigridur Halldorsdottir
School of Health Sciences, University of Akureyri, Akureyri, Iceland

Gabor B. Racz
Department of Anesthesiology, Pain Center, Texas Tech University Health Sciences Center, USA

Carl E. Noe
Department of Anesthesiology and Pain Management, Eugene McDermott Center for Pain Management, University of Texas Southwestern Medical Center, USA

Printed in the USA
CPSIA information can be obtained
at www.ICGtesting.com
JSHW011811301024
72690JS00002B/48

9 781632 422514